Human Kinetics

Human Kinetics

Edited by Newman Wagner

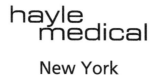

hayle
medical

New York

Hayle Medical,
750 Third Avenue, 9th Floor,
New York, NY 10017, USA

Visit us on the World Wide Web at:
www.haylemedical.com

ISBN: 978-1-63241-451-9

Cataloging-in-Publication Data

Human kinetics / edited by Newman Wagner.
   p. cm.
Includes bibliographical references and index.
ISBN 978-1-63241-451-9
1. Human mechanics. 2. Kinesiology. 3. Human locomotion. I. Wagner, Newman.
QP303 .H86 2017
612.76--dc23

Table of Contents

Preface

This book was inspired by the evolution of our times; to answer the curiosity of inquisitive minds. Many developments have occurred across the globe in the recent past which has transformed the progress in the field.

Human kinetics is the study of the movement in the human body. This book on human kinetics discusses the fundamental principles that govern this field. Human kinetics focuses on the application of the laws of motion on a body that are capable of self-propelled movement. Injury and instability in muscles and joints are caused by the increased displacement of the body that is experiencing motion. This book outlines the processes and applications of human kinetics in detail. As this field is emerging at a fast pace, this book will help the readers to better understand the concepts of human kinetics. With state-of-the-art inputs by acclaimed experts of this field, this book targets students and professionals.

This book was developed from a mere concept to drafts to chapters and finally compiled together as a complete text to benefit the readers across all nations. To ensure the quality of the content we instilled two significant steps in our procedure. The first was to appoint an editorial team that would verify the data and statistics provided in the book and also select the most appropriate and valuable contributions from the plentiful contributions we received from authors worldwide. The next step was to appoint an expert of the topic as the Editor-in-Chief, who would head the project and finally make the necessary amendments and modifications to make the text reader-friendly. I was then commissioned to examine all the material to present the topics in the most comprehensible and productive format.

I would like to take this opportunity to thank all the contributing authors who were supportive enough to contribute their time and knowledge to this project. I also wish to convey my regards to my family who have been extremely supportive during the entire project.

Editor

Definite Differences between *In Vitro* Actin-Myosin Sliding and Muscle Contraction as Revealed Using Antibodies to Myosin Head

Haruo Sugi[1]*, **Shigeru Chaen**[2], **Takakazu Kobayashi**[3], **Takahiro Abe**[3], **Kazushige Kimura**[3], **Yasutake Saeki**[4], **Yoshiki Ohnuki**[4], **Takuya Miyakawa**[5], **Masaru Tanokura**[5], **Seiryo Sugiura**[6]

1 Department of Physiology, School of Medicine, Teikyo University, Tokyo, Japan, 2 Department of Integrated Sciences in Physics and Biology, College of Humanities and Sciences, Nihon University, Tokyo, Japan, 3 Department of Electronic Engineering, Shibaura Institute of Technology, Tokyo, Japan, 4 Department of Physiology, School of Dentistry, Tsurumi University, Yokohama, Japan, 5 Department of Applied Biochemistry, Graduate School of Agriculture and Life Sciences, University of Tokyo, Tokyo, Japan, 6 Graduate School of Frontier Sciences, University of Tokyo, Tokyo, Japan

Abstract

Muscle contraction results from attachment-detachment cycles between myosin heads extending from myosin filaments and actin filaments. It is generally believed that a myosin head first attaches to actin, undergoes conformational changes to produce force and motion in muscle, and then detaches from actin. Despite extensive studies, the molecular mechanism of myosin head conformational changes still remains to be a matter for debate and speculation. The myosin head consists of catalytic (CAD), converter (CVD) and lever arm (LD) domains. To give information about the role of these domains in the myosin head performance, we have examined the effect of three site-directed antibodies to the myosin head on in vitro ATP-dependent actin-myosin sliding and Ca^{2+}-activated contraction of muscle fibers. Antibody 1, attaching to junctional peptide between 50K and 20K heavy chain segments in the CAD, exhibited appreciable effects neither on in vitro actin-myosin sliding nor muscle fiber contraction. Since antibody 1 covers actin-binding sites of the CAD, one interpretation of this result is that rigor actin-myosin linkage is absent or at most a transient intermediate in physiological actin-myosin cycling. Antibody 2, attaching to reactive lysine residue in the CVD, showed a marked inhibitory effect on in vitro actin-myosin sliding without changing actin-activated myosin head (S1) ATPase activity, while it showed no appreciable effect on muscle contraction. Antibody 3, attaching to two peptides of regulatory light chains in the LD, had no significant effect on in vitro actin-myosin sliding, while it reduced force development in muscle fibers without changing MgATPase activity. The above definite differences in the effect of antibodies 2 and 3 between in vitro actin-myosin sliding and muscle contraction can be explained by difference in experimental conditions; in the former, myosin heads are randomly oriented on a glass surface, while in the latter myosin heads are regularly arranged within filament-lattice structures.

Editor: Miklos S. Kellermayer, Semmelweis University, Hungary

Funding: The authors have no support or funding to report.

Competing Interests: The authors have declared that no competing interests exist.

* E-mail: sugi@kyf.biglobe.ne.jp

Introduction

Although more than 50 years have passed since the monumental discovery that muscle contraction results from relative sliding between actin and myosin filaments coupled with ATP hydrolysis [1,2], molecular mechanisms of the myofilament sliding are not yet fully understood. It is generally believed that a myosin head extending from myosin filaments first attaches to actin filaments, undergoes conformational changes to produce unitary myofilament sliding, and then detaches from actin filaments [3,4]. In accordance with this view, biochemical studies on reaction steps of actomyosin ATPase in solution [5] indicate that the myofilament sliding is caused by cyclic interaction between myosin heads and actin filaments; the myosin head (M) first attaches to actin (A) in the form of M·ADP·Pi to undergo a conformational change, i.e. power stroke, associated with release of Pi and ADP, and then forms rigor linkage (AM) with A. Upon binding with a new ATP, M detaches from A to exert a recovery stroke associated with

formation of M·ADP·Pi to again attach to A. Despite extensive studies, the myosin head power stroke still remains to be a matter for debate and speculation [6].

The myosin head (myosin subfragment 1, S1) consists of catalytic domain (CAD) and lever arm domain (LD), which are connected by converter domain (CVD). In 1989, Sutoh, Tokunaga and Wakabayashi [7] prepared monoclonal antibodies; one directed to junctional peptide between 50-kDa and 20 kDa heavy chain segments in the CAD (anti-CAD antibody), while the other directed to reactive lysine residue (Lys83) located close to the junction between the CAD and the CVD (anti-RLR antibody) [8], and succeeded in showing that anti-CAD antibody binds at the distal region of the CAD, while anti-RLR antibody binds at the boundary between the CAD and CVD domains. The gas environmental chamber (EC) enables us to study dynamic structural changes of hydrated biomolecules electron microscopically. Using the EC, we succeeded in recording ATP-induced movement of individual myosin heads, effectively position-marked with anti-CAD or anti-RLR antibody, in hydrated vertebrate myosin filaments in the absence of actin filaments [9,10,11]. On ATP application, myosin heads moved away from the central bare region of myosin filaments with an amplitude of 5–7.5 nm, and after exhaustion of applied ATP, myosin heads returned towards their initial position, indicating our success in visualizing myosin head recovery stroke [10]. More recently, we have further succeeded in recording myosin head power stroke in hydrated mixture of actin and myosin filaments [12,13]. These results constitute the first electron microscopic visualization of myosin head power and recovery strokes producing muscle contraction.

In the present study, we attempted to examine whether or not these site-directed antibodies have influence on ATP-dependent actin-myosin sliding and Ca^{2+}-activated muscle contraction. In addition to anti-CAD and anti-RLR antibodies, we also used another antibody directed to junctional peptides of two regulatory light chains in the LD [11]. Unexpectedly, we have obtained the following results : (1) anti-CAD antibody showed effects neither on in vitro actin-myosin sliding nor on muscle fiber contraction; (2) anti-RLR antibody inhibited in vitro actin-myosin sliding without affecting actin-activated S1 ATPase activity, but had no effect on muscle fiber contraction; and (3) anti-LD antibody showed no significant effect on in vitro actin-myosin sliding, but reduced Ca^{2+}-activated isometric force development without changing the maximum velocity of shortening and MgATPase activity. One interpretation of these results is that, during muscle contraction, rigor actin-myosin linkage AM is absent or at most a transient intermediate . It is also suggested that the mechanism of in vitro actin-myosin sliding definitely differs from muscle contraction, due to random orientation and fixation of myosin heads in vitro motility assay systems [14].

Materials and Methods

Preparation of Monoclonal Antibodies to Myosin Head

Monoclonal antibodies (IgG) directed to the junctional peptide between 50- and 20-kDa segments of myosin heavy chain, located close to the actin binding sites (anti-CAD antibody), and directed to the reactive lysine residue (lys83), located close to the CAD-CVD junction (anti-RLR antibody) were prepared by the method of Sutoh et al. [7]. Monoclonal antibody (IgG) directed to two peptides (Met58~Ala70 and Leu106~Phe120) of the myosin regulatory light chain in the LD (anti-LD antibody) was prepared by the method of Minoda et al. [11]. As shown in Fig. 1, anti-CAD antibody and anti-RLR antibody molecules (IgG) actually attach to the head of myosin molecule (A and B), while anti-LD antibody molecules (IgG) attach to the head-rod junction of myosin molecule, i.e. the myosin LD (C). These antibodies have already been proved to effectively position-mark myosin heads in synthetic myosin filaments [9,10,11].

Measurement of *In Vitro* Sliding Velocity of Actin Filaments on Myosin Heads

Myosin and actin were prepared from rabbit skeletal muscle by the method of Perry [15] and Spudich and Watt [16], respectively. First, myosin in a high salt solution, containing 0.6 M KCl, 50 mM phosphate buffer (pH 6.8) and 0.1 mM DTT, was introduced at a concentration of 0.1 mg/ml into a flow chamber. The chamber was then rinsed with 1 mg/ml BSA, and assay solution containing 10 nM F-actin filaments, labeled with rhodamine-conjugated phalloidin (Molecular Probe), 25 mM KCl, 25 mM imidazole (pH 7.5), 2 mM ATP, 4 mM MgCl₂, 1 mM DTT, 1% β-mercaptoethanol, 4.5 mg/ml glucose, 0.21 mg/ml glucose oxidase, 0.035 mg/ml catalase, and anti-CD antibody or

anti-LD antibody was introduced into a nitrocellulose-coated flow cell. Sliding velocity of actin filaments on myosin heads was determined using a video system (30 frames/s, Hamamatsu Photonics C-7190). Experiments were made at 25°C.

Measurement of Actin-Activated S1 MgATPase Activity

Myosin subfragment 1 (S1) was obtained by digestion of myosin with chymotrypsin following the procedure of Margossian and Lowey [17]. Actin-activated myosin head (S1) Mg-ATPase activity was determined by mixing S1 (0.05 mg/ml) with F-actin (0–50 μM) and measuring release of phosphate (Pi) at 25°C using the malachite green method [18], in an assay buffer containing 25 mM KCl, 25 mM imidazole (pH 7.5), 4 mM MgCl₂, 1 mM DTT. Reaction was initiated by adding 1/5 volume of 6 mM ATP, and stopped by adding 4 volumes of 0.3 M perchloric acid. Data from 2–3 independent S1 samples were averaged.

Determination of Contraction Characteristics of Ca^{2+}-Activated Muscle Fibers

White male rabbits weighing 2 to 2.5 kg were killed by injection of sodium pentobarbital (50 mg/kg) into the ear vein, and psoas muscles were dissected from the animals. The animals were treated in accordance with the Guiding Principles for the Care and Use of Animals in the Field of Physiological Sciences, published by the Physiological Society of Japan. The protocol was approved by the Teikyo University Animal Care Committee (protocol #07-050). Glycerol-extracted muscle fiber strips were prepared from rabbit skeletal muscle as described by Sugi et al. [19]. Single muscle fibers (diameter, 50–80 μm) were dissected from the glycerol-extracted strips, and mounted horizontally in an experimental chamber (0.1 ml) between a force transducer and a servomotor by glueing both ends to the extension of the transducer and the servomotor with collodion. The servomotor contained a displacement transducer (differential capacitor) sensing the motor arm position. Further details of experimental apparatus have been described elsewhere [18]. The fibers were kept at their slack length (L₀, sarcomere length 2.4 μm). Relaxing solution contained 125 mM KCl, 4 mM MgCl₂, 4 mM EGTA, 20 mM Pipes (pH 7.0). Contracting solution was prepared by adding 4 mM CaCl₂ to relaxing solution to maximally activate the fibers. The experiments were made at 20°C.

The servomotor system was operated either in the length clamp mode or in the force control mode [20]. First, the system was in the length clamp mode so that the fiber contracted isometrically in contracting solution. After the fiber developed steady isometric force, the servomotor system was switched to the force control mode, and a ramp decrease in force (= load) from the steady force to zero (complete in 50–100 ms) was applied to the fiber. The resulting fiber shortening was recorded together with the ramp decrease in force, and the force-velocity curve was obtained and displayed on the X-Y plotter. Details of the method have been described elsewhere [19,20,21].

The fiber was first activated maximally with contracting solution, and when the maximum steady isometric force was developed, the force-velocity curve was obtained by applying a ramp decrease in force. Then the fiber was made to relax in relaxing solution containing the antibody, and after 30 min it was again activated with contracting solution containing the antibody.

Measurement of MgATPase Activity of Ca^{2+}-activated Muscle Fibers

Mg-ATPase activity of a small fiber bundle consisting of 2–3 muscle fibers during Ca^{2+}-activated isometric force development

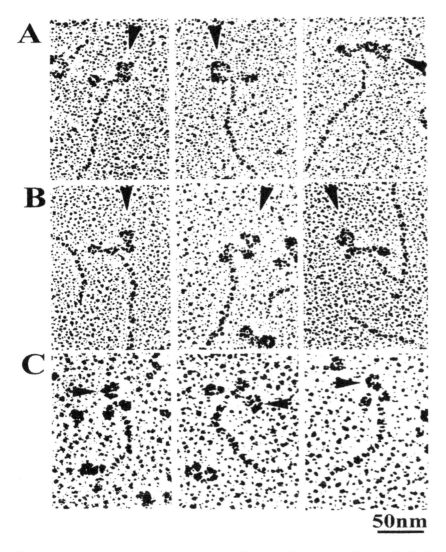

Figure 1. A gallery of electron micrographs of rotary shadowed antibodies (IgG) attached to myosin heads. Anti-CAD antibody-myosin(A), anti-RLR antibody-myosin (B), and anti-LD antibody-myosin (C) complexes are shown in A,B and C, respectively. IgG molecules are indicated by arrowheads. The panels are provided from the published papers (Sutoh et al., 1989; Minoda et al., 2011).

was recorded by the decrease of NADH during cleavage of ATP [19,22]. The fibers were mounted in the sample compartment (0.36 ml) of a dual wavelength spectrophotometer (Nihon Bunko) with a sample monochrometer at 340 nm and a reference monochrometer at 400 nm, so that the decrease of NADH was measured from the difference in absorbance between 340 and 400 nm. To both relaxing and contracting solutions, 0.25 mM NADH, 1.25 mM phosphoenolpyruvate, 50 units/ml pyruvate kinase, 50 units/ml lactic dehydrogenase, 10 mM NaN_3, 50 μM quercetin, 1 μg/ml oligomycin were added. Solutions in the compartment was constantly stirred with a magnetic stirrer. The experiments were performed at 10°C.

Results

Anti-CAD Antibody Has No Effect on Both *In Vitro* Actin-Myosin Sliding and Muscle Fiber Contraction

Prior to the application of anti-CAD antibody, the average velocity of ATP-dependent in vitro actin filament sliding on myosin heads was determined to be 2.3±0.6 μm/s (mean±SD,

n = 380 from 10 independent experiments). Though this value is much smaller than that reported by Harada et al. [23], it has been pointed out by Uyeda et al. [24] that the velocity of actin-myosin sliding is markedly influenced by a number of factors, such as preparation of myosin sample, composition of substratum on which actin-myosin sliding takes place, and density of myosin heads in the assay system. As shown in Fig. 2, the velocity of in vitro actin-myosin sliding did not change appreciably in the presence of anti-CAD antibody at concentrations up to 2 mg/ml. Similar results were obtained from 9 other experiments.

Fig. 3 shows superimposed force-velocity curves of a maximally Ca^{2+}-activated muscle fiber, obtained in the absence and in the presence of anti-CAD antibody at concentrations up to 2 mg/ml. As can be seen in the figure, the two curves were double-hyperbolic in shape [19,21,25], and almost identical with each other. The maximum shortening velocity at zero external load, i.e. the point of intersection of the force-velocity curve with the velocity axis, remained unchanged in the presence of antibody; the small difference in the maximum isometric force was well within the range of variation in skinned fiber preparations [26].

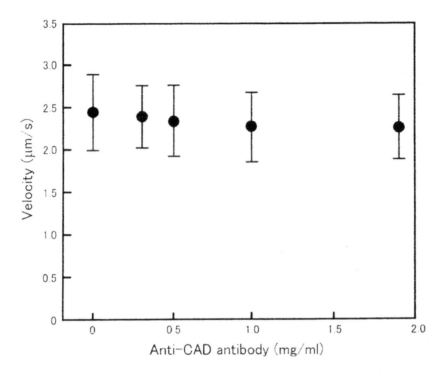

Figure 2. No appreciable effect of anti-CAD antibody on *in vitro* actin filament sliding on myosin heads. In this and Figs. 4 and 5, mean velocities of sliding are plotted against antibody concentration with vertical bars indicating S.D., and each data point is obtained from 80–120 measurements.

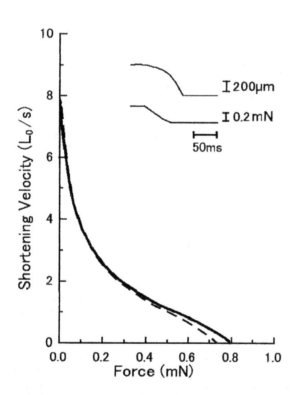

Figure 3. No appreciable effect of anti-CAD antibody on force-velocity curves of Ca^{2+}-activated muscle fiber. In this and Fig. 5, solid and broken lines indicate force-velocity curves before and after application of anti-CAD antibody (2 mg/ml), respectively. Inset shows an example of fiber length (upper trace) and force (lower trace) changes in response to a ramp decrease in force.

Anti-RLR Antibody Inhibits *In Vitro* Actin-Myosin Sliding, but Has No Effect on Muscle Fiber Contraction

As shown in Fig. 4A, anti-RLR antibody showed a marked inhibitory effect on ATP-dependent in vitro actin-myosin sliding. The velocity of actin filament sliding on myosin heads decreased by about 50% with 0.02 mg/ml antibody, and the actin-myosin sliding was completely eliminated with the antibody >1.4 mg/ml. Similar results were obtained on 7 other experiments. On the other hand, actin-activated MgATPase activity of myosin head (S1) did not change appreciably in the presence of anti-RLR antibody >1.4 mg/ml; both the V_{max} (1.98 s^{-1}) and the K_m (81.6 μM) remained unchanged by the antibody (Fig. 4B).

In contrast with its marked inhibitory effect on in vitro ATP-dependent actin-myosin sliding, anti-RLR antibody showed no appreciable effect on contraction of Ca^{2+}-activated muscle fibers at concentrations up to 2 mg/ml. As has been the case with anti-CAD antibody, the force-velocity curves in the presence and absence of anti-RLR antibody were almost identical, so that both the maximum velocity of shortening V_{max} and the maximum isometric force remained unchanged in the presence of anti-RLR antibody (Fig. 5). Similar results were obtained on 8 other experiments obtained from 8 different fibers.

Anti-LD Antibody Has No Significant Effect on *In Vitro* Actin-Myosin Sliding, but Inhibits Ca^{2+}-Activated Force Development of Muscle Fibers without Affecting MgATPase Activity

As shown in Fig. 6, the sliding velocity of actin filaments on myosin heads did not change significantly in the presence of the antibody up to 2 mg/ml. Though the velocity of actin filament sliding exhibited a tendency to decrease slightly with increasing antibody concentration, the difference between the data points was

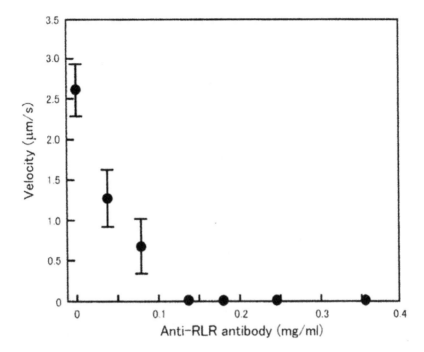

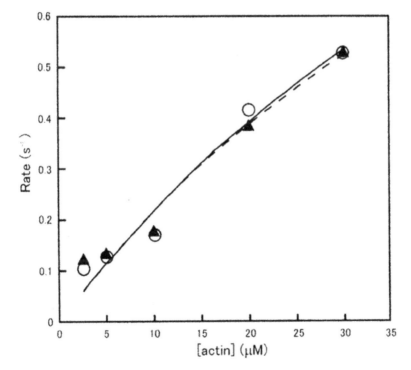

Figure 4. (A) Inhibitory effect of anti-RLR antibody on in vitro actin filament sliding on myosin heads. (B) No appreciable effect of anti-RLR antibody on actin-activated myosin head (S1) MgATPase activity. In B, the ATPase activities in the absence and in the presence of the antibody (0.36 mg/ml) are shown by open circles and black triangles, respectively. Curves are fitted by Michaelis-Menten kinetics.

not statistically significant. Similar results were obtained from 6 other experiments.

In contrast, anti-LD antibody was found to inhibit Ca^{2+}-activated isometric force development of muscle fibers in a concentration-dependent manner (Fig. 7). In the presence of

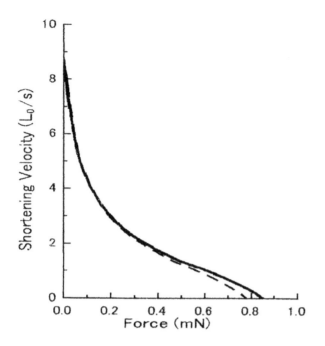

Figure 5. No appreciable effect of anti-RLR antibody on force-velocity curves of Ca²⁺-activated muscle fiber.

2 mg/ml anti-LD antibody, Ca^{2+}-activated isometric force was reduced by 70–80%. The effect of anti-LD antibody was reversible. When the fibers were returned to relaxing solution without antibody and kept in it for 20 min, they completely restored their ability to develop Ca^{2+}-activated isometric force as large as that before application of the antibody. Examples of the force-velocity curves obtained in the absence and in the presence of the antibody obtained from one and the same fiber are

presented in Fig. 8. Despite a marked decrease in Ca^{2+}-activated isometric force in the presence of the antibody (2 mg/ml), the V_{max} remained unchanged (Fig. 8A), and if the force was normalized with respect to the maximum values, the two curves were found to be identical (Fig. 8B).

Fig. 9 shows typical examples of simultaneous recordings of MgATPase activity and isometric force development of a Ca^{2+}-activated muscle fiber. Despite the marked reduction of isometric force, MgATPase activity of the fiber, as measured from the slope of ATPase records during the steady isometric force development, did not change significantly. In 8 different fibers examined, the MgATPase activity in the absence and in the presence of the antibody (2 mg/ml) was 0.55 ± 0.17 mM/s and 0.54 ± 0.16 mM/s (mean$\pm$SD, n = 8), respectively.

Discussion

Evaluation of the Proportion of Myosin Heads Bound to Antibodies in the Present Experiments

Prior to the discussion on the effect of antibodies on in vitro actin-myosin sliding and muscle fiber contraction, it seems necessary to evaluate the proportion of myosin heads bound to antibodies in the present experiments, especially within single skinned muscle fibers. First of all, the possibility that antibodies do not diffuse into muscle fibers can be excluded by the following reasons. (1) Using the confocal microscope, fluorescently labeled dummy antibody (IgG) has been shown to diffuse into skinned muscle fibers, and evenly distribute in the interior of the fiber within 3 min [27]. (2) Anti-LD antibody, which is believed to differ from anti-CAD antibody only at the epitope-binding site, shows reversible inhibitory effect on Ca^{2+}-activated force development (Figs. 4–7), indicating that IgG molecules can diffuse into the fiber to exhibit their inhibitory effect by attaching to their epitope, and can diffuse out of the fiber after its removal from external solution. The same explanation may apply to both anti-CAD antibody and anti-RLR antibody, which has no effect on Ca^{2+}-activated

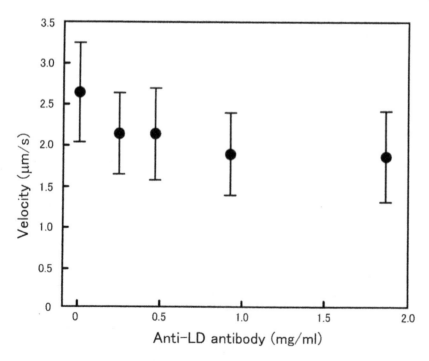

Figure 6. No appreciable effect of anti-LD antibody on *in vitro* actin filament sliding on myosin heads.

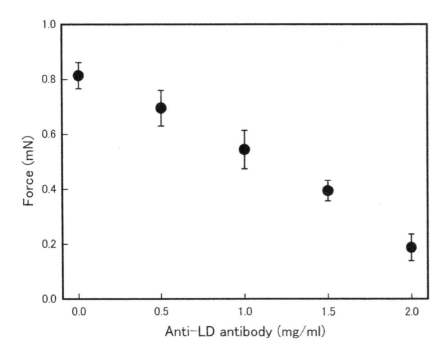

Figure 7. Inhibitory effect of anti-LD antibody on Ca²⁺-activated isometric force development. The magnitude of steady Ca^{2+}-activated isometric force is plotted against the antibody concentration. Vertical bars represent S.E.M. (n = 4~6).

contraction of muscle fibers. (3) In addition, we have recently found that development of rigor force and stiffness in skinned fibers is reversibly slowed down, without appreciably changing their peak values, by all the three antibodies used in the present study [28], again indicating that these antibodies can diffuse into the fiber to bind with their respective epitope. In the case of anti-CAD antibody, its ineffectiveness in inhibiting rigor linkage formation might result from that the antibody (IgG) molecules might first attach to myosin heads, but then would gradually be

overridden by actin filaments which tend to form strong and stable rigor linkages with myosin heads.

On the other hand, our published electron micrographs of hydrated synthetic myosin filaments [10, Fig. 2] give information about the proportion of myosin heads bound with antibodies within a single muscle fiber. Judging from the structure of myosin filaments consisting of myosin molecules, the number of myosin heads in each native myosin filament (diameter, 15 nm, length, 1.6 μm) is estimated to be 300. The synthetic myosin filament

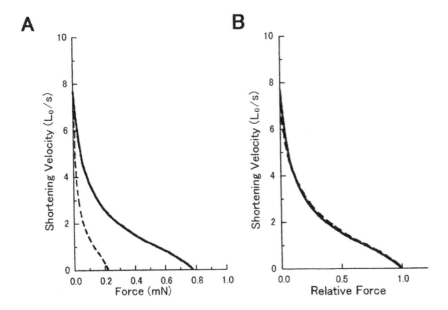

Figure 8. Effect of anti-LD antibody on force-velocity curves of a Ca²⁺-activated muscle fiber. (A) Force-velocity curves before (solid line) and after (broken line) application of the antibody (1.5 mg/ml). (B) The same force-velocity curves with force expressed relative to the maximum value.

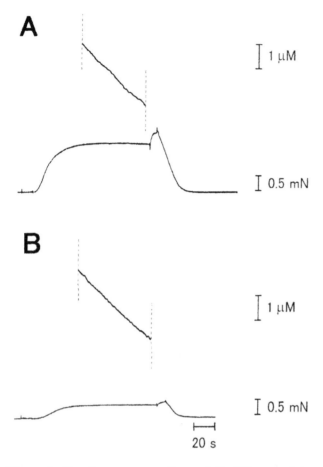

Figure 9. Simultaneous recordings of MgATPase activity (upper traces) and Ca²⁺-activated isometric force development (lower traces) of a small bundle consisting of two fibers. Records A and B are taken before and after application of anti-LD antibody (2 mg/ml), respectively.

(myosin-myosin rod copolymer mixed at a ratio of 1:1) shown in Fig. 2B [10] has a length of ~1.5 µm and a diameter of ~90 nm. As a native myosin filament is 1.6 µm in length and 15 nm in diameter, the size of this particular filament roughly corresponds to a bundle consisting of 6 native myosin filaments running in parallel with one another. Considering that this filament is a 1:1 mixture of myosin and myosin rod, the number of myosin heads in it may be ~900 (300×6×1/2). Since antibodies can attach only one of the two myosin heads in each myosin molecule [10], the number of myosin heads available for antibodies is ~450. In addition, it seems likely that myosin heads located at the filament surface can only bind with externally applied antibodies. If this factor is taken into consideration, the number of myosin heads available for antibodies would be further reduced to <200. In fact, close inspection of the synthetic filament shown in Fig. 2B [10] indicates that the number of gold particles attached to myosin heads via anti-CAD antibody is >200. This may be taken to indicate the high affinity of anti-CAD antibody to myosin head. In the case of a large synthetic filament shown in Fig. 2A [10], however, the number of gold particles attached to myosin heads is not so large, probably because antibodies may not readily accessible to myosin heads due to complex myosin-myosin rod network. We made similar observations on electron micrographs of synthetic filaments, in which myosin heads were position-marked with anti-RLR and anti-LD antibodies [11].

In conclusion, in the case of muscle fibers containing regularly arranged myofilament-lattice, the proportion of myosin heads with bound antibody may be expected to be fairly large, probably at least >50%. The same conclusion may also apply to myosin heads fixed on nitrocellulose membrane.

Evidence for the Absence of Rigor Linkages during Cyclic Actin-myosin Interaction in Muscle Contraction

A most striking result found in the present study is that anti-CAD antibody has appreciable effects neither on ATP-dependent in vitro actin-myosin sliding nor Ca²⁺-activated muscle fiber contraction (Figs. 2 and 4). It has been known that myosin heads have two actin-binding sites, one at residues 700~720 in the 20-kDa segment, while the other at residues towards the C-terminus of the 50-kDa segment of myosin heavy chain. Both binding sites are close to the junctional peptide connecting these two heavy chain segments [29]. If bulky anti-CAD antibody (IgG) binds to the junctional peptide, the two actin-binding sites are completely covered by the antibody molecule, so that myosin heads can no longer form linkages with the myosin-binding sites on actin monomers constituting actin filaments. As already mentioned in this paper, it seems possible that, during cyclic actin-myosin interaction taking place in muscle, rigor myosin head AM may be absent or at most a transient intermediate. This idea is inconsistent with the general view [5] that myosin heads take rigor or rigor-like configuration at the end of their power stroke during muscle contraction.

In this connection, Radocaj et al. [30] attempted to detect rigor or rigor-like myosin heads with the technique of time-resolved X-ray diffraction. They applied ramp-shaped releases to Ca²⁺-activated skinned muscle fibers, in the hope that myosin heads at the end of their power stroke would accumulate transiently. They failed, however, to detect accumulation of rigor myosin heads AM. They suggest that, at the end of power stroke, myosin heads would take the form of AM, which is structurally different from the rigor actin-myosin complex, determined by static crystallographic and electron microscopic studies [6]. In accordance with their suggestion, we have recently obtained evidence that myosin heads in rigor muscle fibers contain two different types of rigor AM linkages, one with somewhat active mechanical property while the other with purely passive property [31]. The former active AM linkages have a long average lifetime, and it seems possible that myosin heads mostly take the form of this active AM linkages during physiological actin-myosin interaction. Of course, much more experimental work is needed to settle this important issue.

Definite Differences Between In Vitro Actin-Myosin Sliding and Muscle Fiber Contraction

Homsher et al. [32] compared the effect of substrate concentration, ionic strength and temperature on the velocity of in vitro ATP-dependent actin-myosin sliding (V_f) and on the maximum unloaded shortening velocity of Ca²⁺-activated muscle fibers (V_u). They found that these factors affected both V_f and V_u in a qualitatively similar manner except for extreme conditions. In contrast, the present study has revealed striking differences in the effect of anti-RLR and anti-LD antibodies between in vitro actin-myosin sliding and muscle fiber contraction. Anti-RLR antibody showed a marked inhibitory effect on in vitro actin-myosin sliding without changing actin-activated myosin head (S1) MgATPase activity (Fig. 4A,B), but had no appreciable effect on Ca²⁺-activated muscle fiber contraction (Fig. 5). The marked inhibitory effect of anti-RLR antibody on in vitro actin-myosin sliding (Fig. 4A) is consistent with the report of Muhlrad et al. [33] that

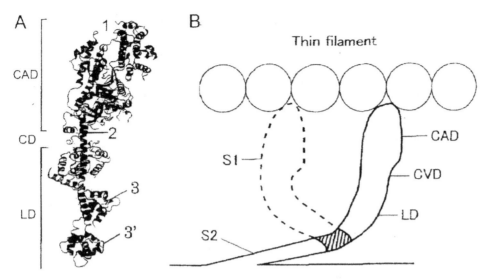

Figure 10. Schematic diagrams showing change in myosin head configuration before and after power stroke. (A) Ribbon diagram of the myosin head showing approximate regions of attachment of anti-CAD, anti-CVD and anti-LD antibodies, indicated by numbers 1, 2 and 3 and 3′, respectively. (B) Myosin head configurations before and after power stroke, indicated by solid and broken lines, respectively. Note rotation of the LD around the LD-S2 junction (shaded area) as well as rotation of the CAD around the CVD.

chemical modification (trinitrophenylation) of the RLR inhibits in vitro actin-myosin sliding. They showed, however, that the chemical modification of the RLR eliminated actin-activated myosin head (S1) MgATPase activity, while in the present study it was not affected by the antibody (Fig. 4B). It may be that the chemical modification of the RLR may change 3D structure of myosin heads to inhibit the ATPase activity of the CAD, whereas the reversible binding of anti-RLR antibody to the RLR do not produce any structural changes in the CAD.

The striking difference in the effect of anti-RLR antibody between in vitro actin-myosin sliding and muscle fiber contraction can be accounted for in terms of difference in the condition, under which myosin heads interact with actin filaments. In the in vitro systems, myosin heads are randomly oriented on a glass surface, and each myosin head should have enough flexibility to interact with an actin filament moving in random directions; if the RLR binds to anti-RLR antibody, or is chemically modified [33], the flexibility of myosin heads around the CVD would be markedly reduced to impair their ability to interact with actin filaments. Meanwhile, in muscle fibers, each myosin filament is surrounded by 6 actin filaments at appropriate distances in the hexagonal myofilament-lattice structure, so that myosin heads on myosin filaments can interact with actin filaments despite the reduced flexibility around the CVD caused by binding of anti-RLR antibody. The explanation stated above is supported by our unpublished observation that the sliding velocity of fluorescently labeled actin filaments along synthetic "mini" myosin filaments (length, ~500 nm) [34] is 2.36 ± 1.26 µm/s (mean±SD, n = 211, at 25°C), and does not change appreciably in the presence of anti-RLR antibody (up to 2 mg/ml), since myosin heads in the filament are regularly arranged with uniform polarity in the synthetic filament.

At present, we reserve further speculations about the role of the myosin head CVD in producing myosin head power stroke, but would like to emphasize that a number of findings obtained using in vitro motility assay systems are interesting, but great care should be taken before relating the results obtained to the mechanism of muscle contraction consisting of hexagonal myofilament-lattice structure.

The discussions stated above, however, rest on the assumption that anti-RLR antibody molecule (IgG) does not bind to nitrocellrose memberane, on which in vitro actin-myosin sliding occurs. If, however, anti-RLR antibody molecule can bind to nitrocellurose membrane unlike the other two antibodies, it might act to inhibit actin-myosin sliding by crosslinking myosin heads to the substratum. This possibility should be kept in mind.

Evidence for Essential Role of Junction between Myosin Head LD and Myosin Subfragment 2 in Producing Muscle Contraction

Figure 10A is a ribbon diagram of the myosin head in which approximate points of attachment of the three different antibodies used in the present experiments are indicated, while Figure 10B shows schematic representation of changes in myosin head configuration before (solid line) and after (broken line) power stroke. As can be seen in Fig. 10B, rotation of the LD around the LD-S2 junction takes place as well as rotation of the CAD around the CVD. Since anti-LD antibody attaches to the peptides of regulatory light chains near the LD-S2 junction, its inhibitory effect on Ca^{2+}-activated force development (Figs.7–9) indicates involvement of this region in the rotation of the LD around the LD-S2 junction producing myosin head power stroke. The above idea may also be consistent with our unpublished observation that the velocity of actin filament sliding along synthetic "mini" myosin filaments with uniform polarity [34], is reduced by ~50% with 0.2 mg/ml ant-LD antibody, and is reduced to zero with anti-LD antibody above 1 mg/ml; the complete elimination of actin filament sliding along "mini" myosin filament may result from that the antibody binds with all the myosin heads available for filament sliding. On the other hand, the ineffectiveness of anti-LD antibody on MgATPase activity of muscle fibers (Fig. 9) may be due to that the CAD, which contains ATP-binding site, is geographically distant from the LD-S2 junction.

The importance of the LD-S2 junction in producing muscle contraction has also been indicated by the report that a polyclonal antibody to the S2 region inhibits muscle fiber contraction without changing MgATPase activity [19]. On the other hand, the ineffectiveness of anti-LD antibody on in vitro actin-myosin sliding (Fig. 6) can also be accounted for by the manner of fixation of myosin heads on a glass surface, As myosin heads are truncated at the LD-S2 junction so that rotation of the LD around the LD-S2 junction can no longer take place. A small tendency of the actin-myosin sliding velocity might result from that, in a small proportion of fixed myosin heads, truncation is incomplete so that the LD rotation around the LD-S2 junction takes place.

Despite the reduction of the maximum Ca^{2+}-activated isometric force by the antibody in a concentration-dependent manner (Fig. 7), the force-velocity curves were scaled according to the maximum force developed, while the V_{max} remained unchanged (Fig. 8A,B). These results indicate that myosin heads, in which rotation of the LD around the LD-S2 junction is impaired by the antibody, provides no appreciable internal resistance against muscle fiber shortening. This also implies that reduction in the number of myosin heads involved in producing contraction may constitute another reason for the reduction of isometric force by anti-LD antibody.

In addition to the structures essential for muscle contraction, including actin and nucleotide binding sites in the CAD and switches I and II linking these sites to the CVD [6], the present results indicate that the CAD-CVD junction and the LD-S2 junction also contribute in producing force and motion in muscle. Much more experimental work is necessary to clarify mechanisms of muscle contraction at the molecular level.

Acknowledgments

We wish to thank Japan Electron Optics Laboratory, Ltd. for generously providing facilities to carry out our work. We are also indebted to Mr. S. Miyazaki for technical help, and Drs. K. Sutoh, M. Tokunaga and T. Wakabayashi for allowing us to use their published electron micrographs of antibody-myosin complexes.

Author Contributions

Conceived and designed the experiments: HS. Analyzed the data: SC TK TA KK YS YO SS. Wrote the paper: HS. Made biochemical experiment: SC. Performed physiological experiment: TK TA KK YS YO SS. Prepared antibody: TM MT.

References

1. Huxley AF, Niedergerke R (1954) Interference microscopy of living muscle fibres. Nature 173: 971–973.
2. Huxley HE, Hanson J (1954) Changes in the cross striations of muscle during contraction and stretch. Nature 173: 973–976.
3. Huxley AF (1957) Muscle structure and theories of contraction. Prog Biophys Biophys Chem 7: 255–318.
4. Huxley HE (1969) The mechanism of muscle contraction. Science 164: 1356–1366.
5. Lymn RW, Taylor EW (1971) Mechanism of adenosine triphosphate hydrolysis by actomyosin. Biochemistry 10: 4617–4624.
6. Geeves MA, Holmes KC (1999) Structural mechanism of muscle contraction. Annu Rev Biochem 68: 687–728.
7. Sutoh K, Tokunaga M, Wakabayashi T (1989) Electron microscopic mappings of myosin head with site-directed antibodies. J Mol Biol 206: 357–363.
8. Mornet D, Pantel P, Bertrand R, Audemard E, Kassab R (1980) Localization of the reactive trinitrophenylated lysyn residue of myosin ATPase site in the NH_2-terminal (27K domain) of S1 heavy chain. FEBS Lett 117: 183–188.
9. Sugi H, Akimoto T, Sutoh S, Chaen S, Oishi N et al. (1997) Dynamic electron microscopy of ATP-induced myosin head movement in living muscle thick filaments. Proc Natl Acad Sci USA 94: 4378–4382.
10. Sugi H, Minoda H, Inayoshi Y, Yumoto F, Miyakawa T et al. (2008) Direct demonstration of the cross-bridge recovery stroke in muscle thick filaments in aqueous solution using the hydration chamber. Proc Natl Acad Sci USA 105: 17396–17401.
11. Minoda H, Okabe T, Inayoshi Y, Miyakawa T, Miyauchi Y et al. (2011) Electron microscopic evidence for the myosin head lever arm mechanism in hydrated myosin filaments using the gas environmental chamber. Biochem Biophys Res Commun 405: 651–656.
12. Sugi H, Minoda H, Miyakawa T, Tanokura M (2011) Electron microscopic recording of the cross-bridge power stroke in hydrated myosin filaments using the gas environmental chamber. J Muscle Res Cell Motil 32: 34.
13. Sugi H (2013) Visualization and measurement of the power stroke in individual myosin heads coupled with ATP hydrolysis using the gas environmental chamber. J Physiol Sci 103 Suppl: S35.
14. Kron SJ, Spudich JA (1986) Fluorescent actin filaments move on myosin fixed to a glass surface. Proc Natl Acad Sci USA 83: 6272–6276.
15. Perry SV (1955) Myosin adenosinetriphosphatase. Methods Enzymol 2: 582–588.
16. Spudich JA, Watt S (1971) The regulation of rabbit skeletal muscle contraction I. Biochemical studies of the interaction of the tropomyosin-troponin complex with actin and the proteolytic fragments of myosin. J Biol Chem 246: 4866–4871.
17. Margossian SS, Lowey S (1982) Preparation of myosin and its subfragments from rabbit skeletal muscle. Methods Enzymol 85: 55–72.
18. Kodama T, Fukui K, Kometani K (1986) The initial phosphate burst in ATP hydrolysis by myosin and subfragment-1 as studied by a modified malachite green method for determination of inorganic phosphate. J Biochem 99: 1465–1472.
19. Sugi H, Kobayashi T, Gross T, Noguchi K, Karr T (1992) Contraction characteristics and ATPase activity of skeletal muscle fibers in the presence of antibody to myosin subfragment 2. Proc Natl Acad Sci USA 89: 6134–6137.
20. Iwamoto H, Sugaya R, Sugi H (1990) Force-velocity relation of frog skeletal muscle fibres shortening under continuously increasing load. J Physiol 422: 185–202.
21. Yamada T, Abe O, Kobayashi T, Sugi H (1993) Myofilament sliding per ATP molecule in rabbit muscle fibres studied using laser flash photolysis of caged ATP. J Physiol 466: 229–243.
22. Chaen S, Shimada M, Sugi H (1986) Evidence for cooperative interactions of myosin heads with thin filaments in the force generation of vertebrate skeletal muscle fibers. J Biol Chem 261: 13632–13636.
23. Harada y, Sakurada K, Aoki T, Thomas DD, Yanagida T (1990) Mechano-chemical coupling in actomyosin energy transduction studied by in vitromovement assay. J Mol Biol 216: 49–68.
24. Uyeda TQP, Kron SJ, Spudich JA (1990) Myosin step size estimation from slow sliding movement of actin over low densities of heavy meromyosin. J Mol Biol 214: 699–710.
25. Edman KAP (1988) Double-hyperbolic force-velocity relation in frog muscle fibres. J Physiol 494: 301–321.
26. Brenner B (1998) Skinned muscle fibers. In: Sugi H, editor. Current Methods in Muscle Physiology. Oxford: Oxford University Press. 33–69.
27. Kraft TM, Messserli M, Rothen-Rutshauser B, Perriad J-C, Wallimann T et al. (1995) Equilibrium and exchange of fluorescently labeled molecules in skinned skeletal muscle fibers visualized by confocal microscopy. Biophys J 69: 1246–1258.
28. Kobayashi H, Abe T, Kimura T, Sugi H (12013) Monoclonal antibodies to myosin head retard formation of rigor actin-myosin linkages in skinned rabbit psoas muscle fibers. IUPS 2013 Abstract Book digital edition, PCD251.
29. Bagshaw CR (1993) Muscle Contraction. London: Chapman & Hall, 155pp.
30. Radcaj A, Weiss T, Helsby WI, Brenner B, Kraft TM (2009) Force-generating cross-bridges during ramp-shaped releases: Evidence for a new structural state. Biophys J 96: 1430–1446.
31. Sugi H, Hajar K, Kimura K, Kobayashi T, Sugiura S (2014) Evidence for the presence of AM-ADP myosin heads in rigor muscle fibers: Its implication of the sate of myosin heads after the end of powerstroke. Abstract of the 2014 Biophysical Society Meeting, In Press.
32. Homsher E, Wang F, Sellers JR (1992) Factors affecting movement of F-actin filaments propelled by skeletal muscle heavy meromyosin. Am J Physiol 262 (Cell Physiol 31): C714–C723.
33. Muhlrad A, Peyser YM, Nili M, Ajtai K, Reisler E et al. (2003) Chemical decoupling of ATPase activation and force production from the contractile cycle in myosin by steric hindrance of lever arm movement. Biophys J 84: 1047–1056.
34. Saito K, Aoki T, Aoki T, Yanagida T (1994) Movement of single myosin filaments and myosin step size on actin filaments suspended in solution by a laser trap. Biophys J 66: 769–777.

2

Incubating Isolated Mouse EDL Muscles with Creatine Improves Force Production and Twitch Kinetics in Fatigue Due to Reduction in Ionic Strength

Stewart I. Head*, Bronwen Greenaway, Stephen Chan

School of Medical Sciences, University of New South Wales, Sydney, New South Wales, Australia

Abstract

Background: Creatine supplementation can improve performance during high intensity exercise in humans and improve muscle strength in certain myopathies. In this present study, we investigated the direct effects of acute creatine incubation on isolated mouse fast-twitch EDL muscles, and examined how these effects change with fatigue.

Methods and Results: The extensor *digitorum longus* muscle from mice aged 12–14 weeks was isolated and stimulated with field electrodes to measure force characteristics in 3 different states: (i) before fatigue; (ii) immediately after a fatigue protocol; and (iii) after recovery. These served as the control measurements for the muscle. The muscle was then incubated in a creatine solution and washed. The measurement of force characteristics in the 3 different states was then repeated. In un-fatigued muscle, creatine incubation increased the maximal tetanic force. In fatigued muscle, creatine treatment increased the force produced at all frequencies of stimulation. Incubation also increased the rate of twitch relaxation and twitch contraction in fatigued muscle. During repetitive fatiguing stimulation, creatine-treated muscles took $55.1 \pm 9.5\%$ longer than control muscles to lose half of their original force. Measurement of weight changes showed that creatine incubation increased EDL muscle mass by 7%.

Conclusion: Acute creatine application improves force production in isolated fast-twitch EDL muscle, and these improvements are particularly apparent when the muscle is fatigued. One likely mechanism for this improvement is an increase in Ca^{2+} sensitivity of contractile proteins as a result of ionic strength decreases following creatine incubation.

Editor: Bradley Steven Launikonis, University of Queensland, Australia

Funding: This work was supported by a grant from the National Health and Medical Research Council of Australia (NHMRC Project Grant #512254, http://www.nhmrc.gov.au). The funders had no role in study design, data collection and analysis, decision to publish, or preparation of the manuscript.

Competing Interests: The authors have declared that no competing interests exist.

* E-mail: S.Head@unsw.edu.au

Introduction

The ingestion of supplementary creatine can increase intramuscular creatine and improve performance, particularly during maximally fatiguing exercise [1,2]. It can also enhance muscle strength in certain myopathies, such as muscular dystrophy [3]. Creatine cannot be synthesized in skeletal muscle cells and is transported into skeletal muscle by a Na^+-dependent transmembrane protein [4]. The creatine(Cr)/phosphocreatine(PCr) cycle acts as a temporal buffer of ATP during the first seconds of intense skeletal muscle contraction before glycolysis and mitochondrial mechanisms can respond to the increased demand for ATP. Without this buffering most skeletal muscles would run out of ATP after less than one second of intense exercise [5]. The Cr/PCr cycle is also an important source and transporter of ATP during the later stages of prolonged muscle activity. The Cr/PCr cycle is catalyzed by creatine kinase (CK), which has two main isoforms in skeletal muscle. Firstly, Mi-CK, the mitochondrial isoform [6], is bound to the inner membrane of the mitochondria [7] and is functionally linked to oxidative phosphorylation [8]. Secondly, MM-CK, the M-line isoform, is localised to the M-line of the A-band of the contractile apparatus and is functionally coupled to

glycolysis [9]. This means that myosin ATPase preferentially uses ATP supplied by CK rather than cytosolic ATP [10]. This arrangement enables the Cr/PCr system to also function as a "spatial energy buffer" termed the "Creatine Phosphate Shuttle" [10,11]. PCr and Cr "shuttle" molecules between the sites of ATP production and utilisation with several significant advantages. PCr and Cr have higher diffusion rates than ATP or ADP and therefore are more efficient as energy shuttles [12]. At the sarcomeres, where large amounts of ATP are hydrolyzed during repetitive contractions, the MM-CK allows for the immediate phosphorylation of ADP. This maintains a low ADP concentration, thus reducing the ADP-mediated leak of Ca^{2+} from the SR, which would reduce the releasable Ca^{2+} and hence reduce the force output of the muscle [13]. It also reduces the free inorganic phosphate (P_i), slowing the entry of P_i into the SR where it precipitates the Ca^{2+} to cause a failure of Ca^{2+} release, reducing the force produced by the muscle [14–16]. Conversely, phosphorylation of Cr by Mi-CK keeps mitochondrial levels of ADP high, which stimulates the respiration rate and reduces the free energy required for ATP synthesis [8]. Mice which lack the MM-CK isoform of creatine kinase have been developed and display an inability to sustain maximal muscle force output during high intensity work [17]. Contractile kinetics are markedly slowed in the MM-CK-deficient mice [18]. Injection of small amounts of creatine into skeletal muscle deficient in all isoforms of creatine kinase restored its fatigue characteristics to wild-type specifications and interestingly also increases the Ca^{2+} concentration in the sarcoplasm [19], demonstrating that creatine can slow fatigue.

In fast-twitch muscles (muscles composed primarily of fast-twitch, or Type 2, fibres), repeated activation depletes stores of high energy phosphates (ATP and PCr) and there is a graded failure of Ca^{2+} release from the sarcoplasmic reticulum that is thought to be primarily responsible for the decline in the maximal force [15]. As mentioned above one mechanism causing this failure of Ca^{2+} release from the SR is the increase of P_i in the myoplasm (due to the increase in high energy phosphate utilisation). This P_i enters the SR and precipitates the free calcium as calcium phosphate [14,15]. A reduction in P_i entering the SR may explain why fast-twitch muscles of creatine-kinase-deficient mice (all isoforms) are markedly more fatigue resistant than wild-types [20].

Creatine has also been reported to increase the Ca^{2+} sensitivity of the contractile proteins, by virtue of the reduction in ionic strength that occurs when water follows creatine osmotically into the muscle fibre [21]. The ability to produce more force for a given intracellular $[Ca^{2+}]$ would enhance muscle performance and alleviate some of the force loss resulting from reduced SR Ca^{2+} release during fatigue.

Despite some of the abovementioned benefits of creatine for muscle performance, several studies [22–25] have reported that oral creatine supplementation has no effect on either twitch or tetanic force in rodent muscles. As these studies used unpaired data sets they would not pick up small changes [21]. In addition they did not examine the effects of creatine supplementation on fatigued muscles. In a recent study, Bassit et al. [26] showed that in fatigued muscle the fall in twitch force was less pronounced in the creatine-supplemented group. Resistance to fatigue during 60 min of contractile activity was significantly greater in the creatine-supplemented group as compared to placebo.

The aim of our present study was to provide further insight into how creatine may enhance muscle performance, by examining the contractile properties of isolated whole muscles before and after the acute application of creatine, in the absence and presence of fatigue. We used an isolated fast-twitch muscle preparation, using the extensor digitorum longus (EDL) muscle from the mouse (composed almost entirely of fast glycolytic and fast oxidative fibres [27]), to examine the rate and extent of the force loss during muscle fatigue before and after incubating the muscle in creatine. In each case the muscle was used as its own control, with the muscle being fatigued in the absence of creatine, allowed to recover, then incubated in creatine, washed, and subjected again to the same fatigue protocol. This use of paired data [21] means that the statistics are very robust in being able to detect small differences as the same muscle is used for both treatment and control conditions; additionally, the topical application of creatine to the muscle removes the variability associated with oral creatine supplementation.

Methods

Ethics statement

Ethical approval was granted by the Animal Ethics Committee of the University of New South Wales (AEC 94\025). 12 mice (C57BL/10) aged 13 to 14 weeks were used. Animals were sacrificed using an overdose of Halothane (Fluothane^{TM}, Zeneca Limited, UK) followed by cervical dislocation.

Water accumulation

In order to assess the water accumulation that resulted from incubation with 10 mM creatine, 7 EDL muscles were dissected out, blotted and weighed, then incubated in oxygenated Krebs solution containing 10 mM creatine for 30 minutes. They were then blotted on filter paper and weighed again. To see whether creatine incubation affects the diameter of muscle fibres, single enzymatically isolated flexor digitorum brevis (FDB) fibres were viewed under a Nikon inverted microscope at ×600, while perfused with oxygenated Krebs solution. A graticule was used to measure the fibre diameter at its widest point. The solution was then switched to one containing 10 mM creatine for 30 minutes, after which the fibres were observed during a washout period for 30 minutes. The isolated fibres were firmly attached to the glass coverslip and the graticule position was monitored throughout the procedure to ensure that its position relative to the fibre did not change during the procedure.

Whole muscle setup and solutions

Details of the muscle set-up procedure have been reported elsewhere [28]. Briefly, the EDL muscles were removed and attached to a force transducer and positioned between two platinum plates so that the muscle could be stimulated electrically and the resultant force response recorded. The muscles were set to their optimal length and were continuously superfused with Krebs solution (in mM): 4.75 KCl, 118 NaCl, 1.18 KH_2PO_4, 1.18 $MgSO_4$, 24.8 $NaHCO_3$, 2.5 $CaCl_2$, 11 glucose, bubbled with 95% O_2 5% CO_2 to maintain the pH at 7.4. The optimal length was termed L_0 and all subsequent measures were made at this muscle length. After determining the set length of the muscle it was allowed to equilibrate for 5 minutes in the bath.

Following this a force-frequency curve was generated using frequencies of 2, 5, 10, 15, 20, 25, 30, 50, 60, 75 and 100 Hz. This served as the "pre-fatigue" force-frequency curve for the muscle. A fatigue run was then carried out using our published fatigue protocol [29,30], stimulating the muscle at 100 Hz, 1 second on, 1 second off for 30 seconds. This protocol typically reduced the force by 70–80%. Immediately following this, a force-frequency curve was generated to measure the extent and nature of fatigue. This served as the "fatigue" force-frequency curve. A 20-minute recovery period followed in which the muscle was stimulated for 200 msec at 100 Hz once every 5 minutes in order to monitor the rate of recovery from fatigue. A force-frequency curve was then generated to determine recovery. This served as the "recovery" force-frequency curve. In our laboratory, we have observed that EDL muscles can be run up to five times through the protocol described above, without any significant deterioration of the muscle (unpublished data).

Following determination of the force-frequency characteristics of untreated muscle (the control condition), the muscle was incubated in a 9.9 mM creatine solution, prepared by dissolving creatine (Creatine Anhydrous from SIGMA) in the Krebs solution described above. The incubation period was 30 minutes and the muscle was stimulated at 100 Hz for 200 msec once every five minutes. The creatine-specific transporter protein CreaT [31] controls cellular creatine uptake. This moves creatine into the cell, against a concentration gradient, in a sodium- and chloride-dependent process [31]. Stimulating the muscle throughout incubation facilitates this uptake as described by Odoom et al. [32]. The rate of creatine uptake into the muscle under these conditions is estimated to be 70 nmol gww^{-1} [4]. The solution containing creatine was then washed out over a 5-min period and the muscle re-perfused with Krebs solution, so that the force produced by the muscle was not secondarily affected by having creatine present in the bathing solutions during the experimental procedures. The protocol from the pre-fatigue force-frequency curve to the post-fatigue force-frequency curve was then repeated. All experiments were undertaken at 22°C.

In the presentation of results, all forces are expressed as specific force (absolute force divided by cross-sectional area). The mean cross-sectional area of each muscle was calculated by dividing the muscle's wet mass by the product of its optimum length and the density of mammalian skeletal muscle (1.06 g cm^{-3}). The wet muscle mass was measured at the end of each experiment and hence represents the muscle mass following creatine incubation. In the water accumulation experiments described above, it was found that creatine incubation resulted in an average 7.3% increase in muscle weight. To allow for this, cross-sectional areas have been reduced by this amount in calculating specific forces before creatine incubation.

Statistical tests and analysis

A two-tailed paired t-test (GraphPad Prism) was used to test the significance of treatments. The significance level was $P<0.05$. However, when comparing control force versus creatine-treated force at each stimulation frequency of the force-frequency curve, a different test was used to reduce the possibility of Type I error arising from the large number of comparisons. Here we used Bonferroni multiple comparison post-tests following two-way repeated measures ANOVA, with an overall significance level of 5% (GraphPad Prism).

One further analysis performed on the force-frequency data was to fit a sigmoidal curve to the forces measured in every force-frequency activation sequence. This curve relates the muscle force P to the stimulation frequency f according to the following equation [33]:

$$P = P_{\min} + \frac{P_{\max} - P_{\min}}{1 + \left(\frac{K_f}{f}\right)^h}$$

where $P_{\max}$ is the maximum force, $P_{\min}$ is the minimum force, K_f is the half-frequency (the frequency at which force is halfway between minimum and maximum) and h is the Hill coefficient (an indication of the steepness of the curve).

Results

Whole muscle mass and single fibre diameter in 10 mM creatine

Creatine enters skeletal muscle by a saturable process, with an accompanying increase in intracellular water that is evidenced by an increase in muscle weight [34]. To show that our incubation procedure results in the successful uptake of creatine, we incubated EDL muscles and FDB fibres for 30 minutes in oxygenated Krebs solution containing 10 mM creatine, and measured resulting changes in muscle weight and fibre diameter. Following incubation, there was an increase in EDL wet weight of 7% (Fig. 1*A*), and an increase in FDB fibre diameter of 9% (Fig. 1*B*). These results demonstrate that our incubation procedure results in the uptake of creatine by the muscles and by the individual fibres [34].

Force-frequency curves from EDL muscles

The effects of creatine incubation on the force-frequency curves are illustrated in Fig. 2. Before fatigue (Fig. 2*A*), creatine treatment resulted in a significantly higher force at 100 Hz. In fatigued muscle (Fig. 2*B*), incubation in a creatine load solution prevented a significant amount of the loss of force seen as a result of repetitive

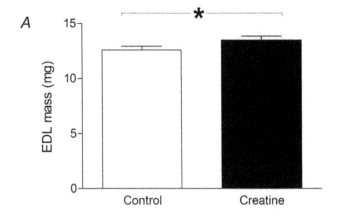

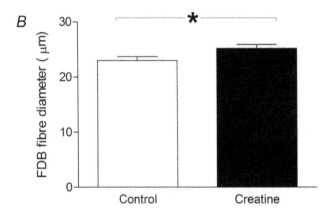

Figure 1. Changes in EDL muscle mass and FDB fibre diameter following creatine incubation. Creatine incubation resulted in a significant increase in the wet weight of whole EDL muscle (*A*) and a significant increase in the diameter of single FDB fibres (*B*), demonstrating the uptake of creatine by these muscles and fibres. Statistically significant differences are indicated by "*" ($P<0.05$).

activation in the same muscle under control (untreated) conditions. In the fatigued state, the creatine-treated muscle was found to produce significantly more force at all frequencies when compared with the muscle before creatine incubation (Fig. 2*B*). Maximal tetanic force in fatigued muscle was 27.0 ± 1.85 N cm^{-2} following creatine incubation compared with 14.9 ± 2.13 N cm^{-2} before creatine treatment (Fig. 2*B*). After recovery from fatigue (Fig. 2*C*), creatine treatment did not significantly affect the force at any frequency when compared with control.

Sigmoidal curves were fitted to the force-frequency data to obtain the half-frequency (the frequency at which force is halfway between minimum and maximum) and the Hill coefficient (a measure of the steepness of the curve). The values of these parameters are shown in Fig. 3. When the muscle was fatigued, creatine incubation resulted in a significant reduction of the half-frequency (Fig. 3*A*). In terms of the force-frequency curves for fatigued muscle shown in Fig. 2*B*, the curve for creatine-treated muscle has shifted to the left by 10.2 Hz compared to the control curve. No significant differences in the Hill coefficient (steepness of the curve) were found between creatine-treated and control conditions (Fig. 3*B*).

Twitch and tetanus in EDL muscles

The rate of relaxation during a muscle twitch, calculated as the fall in force divided by the change in time during the first 50% of

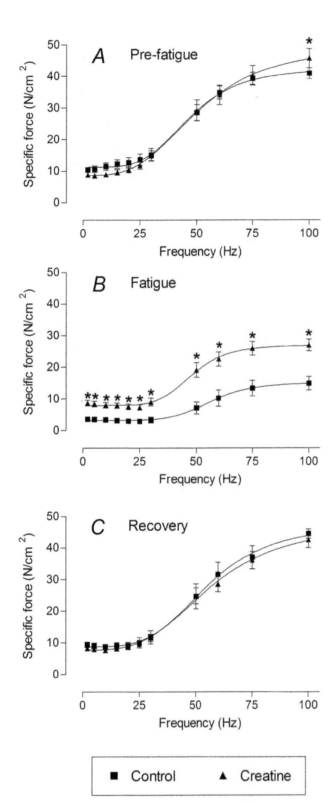

Figure 2. Force-frequency curves for EDL muscles before and after creatine treatment. Each graph shows the force-frequency curves under control and creatine-treated conditions. In the pre-fatigue state (A), creatine significantly increased the force produced at 100 Hz. In the fatigued state (B), creatine incubation significantly increased the force produced at every frequency. In the recovered state (C), creatine had no significant effect on the force at any frequency. Statistically significant differences are indicated by "*" ($P<0.05$). Tests for significance at each frequency were conducted using Bonferroni

multiple comparison post-tests following two-way repeated measures ANOVA (GraphPad Prism).

relaxation, is shown in Fig. 4A. In fatigued muscle, the rate of relaxation following creatine incubation was significantly faster than control. The rate of contraction during a muscle twitch, calculated as the peak twitch force divided by the time taken to reach peak force, is shown in Fig. 4B. In fatigue, the rate of contraction following creatine incubation was significantly faster than control.

The twitch-to-tetanus ratio was unchanged for the creatine-treated condition with respect to the control condition both before fatigue and after recovery. In creatine-treated muscles, however, there was a difference between the ratio in fatigue and the ratios for the pre-fatigue and recovered states. Notably this difference did not occur before creatine treatment. Fig. 5A shows that creatine treatment leads to a comparatively greater increase in twitch to tetanus ratio when the EDL muscles are fatigued compared to controls.

Fig. 5B shows that creatine treatment increases twitch and tetanic force when the muscle is fatigued, but has little effect on twitch and tetanic force when the muscle is recovered.

Rate of fatigue in EDL muscles

Creatine significantly increased the EDL muscle's resistance to fatigue. The parameter measured during the fatigue runs was the time taken for the maximum force produced by the muscle to fall to 50% of the pre-fatigue maximum. Creatine-treated muscle took $55.1\pm9.5\%$ ($P<0.05$) longer than the control for the force to fall to this point (Fig. 6A). Total force decline, as a percentage of initial force, was $84.8\pm2.0\%$ before creatine incubation and $71.1\pm1.8\%$ after creatine incubation ($P<0.05$). Fig. 6B shows the pattern of force decline during the fatigue run, before and after creatine incubation.

Discussion

Creatine and its effects on ionic strength and force production

In the present study we have shown that acute application of creatine enhances force production in isolated fast-twitch EDL muscle, especially during fatigue. In unfatigued muscle, creatine enhanced maximum force production (Fig. 2A). In fatigued muscle, creatine reduced the half-frequency (Fig. 3A), resulting in a left-shifting of the force-frequency relationship and an enhanced force production at every stimulation frequency (Fig. 2B).

We have also shown that acute incubation with creatine increased the weight of intact muscles and increased the diameter of individual fibres (Fig. 1). The most likely mechanism for this is that the uptake of creatine is accompanied by an increase in cellular water which occurs to maintain osmotic balance [35]. Increases in muscle mass along with water retention have frequently been reported as a side effect of creatine ingestion. Studies [36–38] reported increases in fat-free body mass of 1–2 kg which equates with a 7% increase in muscle water in an average human [21]. This is consistent with the 7% increase we observed in the mass of whole muscles following creatine incubation (Fig. 1A).

Our observed effects of creatine on force and muscle mass are consistent with the study of Murphy *et al.* [21], who found that increased creatine concentration, accompanied by a reduction in ionic strength mimicking the osmotic uptake of water, enhanced the Ca^{2+} sensitivity and maximum Ca^{2+}-activated force in

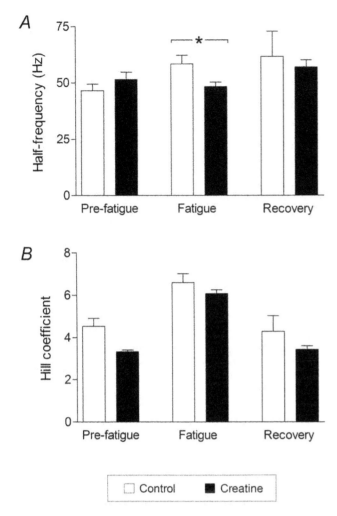

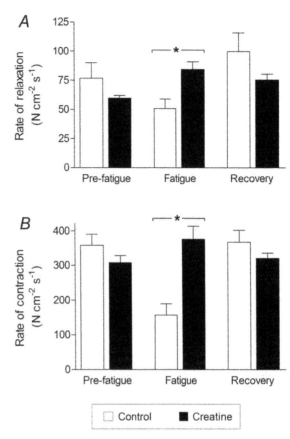

Figure 4. Twitch kinetics of EDL muscles before and after creatine treatment. A, Rate of relaxation. Creatine treatment resulted in significantly faster relaxation in fatigued muscle. B, Rate of contraction. Creatine treatment resulted in significantly faster contraction in fatigued muscle. Statistically significant differences are indicated by "*" (P<0.05).

Figure 3. Half-frequency and Hill coefficient of force-frequency curves. Sigmoidal curves were fitted to the force-frequency data to obtain the half-frequency (A) and Hill coefficient (B). Creatine treatment resulted in a significant reduction in the half-frequency in fatigued muscle. Statistically significant differences are indicated by "*" (P<0.05).

mechanically skinned EDL fibres. Under these conditions, the force-pCa curve for EDL fibres was shifted to the left [21], which is analogous to the left-shifting of the force-frequency curve caused by creatine in our fatigued muscles. Hence an increase in the Ca^{2+} sensitivity of the contractile proteins could underlie the shift of the force-frequency curve that we found when creatine was applied to fatigued muscle.

Murphy *et al.* [21] concluded that the beneficial effects of creatine occurred through the reduction in ionic strength, rather than some direct action of creatine, because creatine actually had an inhibitory effect on force and Ca^{2+} sensitivity when ionic strength was left unchanged. In our present study, we can assume that the ionic strength within our EDL muscles has decreased, since the increase in mass following creatine incubation suggests osmotic water uptake. Hence we postulate that a reduction in ionic strength following creatine incubation is responsible for the enhanced force production of our creatine-treated muscles. The influence of ionic strength on muscle contractility is an established observation in the literature [39–41]; it is possible that a reduction in ionic strength enhances the force production and Ca^{2+} sensitivity of the contractile apparatus because of reduced

competition from monovalent cations such as K^+ and Na^+ for binding sites on the thin-filament regulatory proteins [41].

Creatine and fatiguing stimulation

Fatigue can be defined as the inability of a muscle to maintain maximal force production as a result of repeated activity. Failure of Ca^{2+} release from the SR is considered to be a major cause of fatigue [42,43]. Fatigued muscle also suffers in respect of contractile kinetics and there is a slowing of contraction and relaxation. Using the alteration of these parameters as a measure of fatigue a major finding of this study was that incubation in a creatine solution, followed by a wash before initiating the fatigue protocol, caused an improved resistance to fatigue in mouse fast-twitch EDL muscle (Fig. 6).

Why does creatine have this inhibitory effect on fatigue? One mechanism that can be deduced from earlier studies is that creatine helps to maintain Ca^{2+} release during fatigue. When creatine is transported into the muscle fibre a proportion of it will be phosphorylated and become part of the phosphocreatine cycle [44]. The Cr/PCr cycle is the major provider of ATP during intense activity in skeletal muscle. The failure of Ca^{2+} release is thought to be primarily due to the build up of P_i which occurs due to the high rates of ATP hydrolysis during intense muscle activation. This P_i enters the SR via an ATP-dependent ion channel transport mechanism (the channel is activated by low

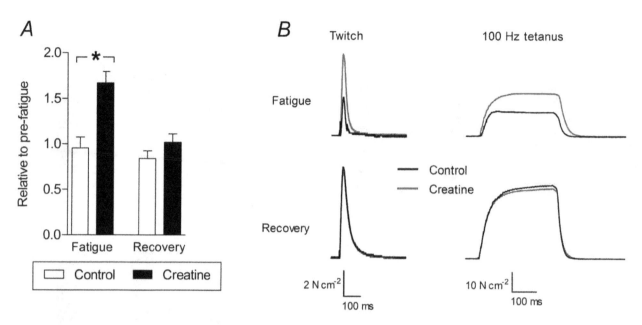

Figure 5. Twitch and tetanus in EDL muscles before and after creatine treatment. *A*, twitch to tetanus ratios expressed relative to the pre-fatigue twitch to tetanus ratio. Before creatine incubation, the twitch to tetanus ratio in fatigued muscle was similar to that in the pre-fatigue state. After creatine incubation however, the twitch to tetanus ratio in the fatigued state was significantly higher than in the pre-fatigue state. Statistically significant differences are indicated by "*" ($P<0.05$). *B*, force tracings of twitches and 100-Hz tetani obtained from one EDL muscle. In the fatigued muscle, creatine incubation increases the twitch force and tetanic force. In the recovered muscle however, creatine incubation makes little difference to the twitch and tetanic forces.

ATP) where it precipitates the free Ca^{2+} resulting in a failure of Ca^{2+} release [42]. Thus increased levels of PCr will keep the P_i levels lower by using the free inorganic phosphate to regenerate ATP from ADP. In addition the open probability of the phosphate transporter in the SR will be reduced as ATP levels are higher. Supporting this, Gallo *et al.* [45] noted that high levels of creatine supplementation which increased intramuscular creatine by 20% improved fatigue resistance in rat EDL muscle by 20% and 7% after 10 and 30 s of stimulation, respectively.

However, another mechanism has been proposed where force is enhanced due to the increased Ca^{2+} sensitivity of the contractile proteins arising from the reduction in ionic strength that accompanies Cr loading [21]. This is a likely mechanism in our current study, given the left-shifting of the force-frequency curve in fatigue following creatine incubation. Thus even if Ca^{2+} release from the SR was impaired during fatigue, creatine incubation may attenuate the resulting loss of force by making the contractile proteins more sensitive to Ca^{2+}.

Creatine and its effect on twitch kinetics

The slowing of contractile kinetics during fatigue is a well established finding in the literature. The decreased speed of relaxation [46] and contraction [47] becomes progressively more pronounced throughout a fatiguing protocol. Relaxation processes account for an important fraction of total energy consumption in muscles during short repeated contractions [48,49]. Relaxation is a

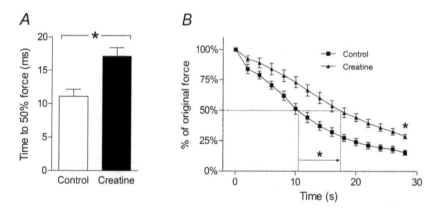

Figure 6. Fatigue run in EDL muscles before and after creatine treatment. *A*, time taken for force to fall to 50% of original force. Creatine incubation resulted in a significant increase in this parameter. *B*, pattern of force decline during the fatigue run, showing the effect of creatine treatment in improving the resistance of muscles to fatigue. It is evident that creatine incubation is associated with an increase in the time taken for force to fall to 50%, as well as a reduction in the total force decline over the whole fatigue run. Statistically significant differences are indicated by "*" ($P<0.05$).

multi-faceted process and different techniques for measurement of changes to the relaxation process have been used. In a review by Gillis [50], relaxation is described as having two distinct phases. The first is the plateau which is a slow linear decline in tension with no change in muscle length. During this phase the intracellular $[Ca^{2+}]$ falls rapidly [51]. In the second phase tension drops rapidly with Ca^{2+} levels relatively constant [51]. Creatine supplementation has been shown to decrease half relaxation time [52] and to improve Ca^{2+} handling in dystrophic muscle [31]. The creatine analogue β-GPA (β-Guanidinopropionoic acid) depletes cellular creatine (and hence phosophocreatine levels) and causes an increase in time to half relaxation [53]. In the absence of the phosphocreatine buffering system (achieved by inhibiting creatine kinase using dinitroflourobenzene) shortening velocity can be up to 30% slower than the control both in mouse skeletal muscle [47] and in frog skeletal muscle [54]. Conversely, mice genetically modified to have an increased expression of creatine kinase demonstrated a faster shortening velocity during a 5 second tetanus [55]. Steeghs *et al.* [56] found that CK-deficient muscle tested *in vivo* displayed an impaired peak tetanic force, a reduced ability to sustain maximal contractions and an increased time to half relaxation. Further, in myotube cultures from the same strain of mouse, both the release and sequestration of Ca^{2+} were negatively affected as measured by a reduced peak and an extended duration of the Ca^{2+} released in a twitch.

In the present study it is possible that the increased rates of contraction and relaxation seen in fatigued muscle pre-incubated in creatine (Fig. 4) is a consequence of lowered ionic strength. However, we cannot rule out an increased supply of PCr as a result of creatine uptake in improving the contractile kinetics. In humans, creatine supplementation increased intramuscular crea- tine by 8% and significantly improved performance during the transition from rest to both moderate- and heavy-intensity exercise, and also improved performance in the transition from moderate-intensity exercise to rest [57].

Conclusions

We have shown that acute incubation with creatine enhances force production in fast-twitch EDL muscle, especially when the muscle is fatigued. Such an effect is likely to occur through an increased Ca^{2+} sensitivity of the contractile proteins due to the reduction in ionic strength that accompanies creatine incubation. The improved resistance to loss of force during fatiguing stimulation is also likely to be explained by an increased Ca^{2+} sensitivity. We have also shown that in fatigued muscle, creatine incubation increases the rate of twitch contraction and relaxation. In fatigued muscle, even small changes in force production and contractile kinetics could be very important in terms of human performance in a race situation. Thus the effects of creatine incubation on isolated muscle demonstrated in our study provide insight into the improved muscle performance observed following creatine supplementation in humans. Providing there are no as yet undiscovered health risks associated with creatine supplementa- tion, creatine may be of great benefit both to athletes and as a therapeutic tool for the treatment of neuromuscular disorders.

Author Contributions

Conceived and designed the experiments: SIH BG. Performed the experiments: SIH BG. Analyzed the data: SIH BG SC. Wrote the paper: SIH BG SC.

References

1. Balsom PD, Ekblom BKS, Sjodin B, Hultman E (1993) Creatine supplemen- tation and dynamic high-intensity intermittent exercise. Scand J Med Sci Sports 3: 143–149.
2. Casey A, Constantin-Teodosiu D, Howell S, Hultman E, Greenhaff PL (1996) Creatine ingestion favorably affects performance and muscle metabolism during maximal exercise in humans. Am J Physiol Endocrinol Metab 271: E31–37.
3. Kley RA, Vorgerd M, Tarnopolsky MA (2007) Creatine for treating muscle disorders. Cochrane Database Syst Rev. CD004760.
4. Willott CA, Young ME, Leighton B, Kemp GJ, Boehm EA, et al. (1999) Creatine uptake in isolated soleus muscle: kinetics and dependence on sodium, but not on insulin. Acta Physiol Scand 166: 99–104.
5. Hultman E, Greenhaff PL (1991) Skeletal muscle energy metabolism and fatigue during intense exercise in man. Sci Prog 75: 361–370.
6. Levine S, Tikunov B, Henson D, LaManca J, Sweeney HL (1996) Creatine depletion elicits structural, biochemical, and physiological adaptations in rat costal diaphragm. Am J Physiol Cell Physiol 271: C1480–1486.
7. Boehm EA, Radda GK, Tomlin H, Clark JF (1996) The utilisation of creatine and its analogues by cytosolic and mitochondrial creatine kinase. Biochim Biophys Acta 1274: 119–128.
8. Wyss M, Smeitink J, Wevers RA, Wallimann T (1992) Mitochondrial creatine kinase: a key enzyme of aerobic energy metabolism. Biochim Biophys Acta 1102: 119–166.
9. Wallimann T, Wyss M, Brdiczka D, Nicolay K, Eppenberger HM (1992) Intracellular compartmentation, structure and function of creatine kinase isoenzymes in tissues with high and fluctuating energy demands: the 'phosphocreatine circuit' for cellular energy homeostasis. Biochem J 281: 21–40.
10. Bessman SP, Geiger PJ (1981) Transport of energy in muscle: the phosphor- ylcreatine shuttle. Science 211: 448–452.
11. Brosnan JT, Brosnan ME (2007) Creatine: endogenous metabolite, dietary, and therapeutic supplement. Annu Rev Nutr 27: 241–261.
12. Jacobus WE (1985) Theoretical support for the heart phosphocreatine energy transport shuttle based on the intracellular diffusion limited mobility of ADP. Biochem Biophys Res Commun 133: 1035–1041.
13. Macdonald WA, Stephenson DG (2001) Effects of ADP on sarcoplasmic reticulum function in mechanically skinned skeletal muscle fibres of the rat. J Physiol 532: 499–508.
14. Allen DG, Lännergren J, Westerblad H (1995) Muscle cell function during prolonged activity: cellular mechanisms of fatigue. Exp Physiol 80: 497–527.
15. Allen DG, Westerblad H (2001) Role of phosphate and calcium stores in muscle fatigue. J Physiol 536: 657–665.
16. Fryer MW, Owen VJ, Lamb GD, Stephenson DG (1995) Effects of creatine phosphate and P_i on Ca^{2+} movements and tension development in rat skinned skeletal muscle fibres. J Physiol 482: 123–140.
17. van Deursen J, Heerschap A, Oerlemans F, Ruitenbeek W, Jap P, et al. (1993) Skeletal muscles of mice deficient in muscle creatine kinase lack burst activity. Cell 74: 621–631.
18. Ventura-Clapier R, Kuznetsov AV, d'Albis A, van Deursen J, Wieringa B, et al. (1995) Muscle creatine kinase-deficient mice. I. Alterations in myofibrillar function. J Biol Chem 270: 19914–19920.
19. Dahlstedt AJ, Katz A, Tavi P, Westerblad H (2003) Creatine kinase injection restores contractile function in creatine-kinase-deficient mouse skeletal muscle fibres. J Physiol 547: 395–403.
20. Dahlstedt AJ, Katz A, Wieringa B, Westerblad H (2000) Is creatine kinase responsible for fatigue? Studies of isolated skeletal muscle deficient in creatine kinase. FASEB J 14: 982–990.
21. Murphy RM, Stephenson DG, Lamb GD (2004) Effect of creatine on contractile force and sensitivity in mechanically skinned single fibers from rat skeletal muscle. Am J Physiol Cell Physiol 287: C1589–1595.
22. Gagnon M, Maguire M, MacDermott M, Bradford A (2002) Effects of creatine loading and depletion on rat skeletal muscle contraction. Clin Exp Pharmacol Physiol 29: 885–890.
23. McGuire M, Bradford A, MacDermott M (2001) The effects of dietary creatine supplements on the contractile properties of rat soleus and extensor digitorum longus muscles. Exp Physiol 86: 185–190.
24. Op't Eijnde B, Lebacq J, Ramaekers M, Hespel P (2004) Effect of muscle creatine content manipulation on contractile properties in mouse muscles. Muscle Nerve 29: 428–435.
25. Robinson DM, Loiselle DS (2002) Effect of creatine manipulation on fast-twitch skeletal muscle of the mouse. Clin Exp Pharmacol Physiol 29: 1105–1111.
26. Bassit RA, Pinheiro CHdJ, Vitzel KF, Sproesser AJ, Silveira LR, et al. (2010) Effect of short-term creatine supplementation on markers of skeletal muscle damage after strenuous contractile activity. Eur J Appl Physiol 108: 945–955.
27. Anderson JE, Bressler BH, Ovalle WK (1988) Functional regeneration in the hindlimb skeletal muscle of the *mdx* mouse. J Muscle Res Cell Motil 9: 499–515.
28. Head SI, Stephenson DG, Williams DA (1990) Properties of enzymatically isolated skeletal fibres from mice with muscular dystrophy. J Physiol 422: 351–367.
29. Chan S, Head SI (2010) Age- and gender-related changes in contractile properties of non-atrophied EDL muscle. PLoS ONE 5: e12345.

30. Chan S, Seto JT, MacArthur DG, Yang N, North KN, et al. (2008) A gene for speed: contractile properties of isolated whole EDL muscle from an alpha-actinin-3 knockout mouse. Am J Physiol Cell Physiol 295: C897–904.
31. Pulido SM, Passaquin AC, Leijendekker WJ, Challet C, Wallimann T, et al. (1998) Creatine supplementation improves intracellular Ca^{2+} handling and survival in *mdx* skeletal muscle cells. FEBS Lett 439: 357–362.
32. Odoom JE, Kemp GJ, Radda GK (1996) The regulation of total creatine content in a myoblast cell line. Mol Cell Biochem 158: 179–188.
33. Motulsky HJ, Christopoulos A (2003) Fitting models to biological data using linear and nonlinear regression. A practical guide to curve fitting. San Diego: Graph Pad Software Inc.
34. Fitch CD, Shields RP (1966) Creatine metabolism in skeletal muscle. I. Creatine movement across muscle membranes. J Biol Chem 241: 3611–3614.
35. Ziegenfuss TN, Lowery LM, Lemon PWR (1998) Acute fluid volume changes in men during three days of creatine supplementation. J Exerc Physiol 1: 1–14.
36. Earnest CP, Snell PG, Rodriguez R, Almada AL, Mitchell TL (1995) The effect of creatine monohydrate ingestion on anaerobic power indices, muscular strength and body composition. Acta Physiol Scand 153: 207–209.
37. van Loon LJC, Oosterlaar AM, Hartgens F, Hesselink MKC, Snow RJ, et al. (2003) Effects of creatine loading and prolonged creatine supplementation on body composition, fuel selection, sprint and endurance performance in humans. Clin Sci 104: 153–162.
38. Volek JS, Duncan ND, Mazzetti SA, Staron RS, Putukian M, et al. (1999) Performance and muscle fiber adaptations to creatine supplementation and heavy resistance training. Med Sci Sports Exerc 31: 1147–1156.
39. April E, Brandt PW, Reuben JP, Grundfest H (1968) Muscle contraction: the effect of ionic strength. Nature 220: 182–184.
40. Ashley CC, Moisescu DG (1977) Effect of changing the composition of the bathing solutions upon the isometric tension-pCa relationship in bundles of crustacean myofibrils. J Physiol 270: 627–652.
41. Fink RH, Stephenson DG, Williams DA (1986) Potassium and ionic strength effects on the isometric force of skinned twitch muscle fibres of the rat and toad. J Physiol 370: 317–337.
42. Allen DG, Lamb GD, Westerblad H (2008) Skeletal muscle fatigue: cellular mechanisms. Physiol Rev 88: 287–332.
43. Westerblad H, Allen DG (1991) Changes of myoplasmic calcium concentration during fatigue in single mouse muscle fibers. J Gen Physiol 98: 615–635.
44. Terjung RL, Clarkson P, Eichner ER, Greenhaff PL, Hespel PJ, et al. (2000) American College of Sports Medicine roundtable. The physiological and health effects of oral creatine supplementation. Med Sci Sports Exerc 32: 706–717.
45. Gallo M, Gordon T, Syrotuik D, Shu Y, Tyreman N, et al. (2006) Effects of long-term creatine feeding and running on isometric functional measures and myosin heavy chain content of rat skeletal muscles. Pflugers Arch 452: 744–755.
46. Westerblad H, Lännergren J (1991) Slowing of relaxation during fatigue in single mouse muscle fibres. J Physiol 434: 323–336.
47. Westerblad H, Dahlstedt AJ, Lännergren J (1998) Mechanisms underlying reduced maximum shortening velocity during fatigue of intact, single fibres of mouse muscle. J Physiol 510: 269–277.
48. Homsher E (1987) Muscle enthalpy production and its relationship to actomyosin ATPase. Annu Rev Physiol 49: 673–690.
49. Homsher E, Kean CJ (1978) Skeletal muscle energetics and metabolism. Annu Rev Physiol 40: 93–131.
50. Gillis JM (1985) Relaxation of vertebrate skeletal muscle. A synthesis of the biochemical and physiological approaches. Biochim Biophys Acta 811: 97–145.
51. Cannell MB (1986) Effect of tetanus duration on the free calcium during the relaxation of frog skeletal muscle fibres. J Physiol 376: 203–218.
52. van Leemputte M, Vandenberghe K, Hespel P (1999) Shortening of muscle relaxation time after creatine loading. J Appl Physiol 86: 840–844.
53. Wakatsuki T, Ohira Y, Nakamura K, Asakura T, Ohno H, et al. (1995) Changes of contractile properties of extensor digitorum longus in response to creatine-analogue administration and/or hindlimb suspension in rats. Jpn J Physiol 45: 979–989.
54. Westerblad H, Lännergren J (1995) Reduced maximum shortening velocity in the absence of phosphocreatine observed in intact fibres of *Xenopus* skeletal muscle. J Physiol 482: 383–390.
55. Roman BB, Foley JM, Meyer RA, Koretsky AP (1996) Contractile and metabolic effects of increased creatine kinase activity in mouse skeletal muscle. Am J Physiol 270: C1236–1245.
56. Steeghs K, Benders A, Oerlemans F, de Haan A, Heerschap A, et al. (1997) Altered Ca^{2+} responses in muscles with combined mitochondrial and cytosolic creatine kinase deficiencies. Cell 89: 93–103.
57. Jones AM, Wilkerson DP, Fulford J (2009) Influence of dietary creatine supplementation on muscle phosphocreatine kinetics during knee-extensor exercise in humans. Am J Physiol Regul Integr Comp Physiol 296: R1078–1087.

3

Functional Relationship between Skull Form and Feeding Mechanics in *Sphenodon*, and Implications for Diapsid Skull Development

Neil Curtis[1]*, **Marc E. H. Jones**[2], **Junfen Shi**[1], **Paul O'Higgins**[3], **Susan E. Evans**[2], **Michael J. Fagan**[1]

1 Medical and Biological Engineering Research Group, Department of Engineering, University of Hull, Hull, United Kingdom, **2** Research Department of Cell and Developmental Biology, University College London, London, United Kingdom, **3** Hull-York Medical School, University of York, York, United Kingdom

Abstract

The vertebrate skull evolved to protect the brain and sense organs, but with the appearance of jaws and associated forces there was a remarkable structural diversification. This suggests that the evolution of skull form may be linked to these forces, but an important area of debate is whether bone in the skull is minimised with respect to these forces, or whether skulls are mechanically "over-designed" and constrained by phylogeny and development. Mechanical analysis of diapsid reptile skulls could shed light on this longstanding debate. Compared to those of mammals, the skulls of many extant and extinct diapsids comprise an open framework of fenestrae (window-like openings) separated by bony struts (e.g., lizards, tuatara, dinosaurs and crocodiles), a cranial form thought to be strongly linked to feeding forces. We investigated this link by utilising the powerful engineering approach of multibody dynamics analysis to predict the physiological forces acting on the skull of the diapsid reptile *Sphenodon*. We then ran a series of structural finite element analyses to assess the correlation between bone strain and skull form. With comprehensive loading we found that the distribution of peak von Mises strains was particularly uniform throughout the skull, although specific regions were dominated by tensile strains while others were dominated by compressive strains. Our analyses suggest that the frame-like skulls of diapsid reptiles are probably optimally formed (mechanically ideal: sufficient strength with the minimal amount of bone) with respect to functional forces; they are efficient in terms of having minimal bone volume, minimal weight, and also minimal energy demands in maintenance.

Editor: Andrew A. Farke, Raymond M. Alf Museum of Paleontology, United States of America

Funding: Funding was provided by the Biotechnology and Biological Sciences Research Council (BBSRC-http://www.bbsrc.ac.uk) - grant numbers: BB/E007465/1, BB/E009204/1 and BB/E007813/1. The funders had no role in study design, data collection and analysis, decision to publish, or preparation of the manuscript.

Competing Interests: The authors have declared that no competing interests exist.

* E-mail: n.curtis@hull.ac.uk

Introduction

There is a longstanding debate as to whether bone in the skull is minimised in relation physiological loading [1,2], or whether skulls are 'over-designed' and constrained by phylogeny, development, and the need to accommodate functions in addition to normal loading [3–5]. The skull provides a structure for jaw and neck muscle attachment and should be rigid enough to withstand the forces these muscles apply, along with accompanying feeding and other forces [6–8]. Exactly how the skull responds to these forces in tandem with accommodating the brain and sense organs is not fully understood. Adaptation to loads consistent with Wolff's law [9] would result in minimisation of bony material with respect to functional loading, and following a long held theory [10] the term *bone functional adaptation* [11–13] is often used to describe the mechanism by which bone is modelled and remodelled. Briefly, it is proposed that bone strain is the stimulus for bone modelling/remodelling [14,15], and there is an *equilibrium window* of strain, above which bone is deposited and below which bone is removed [16–18]. The rules regulating bone adaptation and the exact levels at which bone is remodelled are however likely more complex, being dependent on more than just pure strain magnitudes. Strain rate, load history, bone age, disease, initial bone shape, bone

developmental history, hormonal environment, diet, and genetic factors have all been highlighted as potential factors that could impact bone form [15–25].

The skull of *Sphenodon*, a New Zealand reptile, is not dominated by a large vaulted braincase like mammals, but instead comprises an open arrangement of fenestrae (windows or openings) and bony rods or struts [26,27]. Without the constraint of a large brain and associated forces [28–31], the dominant loads applied to the frame-like skull of *Sphenodon* are most likely linked to feeding (i.e. muscle forces, bite forces, and jaw joint forces). This is probably also true for other diapsids that lack large brains, such as lizards, crocodiles, and theropod dinosaurs, which share comparable skull morphologies (Figure 1). Without the effect of neurocranial expansion, these frame-like skulls may be useful for investigating the correlation between skull form and bone strain under loading. Some insight into this relationship would provide new perspectives towards understanding skull form in other amniotes.

Finite element analysis (FEA) is a virtual technique that is used to predict how a structure will deform when forces and constraints are applied to it, and has been used previously to predict stress and strain distribution within skulls [4,27–29,31–33,35,36]. However, such studies tend to apply limited loading data and are used to investigate particular aspects of skull morphology or the impact of

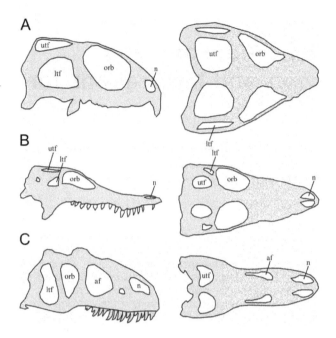

Figure 1. The diapsid skull form. Simplified schematic lateral and dorsal skull views of **A.** *Sphenodon* (redrawn [87]), **B.** *Crocodylus siamensis* (original drawing), **C.** *Allosaurus fragilis* (redrawn [92]). All skulls are scaled to the same length. af – antorbital fenestra; ltf – lower temporal fenestra; n – nasal opening; orb – orbital opening; utf – upper temporal fenestra.

single bites. To fully evaluate skull form it is important to take into account several different load cases, because skull form is most likely to be related to the range of physiological loads experienced by an animal rather than a single load case. We investigated the relationship between skull form and bone strain in *Sphenodon* by carrying out a series of static finite element analyses (FEAs), applying bite forces at several different bite positions. We combine the powerful computational techniques of multibody dynamics analysis (MDA) [32–34] and FEA, to first predict the forces acting on the skull of *Sphenodon*, and in turn analyse the strains within the skull under these forces. This enables us to evaluate the degree of correlation between skull form and three strain modes: tensile (also known as maximum and 1st principal), compressive (also know as minimum and 3rd principal) and von Mises (also known as equivalent and mean). Multibody dynamics analysis has recently been applied to study skull biomechanics [32–38], and was used here to predict muscle forces, joint forces, and bite forces in *Sphenodon* during fifteen separate biting simulations. These simulations covered a range of biting types and locations. They include four bilateral and eight unilateral bites at different tooth positions, a bite on the anterior-most chisel-like teeth, and two ripping bites that incorporate neck muscles (MDA model shown in Figure 2 and a summary of all biting simulations is given in Table 1). A corresponding set of fifteen separate FEAs was carried out to investigate the total mechanical performance of the skull under these predicted forces. Each separate FEA applied a peak static bite force and corresponding muscle and joint forces.

Results

MDA

Total bite and quadrate-articular joint forces (i.e. working and balancing sides combined) are similar whether the animal is biting

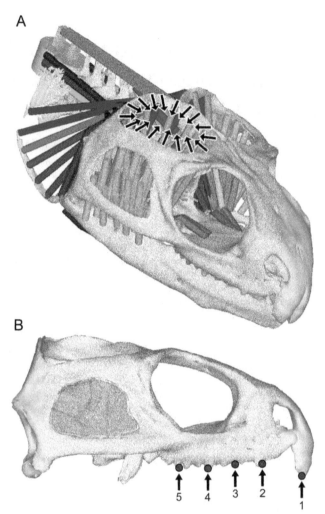

Figure 2. MDA model. A. Multibody computer model used to calculate the muscle, joint and biting forces for a series of biting simulations. Black arrows represent the location and direction of the fascial force vectors applied to the finite element model over one temporal opening. **B.** Bite locations. Bilateral (biting on both sides simultaneously) and unilateral biting (biting on one side only) at locations 2–5; bilateral biting only at location 1; ripping bites at location 2 only. Skull measures approximately 68 mm long from the tip of the premaxilla to the posterior end of the quadrate condyles.

unilaterally or bilaterally. However, the bite force on each side of the skull during bilateral biting is half that of unilateral biting (i.e. the total bite force is shared over both sides of the skull). Also, forces located at the balancing side joint during unilateral biting are always in excess of those at working side joint (Table 2). Bite force at the most posterior bite location (location 5 – Figure 2B) is almost 80% greater than on the chisel-like teeth at the front of the skull (location 1), whereas during unilateral biting the balancing side joint force is approximately 50% greater than the working side joint force at the most posterior bite location (location 5). Total muscle forces applied during the MDA are presented in Table 3.

FEA

Bite location has a considerable effect on the way the skull deforms. During individual bites, strain gradients (or heterogeneous strain magnitudes) are apparent over the skull, with some regions subject to high strains and others subject to low strains

Table 1. The 15 load cases simulated during the MDA and applied in the FEA.

Load case	Type of bite	Side of skull	Bite location	Bite Location
1	unilateral	right	anterior	2
2	unilateral	right	middle	3
3	unilateral	right	posterior	4
4	unilateral	right	posterior-most	5
5	unilateral	left	anterior	2
6	unilateral	left	middle	3
7	unilateral	left	posterior	4
8	unilateral	left	posterior-most	5
9	bilateral	both	anterior	2
10	bilateral	both	middle	3
11	bilateral	both	posterior	4
12	bilateral	both	posterior-most	5
13	bilateral	both	chisel-like tooth	1
14	neck ripping bite (left)	both	anterior	2
15	neck ripping bite (right)	both	anterior	2

See Figure 2 for explanation of bite locations.

(example von Mises strain plots are presented in Figure 3). As the skull deforms it experiences both compressive and tensile strains (dominant strains over all bites at specific skull locations is presented in Figure 4), and during unilateral biting these strains tend to reach their peak magnitudes (Figure 5A). In addition to the peak strains generated during unilateral bites, high strain also occurs in the nasal bone when biting on the large anterior-most chisel-like teeth, a distinctive feature of *Sphenodon* ([39]; Figure 5B, bilateral location 1). Ripping bites in which the neck muscles are highly active also strain the posterior aspects of the skull and braincase more than non-ripping bites (Figure 5B, ripping location 2). Across all simulations unilateral bites account for approximately 79% of the peak strains generated across the skull, with the posterior-most unilateral bite accounting for 60% of peak strains. Biting on the anterior-most chisel-like teeth generates approximately 9% of the peak strains in the skull, while the ripping bites were attributable for 10%. Bilateral bites (excluding biting on the anterior-most teeth) accounted for less than 2% of peak strains

across the skull when all biting simulations were assessed. Strains vary over the skull at any one bite location (including those yielding the highest strains), with approximately 30% of the skull at low levels of strain below 200 microstrain, and 65% of the skull at strains of below 500 microstrain during separate bites (Figure 6).

When the individual peak element strains (i.e. the highest strain any one element ever experienced) are extracted from all fifteen individual biting analyses to generate a combined loading peak strain map, the obvious strain gradients (or heterogeneous strain magnitudes) noted during separate bites are considerably reduced (Figure 7). During combined loading 94.6%, 96.7%, and 98.0% of the skull experiences tensile, compressive, and von Mises strains of above 200 microstrain respectively when the peak element strains over all bites are considered (Figure 6). This compares to an average of approximately 70% during separate bites for all strain modes. Moreover, during combined loading 85.3%, 87.9%, and 91.1% of the skull in our model is at strains of between 400 and 2500 microstrain for tensile, compressive, and von Mises strain

Table 2. Bite forces and jaw joint forces predicted by the MDA.

Bite Type	Bite Location	Bite Force (N)	Working Joint Force (N)	Balancing Joint Force (N)
bilateral	1	121	540	-
bilateral	2	150	524	-
bilateral	3	165	510	-
bilateral	4	185	490	-
bilateral	5	214	462	-
unilateral	2	150	249	276
unilateral	3	166	232	276
unilateral	4	187	212	277
unilateral	5	216	183	278

Total forces are shown for bilateral bites, therefore the force on each side of the skull is approximately half that presented. Working refers to the force on the same side as the bite occurs, while balancing refers to the opposite side to which biting occurs. See Figure 2 for explanation of bite locations.

Table 3. Total muscle forces applied to each side of the skull during the MDA.

Muscle	Total Muscle Force (N)
Depressors (defined as 2 groups)	40
Adductors (defined as 14 groups)	448
Neck (defined as 11 groups)	158

The depressor muscles were represented by two muscle groups, the adductor muscles were represented by fourteen muscle groups, and the neck muscles were represented by eleven muscle groups. This arrangement of muscles accurately depicts the anatomy of *Sphenodon*. Muscle sections are visually presented in Figure 3A, while detailed descriptions of all muscle groups are published elsewhere [18,39].

respectively, implying that the majority of the skull is shaped (remodelled) to keep strains within a specific tolerance range (Figure 6). Mean tensile, compressive, and von Mises strain over the entire skull (average strain across all individual finite elements in the model) is 784 microstrain, 887 microstrain, and 1140 microstrain when peak strains over all load cases are assessed. This value is typically only 500 microstrain during separate bites.

Overall strain distributions over the skull remain largely unchanged with the addition of a fascial sheet over the upper temporal fenestra, but there were some striking reductions in localised peak strains, as highlighted in Figure 8. In particular, there is a reduction of peak strain on the lateral aspect of the postorbital bar where the jugal and postorbital meet, but the most obvious reductions in peak strains are on the posterior surface of the quadrate (encircled in Figure 8B), the temporal bar (squamosal and parietal, encircled in Figure 8B) and the posterior edges of the parietals where they meet in the midline (also encircled in Figure 8B). Localised peak strain areas around the perimeter of the upper fenestra were unaffected, with the exception of a small region on the posterior part of the postorbital.

Discussion

The results of our comprehensive analysis implies that the form of the diapsid skull of *Sphenodon* is strongly linked to feeding forces. We show that both tensile and compressive peak strains are relatively evenly distributed throughout the skull when several loading cases are analysed (Figure 7). Although tensile strains are dominant in some regions of the skull, compressive strains are dominant in others (Figure 4). However, when analysing von Mises strain, which takes into account all principal strains, the distribution of strain is even more uniform when compared to tensile and compressive strains alone (Figure 7).

Our analyses show that over 91% of the skull is at von Mises strains of between 400 and 2500 microstrain when peak biting forces were analysed (Figure 6). While von Mises strain does not show which principal strain mode is dominant, making it difficult to interpret the exact response of the structure (e.g. whether or not it might fracture under tensile forces), von Mises strain does appear to be a good indicator of bone adaptation. *In vivo* studies predominantly on long bones have shown that both tensile and compressive strains are frequently experienced by bones during normal use, with peak strain during forceful loading ranging from 900 to 5200 microstrain [40–52]. In our analyses we find both high compressive and tensile strains over the skull, comparable in magnitude to those recorded experimentally in other animals (Figure 7), where compressive strains are dominant in approximately 60% of the skull (Figure 4). Focusing specifically on skulls, Herring et al. [53,54] recorded strains of 2000–3000 microstrain when the masseter muscle was maximally contacted in a pig skull, peak values very similar to those predicted in our study.

Most literature on bone adaptation only refers to strain without inferring a particular mode, or even magnitude to this regard. What we do know is that bone adapts to mechanical loading, for example in experimental studies on adult rats, Robling et al. [55] showed bone to be deposited on both the tensile and compressive sides of artificially loaded forearms. Also under 'normal' loading situations, Haapassalo et al. [56] used peripheral quantitative computed tomography to show mean bilateral asymmetries (between the racket holding arm and non-racket holding arm) in second moments of area of the humeral midshaft in male tennis players. Although such studies show bone adaptation to functional loading, it is difficult to infer the exact strain magnitudes that initiate a particular bone remodelling effect. A figure published in Martin [57] does provide some suggestion into the approximate strain magnitudes that could cause bone adaptation. In this case, strains of below 50 microstrain are thought to represent disuse and thus bone resorption, whereas strains of between 1500 and 3000

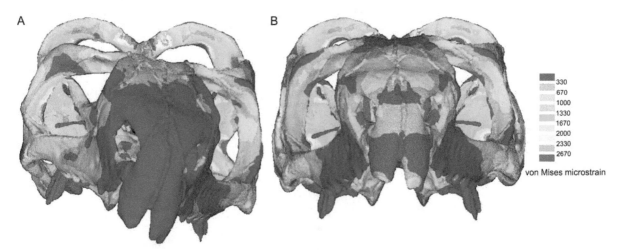

■	330
	670
	1000
	1330
	1670
	2000
	2330
■	2670

von Mises microstrain

Figure 3. von Mises FEA plots during two single bites. Deformation and von Mises strain plots of the skull of *Sphenodon* during **A.** right unilateral biting and **B.** during bilateral biting on the anterior-most chisel-like teeth; (note the displacements are scaled by a factor of 50).

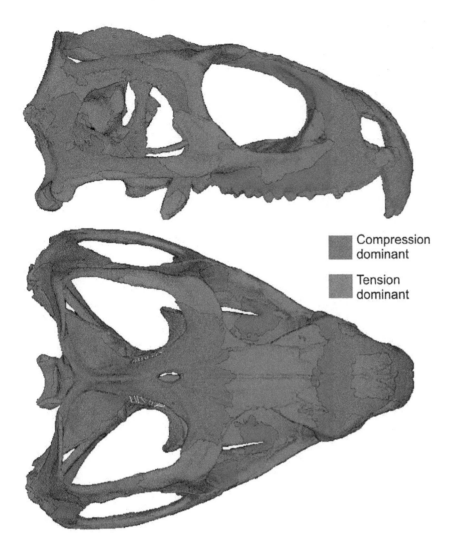

Compression
dominant

Tension
dominant

Figure 4. Plot of dominant strain regions. Cumulative map of peak dominant strains over all bites. Red represents regions of the skull where tensile strains are in excess of compressive strains (i.e. tensile strains are dominant), and blue represents regions where compressive strains are in excess of tensile strains (i.e. compressive strains are dominant).

cause some bone formation. Levels above 3000 microstrain are recognised as pathological overload and strains of between 50 and 1500 microstrain would generate equal bone resorption and formation rates (i.e. homeostasis). These values are only speculative and the strain mode or frequency is not specified, but our predicted von Mises strains in the skull of *Sphenodon* are comparable.

We simulated peak bite forces in our study (i.e. ~140 N at an anterior bite position [36,58]), and although bone needs to be able to withstand such forces without risk of failure, the majority of feeding forces will be significantly lower than these applied peak bite forces. For example, Aguirre et al. [59] showed that the approximate force needed to crush a beetle was 34 N, while Herrel et al. [60] recorded a value of 27 N to crush an egg. *Sphenodon* has a varied diet but it frequently includes beetles and occasionally sea bird eggs [61–63]. Thus, the force required to crush these foods is over four times lower than the peak bite force in *Sphenodon*. Scaling skull strains by a factor of four (i.e. in line with bite forces being four times lower) we show that over 91% of the skull is at strains of between 100 and 625 microstrain, well within the equilibrium window (i.e. equal bone resorption and deposition) as inferred by Martin [57].

The findings of this study imply that the skull of *Sphenodon* is adapted to feeding forces, with some regions adapted to tensile forces and others to compressive forces. Tendons and ligaments provide little resistance to compressive strains, and bone is necessary to provide compressive stability. We show that all regions of the skull experience compressive strain when all biting load cases are analysed, suggesting that it is mechanically necessary. However, while bone is necessary to resist compression, it must also be strong enough not to fail under tension. Therefore, once formed, bone must also adapt to tensile strains, and our results support this. Previous analyses, which include *in vivo* experimentation and FEAs suggest different functions for different regions of the skull based on stress and strain recordings/ predictions [5,64–69] (i.e. specific regions seem better suited to biting forces, bending strains, impact loads etc.). While our findings agree with this to some extent (e.g. a specific area of the skull may be linked to a specific bite point, or the forces generated at the jaw joints), they are not consistent with the conclusion that some regions of the skull are formed in relation to factors unrelated to functional strains (e.g. the idea that bone is formed to protect the brain and/or sensory organs from potential impact forces that have not yet occurred [5]). Previous studies did not take into

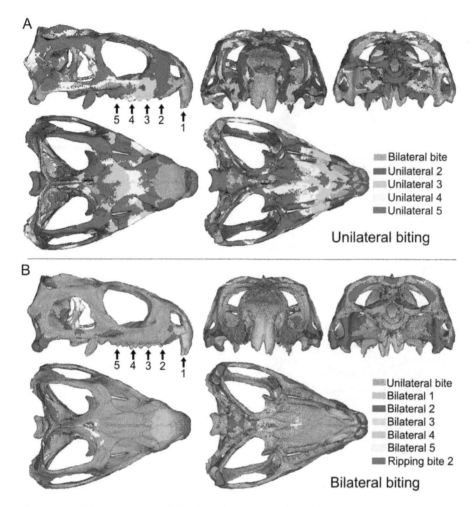

Figure 5. Models showing which bite location generated the highest strains in particular areas of the skull. Results based on von Mises strains. **A.** Unilateral bites and **B.** bilateral bites. (For example, in **A.** unilateral biting at location 2 was responsible for the highest strains in those areas coloured blue).

account the full range of possible and potential loadings, a point made by Mikic and Carter [70] "one difficulty that is encountered when using bone strain data in studies of functional adaptation is the reported data are often far from a complete record of strain over an experimental period". In relation to *in vivo* strain data, these authors further note that "reported results generally consist of a few average cyclic strain parameters that are extracted from a short period of recordings while an animal performs a very restricted task. Most investigators agree, however, that a much more complete record of strain history is required to relate bone biology and morphology to strain".

In our study of skull function we found that strains resulting from a single bite do provide a limited view of overall skull performance (Figure 3 and Figure 6). When we considered a more complete range of physiological loads we showed strains to be more uniform over the entire skull (Figure 7). This finding suggests that the skull is well adapted to a range of functional strains. Although some regions appear to be adapted to tensile strains and others to compressive strains, all regions of the skull seem to be equally important with respect to overall feeding forces. We have shown that unilateral bites, in particular the more posterior unilateral bites, generate the highest strains across the skull. This suggests that such bites are more important to the morphology of the skull of *Sphenodon* than the bilateral ones.

The extent to which general skull form is determined by selection or growth remains uncertain, but our findings show that the skull of *Sphenodon* is optimally suited (mechanically ideal - or at least very well suited) to deal with the full range of loadings applied here. The term 'optimally' refers to the minimum amount of material (i.e. bone) necessary to ensure sufficient skull strength. An optimally formed skull as defined here will be more efficient than a sub-optimal, e.g. heavier skull form, in ensuring minimal bone volume, minimal weight, and also minimal energy demands in maintenance. For clarity, we would predict a non-optimised skull to display one of two contrasting conditions. It would either appear weak in relation to the normal forces applied to it, and experience very high and potentially damaging stresses and strains during normal loading, or, conversely, it might appear overly robust, with very low stresses and strains during normal loading and with excess bone mass that is not mechanically necessary. Since our findings infer that the skull of *Sphenodon* is well formed to resist the everyday forces applied to it, it is not unreasonable to suggest this may also be true for other diapsids with a frame-like skull.

Within our analyses a few small regions of high and low strain are present even when all fifteen biting load cases were accounted for. However, although the muscle representation is detailed in our models, some additional soft tissue structures, such as fascia and ligaments, were not included. At first consideration these

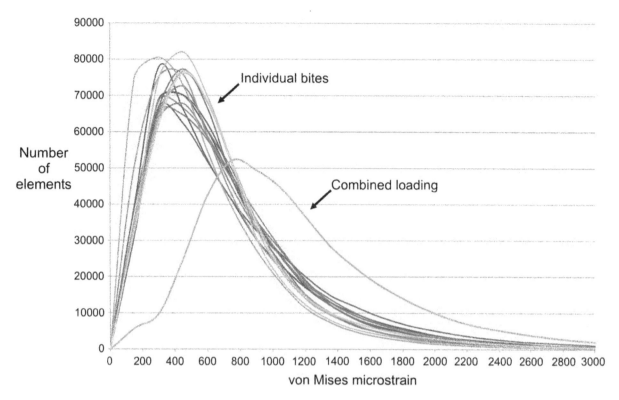

Figure 6. von Mises element strain distribution plots. Plot represents the number of elements within the finite element model that experience a specific strain magnitude. The plot shows the element strains from all fifteen biting simulations (labelled individual bites) and the combined loading model.

structures may appear unimportant, but a recent study investigating the influence of the temporal fascia in primates has revealed that it might play a major role in the function of the skull [71]. Our analyses indicate that the fascial sheet stretched over the upper temporal fenestra in *Sphenodon* may also be significant (Figure 8). This fascial sheet is apparently tensed by upward bulging of the jaw adductor muscles (notably pseudotemporalis superficialis and adductor mandibulae externus medialis) as *Sphenodon* bites down on food (personal observations at Chester Zoo, UK; Dallas Zoo, USA). In this case the fascia serves to reduce peak strains (Figure 8), creating a more uniform strain distribution throughout the skull. The finding that the muscles (including the neck muscles), other soft tissue structures (e.g. upper temporal fascia), bite location, and joint forces all influence the strains within the skull suggests that modifications to any of these anatomical structures has the potential to affect skull form. This may even be somewhat applicable to the formation of unusual skull features, such as crests in chameleons, ceratopsians, and theropod dinosaurs [72–75].

The skull of *Sphenodon*, and probably other non-avian diapsid reptiles without a vaulted braincase (both extant and extinct), is adapted (in the sense of bone adaptation, rather than evolutionary development) to resist a range of load cases, not just single biting loads. The lower temporal bar, secondarily acquired in *Sphenodon* [66,76–80] as well as in the common ancestor of archosaurs like crocodiles [66,80,81], is under compressive strain during all bites. This is consistent with previous suggestions that it provides a brace [66,79,82] that contributes to skull robusticity, and in large theropods such as *Tyrannosaurus rex* Osborn, 1905 and *Allosaurus fragilis* Marsh, 1877 this would be important as they would likely generate extremely large biting forces and experience heavy

cranial loading [4,83]. The corollary is that reptiles that lack a lower bar do not need a brace in this location. Early relatives of *Sphenodon* lack a lower temporal bar, the primitive condition for the group [76–79], but the dorsal position of the jaw joint in these small reptiles suggests that reaction forces would not have been directed along the lower temporal bar, had one existed [78,84].

To conclude, our analysis of the skull of *Sphenodon* indicates that the bone has adapted to tensile and compressive strains generated during normal feeding activities. The combined peak von Mises strain distribution over the skull is relatively uniform, showing that all regions are strong enough mechanically to withstand normal everyday forces, while no region is overly robust and 'over-designed'. Based purely on this finding, the skull form of *Sphenodon* can be considered optimal (mechanically ideal) in the sense that it comprises the minimal amount of bone material for the required skull strength. This optimal form is more efficient in terms of minimal bone volume, minimal weight, and minimal energy demands in maintenance over a sub-optimal, heavier skull form. While this study has not investigated potential forces associated with the brain, sense organs, and non-biting activities such as swallowing and tongue movements, its results are relevant to a broader understanding of skull form and not just to the skulls of diapsid reptiles. However, to test whether all skulls are optimally formed (sufficient strength with the minimal amount of material) with respect to bone strains (both tensile and compressive) would require the application of similar methods to other animal groups. Preliminary findings in macaques are encouraging in this regard (personal observations) but skulls with large vaulted braincases may be subject to additional quasi-static or high frequency low loads (e.g. associated with the brain) that could impact on skull form [28–30,85].

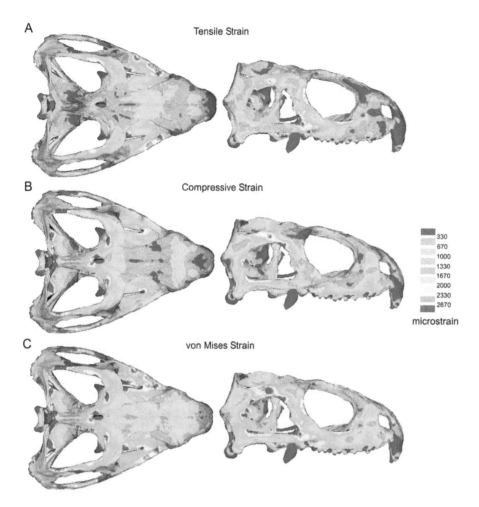

A Tensile Strain

B Compressive Strain

330
670
1000
1330
1670
2000
2330
2670

microstrain

C von Mises Strain

Figure 7. Combined loading tensile, compressive, and von Mises strain plots. Peak combined loading **A.** tensile, **B.** compressive, and **C.** von Mises strain plots.

Materials and Methods

MDA

Detailed descriptions of the MDA model development have been presented elsewhere [33,36,86]. Briefly, the skull and lower jaws (left and right parts) of a *Sphenodon* specimen (specimen LDUCZ x036; Grant Museum of Zoology, UCL, London, UK) were scanned in-house by micro-computed tomography (micro-CT), from which three-dimensional (3D) geometries were constructed using AMIRA image segmentation software (AMIRA 4.1, Mercury Computer Systems Inc., USA). Neck vertebral geometries were generated from additional micro-CT scans (specimen YPM 9194; Yale Peabody Museum of Natural History, New Haven, USA). These 3D geometries were imported into ADAMS multibody analysis software (version 2007 r1, MSC Software Corp., USA) in preparation for an MDA. Within ADAMS detailed muscle anatomy was incorporated onto the geometries, and accurate jaw joint and tooth contact surfaces were specified. Where the neck meets the skull a spherical joint was assigned that permitted the skull to rotate freely about all axes while constraining translational movements. The major adductor (jaw closing), depressor (jaw opening), and neck musculature were included, with each muscle group split into several sections and defined over the anatomical origin and insertions areas on the skull and lower jaws respectively [33,86,87] (Figure 2A). To permit biting, a food bolus was modelled that could be located at any position along the jaw, and a specially developed motion technique, named dynamic geometric optimisation (DGO), was utilised to open the jaw and to simulate peak biting. This motion technique, along with the muscle forces and biting performance, has been described and validated elsewhere [33,36] (in reference to work carried out *in vivo* [58,88]).

The biting simulations covered a range of biting types and locations, including four bilateral and eight unilateral bites at different tooth positions, a bite on the anterior-most chisel-like teeth, and two ripping bites that incorporate neck muscles (MDA model shown in Figure 2 and a summary of the simulations is shown in Table 1). During the ripping bites the jaws closed on a fixed food bolus, upon which and neck muscles were activated to lift (or try to lift) the head up and to the left, and up and to the right. These two ripping simulations ensured full activation of the neck muscles. During each simulation peak bite force, quadrate-articular joint forces, and muscle forces were predicted.

FEA

The same 3D geometry constructed for the MDA skull was converted into a tetrahedral mesh consisting of 640,000 elements. The model was constructed from solid (ten node) higher order elements, which were specified with a Young's modulus of 17 GPa and a Poisson's ratio of 0.3 (consistent with direct

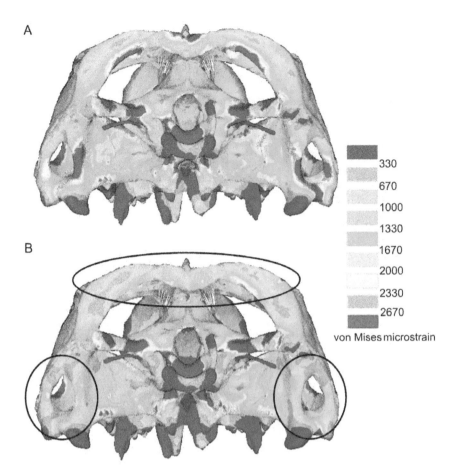

330
670
1000
1330
1670
2000
2330
2670

von Mises microstrain

Figure 8. von Mises FEA plots with and without fascia forces. Posterior views of the skull showing von Mises strains predicted by the combined loading model. **A.** Without including fascial forces and **B.** including modelled fascial forces (see Figure 2A). Encircled regions highlight areas where strains have changed significantly due to the inclusion of the fascial forces.

measurements and within the ranges applied by others [1,89–91]. Using the MDA predicted forces, a series of fifteen FEAs were carried out. Although theoretically all forces within the system should be in equilibrium, due to the large number of individual forces even small variations from the exact MDA locations of these applied forces causes instability within the FEAs (i.e. there would be unconstrained full body motion of the model). To ensure a stable FE solution, fixed constraints were included at the joint and bite contacts as defined by the MDA (i.e. neck joint, jaw joints, and bite point). One node at the neck location was constrained in the medial-lateral and anterior-posterior directions (x and z axes), one node at each jaw joint and bite point was constrained in the vertical direction (y axis). These constraints were considered minimal, and restricted rigid body motion but not deformations of the skull. For example, the neck, bite, and joint contact locations could all deform with respect to each other, and both jaw joint contact locations could deform relative to each other. After the FE solutions were complete, tensile (also known as maximum and 1st principal), compressive (also known as minimum and 3rd principal), and von Mises (also known as equivalent and mean) element strains of all 640,000 elements in the model were stored in element tables. In addition, the peak strain recorded in any one particular element during the fifteen separate simulations was extracted and combined to map the peak strains across the skull. This is referred to as a combined loading model.

An additional investigation was carried out to understand the influence of other *non-bone* structures. To this end we simulated an upper temporal fascial sheet, which is likely tensioned by large superior bulging of the jaw adductor muscles during biting (personal observations from animals at Chester Zoo, UK; Dallas Zoo, USA). Here we applied a total force of 133 N around the perimeter of each upper temporal fenestra (7 N over 19 force vectors – see Figure 2A). This magnitude was based on an unrelated investigation [71], where the total fascial force was found to be approximately 85% of the muscle force applied by an associated muscle group(s). In this case the associated muscles were pseudotemporalis superficialis and adductor mandibulae externus medialis [36,87].

Acknowledgments

The authors thank Chester Zoo (UK) and Dallas Zoo (USA) for allowing us access to *Sphenodon* for filming and observation, and the Grant Museum of Zoology (UCL) for access to specimens.

Author Contributions

Conceived and designed the experiments: NC MEHJ JS PO SEE MJF. Performed the experiments: NC. Analyzed the data: NC MEHJ JS PO SEE MJF. Contributed reagents/materials/analysis tools: NC JS. Wrote the paper: NC. Contributed significantly to editing of the submitted manuscript: MEHJ JS PO SEE MJF. Created the computational models: NC MEHJ. Developed analysis techniques: NC JS.

References

1. Witzel U, Preuschoft H (2005) Finite-element model construction for the virtual synthesis of the skulls in vertebrates: case study of *Diplodocus*. The Anatomical Record 283: 391–401.

2. Witzel U (2011) Virtual synthesis of the skull in Neanderthals by FESS. In: Condemi S, Weniger G-C, eds. Continuity and discontinuity in the peopling of Europe: one hundred fifty years of Neanderthal study (vertebrate paleobiology and paleoanthropology). Verlag Berlin Heidelberg: Springer. pp 203–211.

3. Ross CF, Metzger KA (2004) Bone strain gradients and optimization in vertebrate skulls. Annals of Anatomy 186: 387–396.

4. Rayfield EJ, Norman DB, Horner CC, Horner JR, Smith PM, et al. (2001) Cranial design and function in a large theropod dinosaur. Nature 409: 1033–1037.

5. Hylander WL, Johnson KR (1997) *In vivo* strain patterns in the zygomatic arch of macaques and the significance of these patterns for functional interpretations of craniofacial form. American Journal of Physical Anthropology 102: 203–232.

6. Olson EC (1961) Jaw mechanisms in rhipidistians, amphibians, reptiles. American Zoologist 1: 205–215.

7. Moore WJ (1965) Masticatory function and skull growth. Journal of Zoology 146: 123–131.

8. Frazzetta TH (1968) Adaptive problems and possibilities in the temporal fenestration of tetrapod skulls. Journal of Morphology 125: 145–158.

9. Wolff J (1882) Das gesetz der transformation der Knochen: Hirchwild, Berlin. Translated as 'The Law of Bone Remodelling', Springer-Verlag Berlin 1986.

10. Roux W (1881) Der zuchtende Kampf der Teile, oder die "Teilauslee". Organismus (Theorie der "funktionellen Anpassung"). Leipzig: Wilhelm Engelmann.

11. Churches AE, Howlett CR (1982) Functional adaptation of bone in response to sinusoidally varying controlled compressive loading of the ovine metacarpus. Clinical Orthopaedics and Related Research 168: 265–280.

12. Cowin SC, Hart RT, Balser JR, Kohn DH (1985) Functional adaptation in long bones: establishing *in vivo* values for surface remodeling rate coefficients. Journal of Biomechanics 18: 665–684.

13. Lanyon LE, Rubin CT (1985) Functional adaptation in skeletal structures. In: Hildebrand M, Bramble DM, Liem KF, Wake DB, eds. Functional vertebrate morphology. Cambridge, MA: Belknap Press.

14. Lanyon LE (1982) Mechanical function and bone remodeling. In: Sumner-Smith G, ed. Bone in clinical orthopaedics. Philadelphia: Saunders.

15. Lanyon LE, Skerry T (2001) Postmenopausal osteoporosis as a failure of bone's adaptation to functional loading: a hypothesis. Journal of Bone and Mineral Research 16: 1937–1947.

16. Carter DR (1984) Mechanical loading histories and cortical bone remodeling. Calcified Tissue International 39: 19–24.

17. Frost HM (1987) Bone "mass" and the "mechanostat": a proposal. The Anatomical Record 219: 1–9.

18. Turner CH (1998) Three rules for bone adaptation to mechanical stimuli. Bone 23: 399–407.

19. Hsieh YF, Robling AG, Ambrosius WT, Burr DB, Turner CH (2001) Mechanical loading of diaphyseal bone *in vivo*: the strain threshold for an osteogenic response varies with location. Journal of Bone and Mineral Research 16: 2291–2297.

20. Lieberman DE, Devlin MJ, Pearson OM (2001) Articular area responses to mechanical loading: effects of exercise, age, and skeletal location. American Journal of Physical Anthropology 116: 266–277.

21. Currey JD Bones: structure and mechanics: Princeton University Press.

22. Lee K, Jessop H, Suswillo R, Zaman G, Lanyon LE (2003) Endocrinology: bone adaptation requires oestrogen receptor-alpha. Nature 424: 389.

23. Pearson OM, Lieberman DE (2004) The aging of Wolff's "law:" ontogeny and responses to mechanical loading in cortical bone. Yearbook of Physical Anthropology 47: 63–99.

24. Suuriniemi M, Mahonen A, Kovanen V, Alen M, Lyytikainen A, et al. (2004) Association between exercise and pubertal BMD is modulated by estrogen receptor alpha genotype. Journal of Bone and Mineral Research 19: 1758–1765.

25. Burr DB, Robling AG, Turner CH (2002) Effects of biomechanical stress on bones in animals. Bone 30: 781–786.

26. Preuschoft H, Witzel U (2002) Biomechanical investigations on the skulls of reptiles and mammals. Senckenbergiana Lethaea 82: 207–222.

27. Jones MEH, Curtis N, Fagan MJ, O'Higgins P, Evans SE (2011) Hard tissue anatomy of the cranial joints in *Sphenodon* (Rhynchocephalia): sutures, kinesis, and skull mechanics. Palaeontologia Electronica 14: 17A.

28. Moss ML (1954) Growth of the calvaria in the rat, the determination of osseous morphology. American Journal of Morphology 94: 333–361.

29. Moss ML, Young RW (1960) A functional approach to craniology. American Journal of Physical Anthropology 74: 305–307.

30. Heifetz MD, Weiss M (1981) Detection of skull expansion with increased intracranial pressure. Journal of Neurosurgery 55: 811–812.

31. Sun Z, Lee E, Herring SW (2004) Cranial sutures and bones: growth and fusion in relation to masticatory strain. The Anatomical Record 276A: 150–161.

32. Curtis N, Kupczik K, O'Higgins P, Moazen M, Fagan MJ (2008) Predicting skull loading: applying multibody dynamics analysis to a macaque skull. The Anatomical Record 291: 491–501.

33. Curtis N, Jones MEH, Evans SE, Shi J, O'Higgins P, et al. (2010) Predicting muscle activation patterns from motion and anatomy: modelling the skull of

34. Curtis N (2011) Craniofacial biomechanics: an overview of recent multibody modelling studies. Journal of Anatomy 218: 16–25.

35. Curtis N, Jones MEH, Evans SE, O'Higgins P, Fagan MJ (2010) Feedback control from the jaw joints during biting: an investigation of the reptile *Sphenodon* using multibody modelling. Journal of Biomechanics 43: 3132–3137.

36. Curtis N, Jones MEH, Lappin AK, O'Higgins P, Evans SE, et al. (2010) Comparison between *in vivo* and theoretical bite performance: using multi-body modelling to predict muscle and bite forces in a reptile skull. Journal of Biomechanics 43: 2804–2809.

37. Koolstra JH, van Eijden TMGJ (2004) Functional significance of the coupling between head and jaw movements. Journal of Biomechanics 37: 1387–1392.

38. Moazen M, Curtis N, Evans SE, O'Higgins P, Fagan MJ (2008) Rigid-body analysis of a lizard skull: modelling the skull of *Uromastyx hardwickii*. Journal of Biomechanics 41: 1274–1280.

39. Robinson PL, ed. Morphology and biology of the reptiles; how *Sphenodon* and *Uromastix* grow their teeth and use them: Academic Press, London. pp 43–64.

40. Nunemaker DM, Butterweck DM, Provost MT (1990) Fatigue fractures in thoroughbred racehorses: relationships with age, peak bone strain and training. Journal of Orthopaedic Research 8: 604–611.

41. O'Connor JA, Lanyon LE, MacFie H (1982) The influence of strain rate on adaptive remodeling. Journal of Biomechanics 15: 767–781.

42. Rubin CT, Lanyon LE (1982) Limb mechanics as a function of speed and gait: a study of functional strains in the radius and tibia of horse and dog. Journal of Experimental Biology 101: 187–211.

43. Biewener AA, Thomason JJ, Lanyon LE (1983) Mechanics of locomotion and jumping in the forelimb of the horse (*Equus*): *in vivo* stress developed in the radius and metacarpus. Journal of Zoology, London 201: 67–82.

44. Biewener AA, Thomason JJ, Lanyon LE (1988) Mechanics of locomotion and jumping in the horse (*Equus*): *in vivo* stress in the tibia an metatarsus. Journal of Zoology, London 214: 547–565.

45. Biewener AA, Taylor CR (1986) Bone strain: a determinant of gait and speed? Journal of Experimental Biology 123: 383–400.

46. Lanyon LE, Bourne S (1979) The influence of mechanical function on the development of remodeling of the tibia: an experimental study in sheep. Journal of Bone and Joint Surgery 61-A: 263–273.

47. Hylander WL (1979) Mandibular function in *Galago crassicaudatus* and *Macaca fascicularis*: an *in vivo* approach to stress analysis of the mandible. Journal of Morphology 159: 253–296.

48. Rubin CT, Lanyon LE (1984) Regulation of bone formation by applied dynamic loads. Journal of Bone and Joint Surgery 66-A: 397–402.

49. Swartz SM, Bennett MB, Carrier DR (1992) Wing bone stresses in free flying bats and the evolution of skeletal design for flight. Nature 359: 726–729.

50. Biewener AA, Dial KP (1992) *In vivo* strain in the pigeon humerus during flight. American Journal of Zoology 32: 155A.

51. Burr DB, Milgrom C, Fyrhie D, Forwood M, Nyska M, et al. (1996) *In vivo* measurement of human tibial strains during vigorous activity. Bone 18: 405–410.

52. Blob RW, Biewener AA (1999) *In vivo* locomotor strain in the hindlimb bones of *Alligator mississipiensis* and *Iguana iguana*: implications for the evolution of limb bone saftey factor and non-sprawling limb posture. Journal of Experimental Biology 202: 1023–1046.

53. Herring SW, Mucci RJ (2000) *In vivo* strain in cranial sutures: the zygomatic arch. Journal of Morphology 207: 225–239.

54. Herring SW, Pedersen SC, Huang X (2005) Ontogeny of bone strain: the zygomatic arch in pigs. Journal of Experimental Biology 208: 4509–4521.

55. Robling AG, Hinant FM, Burr DB, Turner CH (2002) Improved bone structure and strength after long-term mechanical loading is greatest if loading is separated into short bouts. Journal of Bone Mineral Research 17: 1545–1554.

56. Haapasalo H, Kontulainen S, Sievanen H, Kannus P, Jarvinen M, et al. (2000) Exercise-induced bone gain is due to enlargement in bone size without a change in volumetric bone density: a peripheral quantitative computed tomography study of the upper arms of male tennis players. Bone 27: 351–357.

57. Martin RB (2000) Toward a unifying theory of bone remodeling. Bone 26: 1–6.

58. Jones MEH, Lappin AK (2009) Bite-force performance of the last rhynchocephalian (Lepidosauria: *Sphenodon*). Journal of the Royal Society of New Zealand 39: 71–83.

59. Aguirre LF, Herrel A, van Damme R, Matthysen E (2003) The implications of food hardness for diet in bats. Functional Ecology 17: 201–212.

60. Herrel A, Wauters P, Aerts P, De Vree F (1997) The mechanics of ovophagy in the beaded lizard (*Heloderma horridum*). Journal of Herpetology 31: 189–393.

61. Ussher GT (1999) Tuatara (*Sphenodon punctatus*) feeding ecology in the presence of kiore (*Rattus exulans*). New Zealand Journal of Zoology 26: 117–125.

62. Walls GY (1978) Influence of the tuatara on fairy prion breeding on Stephens Island, Cook Strait. New Zealand Journal of Ecology 1: 91–98.

63. Walls GY (1981) Feeding ecology of the tuatara (*Sphenodon punctatus*) on Stephens Island, Cook Strait. New Zealand Journal of Ecology 4: 89–97.

64. Dumont ER, Davis JL, Grosse IR, Burrows AM (2011) Finite element analysis of performance in the skulls of marmosets and tamarins. Journal of Anatomy 218: 151–162.

65. McHenry CR, Wroe S, Clausen PD, Moreno K, Cunningham E (2007) Supermodeled sabercat, predatory behavior in *Smilodon fatalis* revealed by high-

resolution 3D computer simulation. Proceedings of the National Academy of Sciences 104: 16010–16015.

66. Moazen M, Curtis N, O'Higgins P, Evans SE, Fagan MJ (2009) Biomechanical assessment of evolutionary changes in the lepidosaurian skull. Proceedings of the National Academy of Sciences 106: 8273–8277.

67. Ross CF, Berthaume MA, Dechow PC, Iriarte-Diaz J, Porro LB, et al. (2011) *In vivo* bone strain and finite-element modeling of the craniofacial haft in catarrhine primates. Journal of Anatomy 218: 112–141.

68. Degrange FJ, Tambussi CP, Moreno K, Witmer LM, Wroe S (2010) Mechanical analysis of feeding behavior in the extinct "terror bird" *Andalgalornis steulleti* (Gruiformes: Phorusrhacidae). PLoS ONE 5: doi:10.1371/journal.pone.0011856.

69. Ravosa MJ, Noble VE, Hylander WL, Johnson KR, Kowalski EM (2000) Masticatory stress, orbital orientation and the evolution of the primate postorbital bar. Journal of Human Evolution 38: 667–693.

70. Mikic B, Carter DR (1995) Bone strain gauge data and theoretical models of functional adaptation. Journal of Biomechanics 28: 465–469.

71. Curtis N, Witzel U, Fitton L, O'Higgins P, Fagan MJ (in press) The mechanical significance of the temporal fasciae in *Macaca fascicularis*: an investigation using finite element analysis. The Anatomical Record.

72. Hammer WR, Hickerson WJ (1994) A crested theropod dinosaur from Antarctica. Science 264: 828–830.

73. Rieppel O, Crumly C (1997) Paedomorphosis and skull structure in Malagasy chamaeleons (Reptilia: Chamaeleoninae). Journal of Zoology 243: 351–380.

74. Bickel R, Losos JB (2002) Patterns of morphological variation and correlates of habitat use in chameleons. Biological Journal of the Linnean Society 76: 91–103.

75. Farlow JO, Dodson P (1975) The behavioral significance of frill and horn morphology in ceratopsian dinosaurs. Evolution 29: 353–361.

76. Evans SE (2008) The skull of lizards and tuatara. In: Gans C, Gaunt AS, Adler K, eds. Biology of the Reptilia. IthacaNew York: Society for the Study of Amphibians and Reptiles. pp 1–344.

77. Evans SE, Jones MEH, eds (2010) The origin, early history and diversification of lepidosauromorph reptiles. Verlag Berlin Heidelberg: Springer. pp 27–44.

78. Jones MEH (2008) Skull shape and feeding strategy in *Sphenodon* and other Rhynchocephalia (Diapsida: Lepidosauria). Journal of Morphology 269: 945–966.

79. Whiteside DI (1986) The head skeleton of the Rhaetian sphenodontid *Diphydontosaurus avonis* gen. et sp. nov., and the modernising of a living fossil.

Physiological Transactions of the Royal Society of London, Series B 312: 379–430.

80. Müller J (2003) Early loss and multiple return of the lower temporal arcade in diapsid reptiles. Naturwissenschaften 90: 473–476.

81. Nesbitt SJ (2011) The early evolution of archosaurs: relationships and the origin of major clades. Bulletin of the American Museum of Natural History 352: 1–292.

82. Rieppel O, Gronowski RW (1981) The loss of the lower temporal arcade in diapsid reptiles. Zoological Journal of the Linnean Society 72: 203–217.

83. Erickson GM, Van Kirk SD, Su J, Levenston ME, Caler WE, et al. (1996) Bite-force estimation for *Tyrannosaurus rex* from tooth-marked bones. Nature 382: 706–708.

84. Jones MEH, Curtis N, Evans SE, O'Higgins P, Fagan MJ (2010) Cranial joints in *Sphenodon* (Rhynchocephalia) and its fossil relatives with implications for lepidosaur skull mechanics. Journal of Vertebrate Paleontology, Program and Abstracts 2010: 113A.

85. Sun Z, Lee E, Herring SW (2004) Cranial sutures and bones: growth and fusion in relation to masticatory strain. The Anatomical Record 276A: 150–161.

86. Curtis N, Jones MEH, Evans SE, O'Higgins P, Fagan MJ (2009) Visualising muscle anatomy using three-dimensional computer models - an example using the head and neck muscles of *Sphenodon*. Palaeontologia Electronica 12.3.7T.

87. Jones MEH, Curtis N, O'Higgins P, Fagan MJ, Evans SE (2009) The head and neck muscles associated with feeding in *Sphenodon* (Reptilia: Lepidosauria: Rhynchocephalia). Palaeontologia Electronica 12.

88. Gorniak GC, Rosenberg HI, Gans C (1982) Mastication in the tuatara, *Sphenodon punctatus* (Reptilia: Rhynchocephalia): structure and activity of the motor system. Journal of Morphology 171: 321–353.

89. Strait DS, Wang Q, Dechow PC, Ross CF, Richmond BG, et al. (2005) Modeling elastic properties in finite element analysis: how much precision is needed to produce an accurate model? The Anatomical Record 283: 275–287.

90. Dumont ER, Grosse IR, Slater GJ (2009) Requirements for comparing the performance of finite element models of biological structures. Journal of Theoretical Biology 256: 96–103.

91. Wang Q, Wright BW, Smith A, Chalk J, Byron CD (2010) Mechanical impact of incisor loading on the primate midfacial skeleton and its relevance to human evolution. The Anatomical Record 293: 607–617.

92. Madsen JH (1976) *Allosaurus fragilis*: a revised osteology: Utah Geological Survey Bulletin 109: 1–163.

4

The Energetic Cost of Walking: A Comparison of Predictive Methods

Patricia Ann Kramer[1]*, **Adam D. Sylvester**[2]

1 Departments of Anthropology and Orthopaedics and Sports Medicine, University of Washington, Seattle, Washington, United States of America, **2** Max Planck Institute for Evolutionary Anthropology, Leipzig, Germany

Abstract

Background: The energy that animals devote to locomotion has been of intense interest to biologists for decades and two basic methodologies have emerged to predict locomotor energy expenditure: those based on metabolic and those based on mechanical energy. Metabolic energy approaches share the perspective that prediction of locomotor energy expenditure should be based on statistically significant proxies of metabolic function, while mechanical energy approaches, which derive from many different perspectives, focus on quantifying the energy of movement. Some controversy exists as to which mechanical perspective is "best", but from first principles all mechanical methods should be equivalent if the inputs to the simulation are of similar quality. Our goals in this paper are 1) to establish the degree to which the various methods of calculating mechanical energy are correlated, and 2) to investigate to what degree the prediction methods explain the variation in energy expenditure.

Methodology/Principal Findings: We use modern humans as the model organism in this experiment because their data are readily attainable, but the methodology is appropriate for use in other species. Volumetric oxygen consumption and kinematic and kinetic data were collected on 8 adults while walking at their self-selected slow, normal and fast velocities. Using hierarchical statistical modeling via ordinary least squares and maximum likelihood techniques, the predictive ability of several metabolic and mechanical approaches were assessed. We found that all approaches are correlated and that the mechanical approaches explain similar amounts of the variation in metabolic energy expenditure. Most methods predict the variation within an individual well, but are poor at accounting for variation between individuals.

Conclusion: Our results indicate that the choice of predictive method is dependent on the question(s) of interest and the data available for use as inputs. Although we used modern humans as our model organism, these results can be extended to other species.

Editor: Alejandro Lucia, Universidad Europea de Madrid, Spain

Funding: The authors have no support or funding to report.

Competing Interests: The authors have declared that no competing interests exist.

* E-mail: pakramer@u.washington.edu

Introduction

Determining the amount of energy that animals devote to movement in their environment has been an area of intense interest to biologists for decades (e.g. [1]) and much research effort has been devoted to teasing apart the many and varied possible causative agents. The principal reason for this scrutiny is that energy is a finite, non-recyclable resource [2]—energy used to move is lost to reproduction, an activity that is both energetically intensive for mothers (e.g. [3]) and sensitive to energetic restriction as reflected in maternal body mass (e.g. [4,5,6,7,8,9,10]). Consequently, those animals that use less locomotor energy to accomplish their activities of daily living should leave more offspring [11].

Understanding energetic expenditure in the body is complicated, because the body is a machine that is capable of performing a complex conversion of energy [12]. Chemical energy enters the body in the form of nutrients (usually obtained through ingestion) and oxygen (through respiration) and is used by the body to fuel internal chemical processes, to move (mechanical energy), and to create heat (thermal energy) [12]. The system is not 100% efficient and some wastage occurs [13]. Energy can also be stored over the short-term (e.g. elastic energy in tendons) or long-term (e.g. fat mass). Although the fundamentals of this transformation are understood (e.g. the conservation of energy dictates that energy input must equal energy output plus storage), the manner in which energy is distributed among the muscles and other tissues to produce stability and movement are not currently fully understood [14] or capable of being monitored [15], i.e., the system remains something of a "black box." Nonetheless, both the amount of tissue activated (muscle volume) and the intensity of the movement seem to affect the amount of metabolic energy used and over the decades of research, two basic methods to understand locomotor energy expenditure have emerged: those based on metabolic energy and those based on mechanical energy.

Metabolic energy

Metabolic approaches are the most direct of the two methods because they predict metabolic function from proxies of it, such as the body's demand for ATP. The most commonly used proxy of metabolic function is the volumetric rate of oxygen consumption ($\dot{V}O_2$), which serves as an estimate for ongoing cellular respiration and thus the body's use of energy; we will employ this proxy here. At this time, metabolic energy consumption approaches to the study of locomotor energy expenditure are inherently empirical and they employ statistical techniques to predict the dependent variable oxygen consumption from independent covariates (e.g. [16,17,18,19,20]). The classic papers of Taylor and his many colleagues (e.g. [21,22,23,24,25]) established that the independent variables velocity (a proxy for movement intensity) and body mass (a proxy for muscle volume) are predictive of oxygen consumption across a wide range of animal orders [13,26].

The independent covariates of "mouse-to-elephant" relationships have also been shown to be predictive of oxygen consumption over groups with less variability (e.g. within a species), but the predictive relationships are different (e.g. [16,19,27]). For instance, Figure 1 describes the general mammalian, primate, and human patterns that relate velocity and the volumetric rate of oxygen consumption per kg of body mass (from [16,20,24]). As is apparent, as velocity increases, energy expenditure per kg body mass increases, but how fast that increase occurs depends on the group and, for humans at least, the gait of interest. Consequently, while it is true to say that velocity is a significant predictor of energy expenditure in all these groups, knowing the relationship across primate genera does not necessarily lead to accurate predictions within a single species like *Homo sapiens*. The same is true for body mass—body mass is a statistically significant predictor of energy expenditure intra-(within *Homo sapiens*) and inter-specifically (within *Primates*), but the intra-specific relationships are different from the inter-specific ones (Figure 2) [17].

Consequently, a predictive equation for energy expenditure, developed from the data of one species, cannot be assumed to be accurate to predict the energy expenditure of another. The same is true in reverse: predictive equations developed from multiple species may lead to inaccuracies in prediction within single species. This same phenomena may also be at work at scales other than species, such as populations or groups (e.g. the differences in basal or resting metabolic rates between populations living in cold and hot climates [28]). Simply extrapolating equations developed from empirical studies of one group can, therefore, lead to wrong results in another, necessitating that metabolic approaches be grounded by a theoretical underpinning that delineates how the differences in morphology and physiology affect energy expenditure.

Mechanical energy

If all groups of interest were amenable to direct metabolic testing, mechanical approaches would be unnecessary. Such is not the case, however, so mechanical energy approaches are important because they may offer some insight into how energy

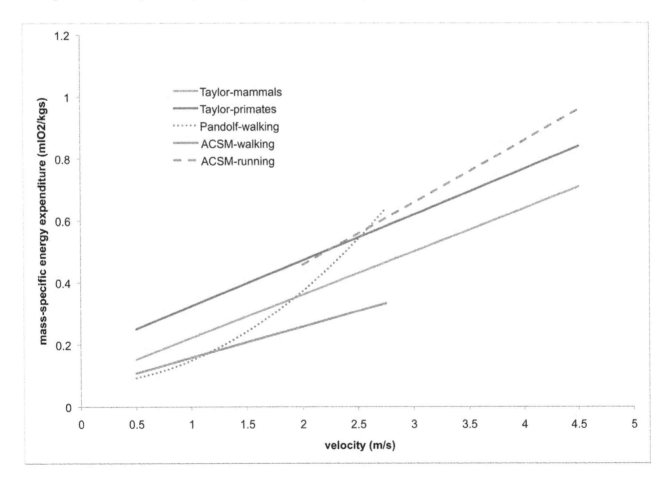

Figure 1. Relationship between velocity and locomotor energy expenditure. The equations for mammals (blue line) and primates (red line) are from Taylor and colleagues (1982); the ACSM equations for human walking (green line) and running (green dashed line) are from the ACSM handbook [20]; the curvilinear human walking equation (green dotted line) is from Pandolf and colleagues [16]. All calculations assumed a body mass of 70 kg.

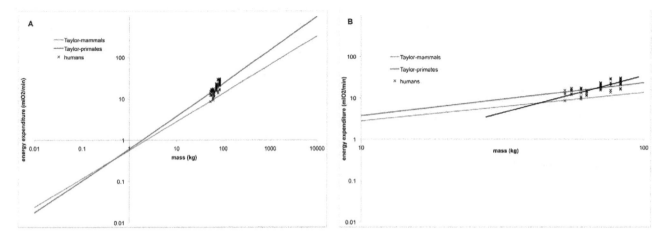

Figure 2. Relationship between body mass and locomotor energy expenditure. A) "Mouse-to-elephant" scale for body mass. B) Human scale for body mass. Equation for mammals (blue line) and primates (red line) from Taylor and colleagues (1982). Individual human data from the current study. Linear regression line through human data (black line) provided fro reference only.

expenditure changes with morphology and gait characteristics and can help explain why equations are not universally applicable across and between species and populations.

The mechanical approaches have focused on the energy output side of the equation (specifically, the energy of movement). All mechanical energy solutions utilize first principles, namely, the Newtonian laws of motion and conservation of energy, to calculate mechanical energy expenditure. These calculations can, therefore, be completely theoretical. Most researchers, however, employ theoretical constructs that are tested empirically, often using statistics. Mechanical energy approaches can address the problem of predicting locomotor energy expenditure from many different angles. This fundamental difference between metabolic and mechanical approaches makes mechanical approaches attractive to study extinct creatures and those difficult to study in the laboratory [29,30,31,32], even though mechanical approaches cannot represent non-mechanical phenomena (e.g. efficiency differences in cardiovascular function among individuals).

Energy of motion. One approach to predict the energy expenditure of walking is to assess the change in the body's potential and kinetic energy. Margaria, Cavagna and colleagues were among the first researchers to combine body mass with the movement of the body's center of mass to assess energy expended, or work done [33]. The movement of the body's center of mass was determined either using a recording of the movement of a marker placed near the center of mass [34] or from the force that the body exerted against the ground [33], i.e., the ground reaction force. These methods can be shown to be equivalent [35] and their choice depends on the availability of equipment to record the motion or the force. Both of these methods address the effect of the amount of tissue activated and intensity of motion.

A second approach is to model the lower body as rigid links that move together to produce the motion of the whole body. In inverse dynamic solutions, the model is driven by motions, while in forward dynamic solutions, external forces are used. Inverse and forward dynamic models have been used to calculate the energy required to move the limbs (dubbed internal work while that of the whole body is designated external work) at the same time as the external work either by using joint moments [36] or by combining segmental energy changes with calculated external work [37]. It is also possible to use a looping process where inverse dynamics is informed by forward dynamics [38].

Muscular energy. Another approach that uses mechanics to predict metabolic function has focused on the production of muscular force using several different methods. One method, force production which was originally developed for running [39], but later extended to walking [40], begins with the hypothesis that the primary cost of locomotion is the cost of generating the muscular force necessary to move the animal. These approaches are theoretically similar to center of mass motion or ground reaction force approaches. Several assumptions are used to operationalize the muscular force production methods: 1) that most of the force generated by the muscles is used to oppose gravity, 2) that a volume of muscle exerts the same force against the ground regardless of an animal's size, shape or speed, and 3) that muscles operate over the same range of the force-velocity curve [39]. With these assumptions in place, the authors develop an equation that makes energy expenditure proportional to body weight divided by contact time ([39], equation 1, p. 265). This method, with the simplifying assumptions in place, becomes a restatement of the empirical result that mass (= weight/gravitational constant) and velocity (as measured by time) are predictive of locomotor energy expenditure.

A second method used to predict muscular force is to model muscles as elements in a multi-segment dynamic model. Dynamic (usually forward dynamic) models are used to create/predict muscle activation sequences that can then be used to calculate muscular energy usage [32,41,42,43]. Another method that uses activated muscle volume (as a proxy of muscular energy use) to predict metabolic energy has recently become available [44], but the technique is applicable only at the species-level because it relies on muscle volume from dissection.

Approaches that emphasize the prediction of muscular forces and energy are different from those that utilize segment and/or whole body potential and kinetic energy, because they are based on creating activation in muscles which can be translated to metabolic energy use. Given that muscular processes are intermediate steps between the intake of nutrients and movement in the environment, methods to predict the force in specific muscles are exciting advances in the field of biomechanics, with the ability to predict 85-90% of the variability in the energy expenditure of walking [45]. In addition to probing deeper into the "black box" of whole-body energy conversion, they have the potential to address the energy expended by non-motion, e.g. joint

Table 1. Predictive methods, input variables and critical equations.

Method	Variable name	Methodology	Input variables	Critical equations
ACSM-walk	ACSM	Statistical	Velocity (v), body mass (m), regression coefficients	$\dot{V}O_2 = (0.1v+0.0583)m$
Force production	EXT-FP	Measured, calculated, statistical	Body mass, velocity, ground contact time	$\dot{V}O_2 = f$ (vm/contact time)
CoM-GRF	EXT-GRF	Measured, calculated	Ground reaction forces, body mass, acceleration (a)	$F = ma$ $v = \int a\,dt$ $Energy = mgh+0.5mv^2$ External work $= \sum dEnergy$ (time)
CoM-sacrum-model	EXT-MAT	Simulated	Velocity, body mass, segment lengths, angles	$\mathbf{x} = f$ (segment length, angles) $v = d\mathbf{x}/dt$ $Energy = mgh+0.5mv^2$ External work $= \sum dEnergy$ (time)
CoM- sacrum-measured	EXT-SAC	Measured, calculated	Motion of sacrum (**x**), body mass	$v = d\mathbf{x}/dt$ $Energy = mgh+0.5mv^2$ External work $= \sum dMEnergy$ (time)
Internal work	INT-MAT	Simulated	Velocity, angular velocity (ω), segment lengths, angles, segment mass and moments of inertia (I)	$Energy = \sum 0.5 (mv^2 + I\omega^2)$ (of segments) Internal work $= \sum dEnergy$ (time)
Joint moments	COMB-JM	Measured, calculated	Ground reaction forces (F), joint shape (r/R), motion of ankle, knee and hip joints	Muscle force $= r/R$ F Power $=$ Muscle force $*$ v Combined work $= \sum$ Power/time (of joints)
Model (int + ext work)	COMB-MAT	Simulated, calculated	Internal (INT-MAT) and external (EXT-MAT) work	Combined work $=$ internal +external work

Note that the ACSM method is a metabolic energy approach while others are mechanical energy approaches. The mechanical energy approaches are grouped into those the approximate external work (the energy required to move the body), internal work (the energy required to move the legs relative to the body) and combined work (external and internal work).

stabilization via co-contraction. Given the complexity of the calculations that underlie these approaches, a software platform is necessary to organize the input and output data and several commercial and public systems are under-development. The implementation of the software is, however, still incomplete. For instance, co-contraction is not yet possible [42] and it not currently possible to model the potential differences in muscle activation among individuals seen in recent electromyography studies (e.g [46,47]). When muscle force models can be tailored to individuals, we look forward to extending this work to these models.

Generalizations about mechanical approaches. All the mechanical calculations are based on the same theoretical underpinnings and consequently, the same limitations apply to all: mechanical calculations require knowledge of the motions or forces involved and the physical characteristics of the system (e.g. mass and lengths). Table 1 indicates the critical equations and variables needed to make the calculations using the various schemes. The upshot is that all of these methods require assumptions about the characteristics of the system that are needed as inputs in order to calculate energy and some variables are easier to measure than others. For instance, total body mass can be measured with a readily available instrument that has low error. The movement of an anatomical landmark, however, requires sophisticated equipment that has higher error. Some variables, like mass moment of inertia, are impossible to measure in living creatures and have to be estimated. Because any mechanical simulation of reality is only as good as the assumptions and simplifications that go into running it, the quality of the inputs are a critical component in the choice of methodology. The underlying theory can be correct, but produce seemingly incorrect results simply because the system was not modeled accurately. The choice among the methods is, then,

made by evaluating which method requires the type (including accuracy) of inputs one has available and provides the output data to answer the questions in which one is interested.

We should note that although modern humans and their ancestors have received the lion's share of attention and most of the examples used herein are drawn from that arena, the methods we discuss are as appropriate for use in other species. For instance, the locomotion of gibbons [48], Japanese macaques [49,50], horses [51,52], cockroaches [53], salamanders and tuataras [54], and extinct non-avian dinosaurs [55] have been evaluated using some of the general methods discussed here. Modern humans are not special, but merely convenient, organisms in which to study the energetics of locomotion.

Summary

When the creatures of interest are suitable for direct observation and study, the metabolic approach seems appropriate. Unfortunately, because no general statistical formula has been establish (i.e., there are different equations for different situations), equations are only valid for the group from which they were developed. If these group-appropriate equations are developed, then direct calculation of actual energy requirements might be obtainable. This seems to be particularly important for studies where the goal is to assess the absolute total daily energy expenditure for a group as in situations where caloric supplementation (due to high energy requirements and low reserves) or restriction (due to high reserves or low energy requirements) is necessary.

When the creatures cannot be directly studied, as is the case with extinct creatures, the best that can be done is to rely on the theoretically-based mechanical energy approaches, where one can vary the assumptions, variables of interest, and/or methodology.

Actual, or absolute levels of, energy expenditure cannot be assessed, but it should be possible to compare relative values. This allows investigation of the effect of different morphologies or to assess the effect of one variable on another. Examples of this might be to compare the effect of different crural indices or of segment length and circumference combinations on the cost of locomotion in modern humans and neandertals, in which direct experimentation is impossible [56,57]. Mechanical models also offer the ability to explore hypothetical morphologies. An example of this scenario would be the suggestion by Lovejoy and colleagues [58,59,60] that hominin bipedalism evolved from a monkey-like quadrupedal ancestor rather than from a knuckle-walking ape-like ancestor.

A logical initial step, however, is to assess the effect of choice of methodology on the prediction of energy expenditure. In order to do this, the detailed morphological, metabolic, kinematic and kinetic data of individuals are needed. The inherent assumption here is that the variability expressed by individuals within a species is sufficient to represent the effect of methodological choice across species. Modern human adults were chosen for the study detailed herein, because as noted above they are readily available as test subjects, they are generally compliant with the testing conditions, and their metabolic and mechanical energy expenditure has been extensively studied. Our techniques and findings are, however, generalizable and applicable to other groups. Consequently, our goals in this paper are 1) to establish the degree to which the various methods of calculating mechanical energy are correlated, and 2) to investigate whether or not, and if so to what degree, do the prediction methods explain the variation in metabolic energy expenditure.

Materials and Methods

In order to relate metabolic energy consumption to mechanical energy calculations, eight people (4 men; 4 women) were recruited. Their volumetric rate of oxygen consumption ($\dot{V}O_2$) was determined as described in detail below. Although other empirically-determined methods are available (e.g. [16,19]), the equation endorsed by the American College of Sports Medicine [20] was used as the representative method to predict metabolic energy for walking (ACSM-walk). Mechanical energy was calculated using the methods detailed in Table 1 and included methods that calculate the external, internal and combined work required to move the body. Mechanical energy approaches included those based on sacral motion, ground reaction force profiles, force production assessed via ground contact time, joint moments (via forward dynamics), and an inverse dynamics

simulation developed in SimMechanics, a module within Matlab (R2010a, The Math Works, Natick, MA), which is detailed below. Prediction of metabolic energy using dynamic models with muscles modeled as spring elements was not evaluated, because individual variation cannot be modeled at this time.

Subjects

The premise behind our sampling scheme was to represent within our sample typical variability in adult humans. Consequently, the only exclusion criterion for this study was the presence of inherent gait pathology (e.g. leg length discrepancy) or substantial injury to the lower extremity (e.g. that requiring surgical repair). Table 2 provides subject-specific values used in the analyses described below. Mass was assessed with a standard scale, calibrated and read to the nearest 0.1 kg. Stature was assessed to the nearest cm. Crural index was calculated from the marker positions that are described below and equaled the ratio of calf length (center of lateral knee to lateral malleolus) and thigh length (vertical distance from greater trochanter to center of lateral knee). Note that calculating crural index in this way will yield higher values than the traditional method based on measuring disarticulated bones. Body mass index (BMI) was calculated as body mass divided by the square of stature. The Institutional Review Board, Committee EG of the University of Washington approved this study and all subjects provided written informed consent before participating.

Metabolic data collection and analysis

Subjects walked on a level treadmill while their $\dot{V}O_2$ (in $mlO_2/$ min) was determined by a VO_{2000} oxygen analyzer (Medgraphics, Minneapolis, MN). The subjects wore a neoprene mask that was attached to the oxygen analyzer via a pneumatach and plastic tubing. Breath-by-breath measurements of $\dot{V}O_2$ and $\dot{V}CO_2$ were obtained and all respiratory quotients were <1.0 to ensure that the exercises were conducted in aerobic conditions.

Resting metabolic rate while standing (stRMR) was determined at the beginning of the exercise session. Subjects were then asked to determine their self-selected slow, normal and fast walking velocities and given time to accommodate to the treadmill and the mask prior to data collection. Individual trials at a velocity lasted for 4 min with 4 minutes of standing at rest between trials. Four minutes was chosen because this gave sufficient time to establish a plateau while exercising and allowed $\dot{V}O_2$ to return to resting values between trials. The order of the trials was randomly determined.

One minute averages of the raw breath-by-breath data were computed. The average from minutes 3 and 4 of each trial were

Table 2. Subject characteristics.

Subject id	Sex	Age (yr)	stRMR (mlO$_2$/s)	Mass (kg)	Stature (m)	Thigh length (m)	Calf length (m)	Foot length (m)	Pelvic width (m)	BMI (kg/m^2)	Crural index
6	M	22.0	205	52.4	1.60	0.371	0.345	0.104	0.253	20.5	0.92
10	F	53.1	250	70.0	1.52	0.353	0.346	0.098	0.288	30.3	0.98
11	M	25.5	255	59.7	1.70	0.380	0.371	0.116	0.289	20.7	0.98
13	M	23.2	353	84.2	1.85	0.470	0.445	0.127	0.268	24.1	0.95
15	F	32.3	169	62.4	1.68	0.435	0.387	0.124	0.235	22.1	0.89
27	M	26.2	371	84.2	1.75	0.424	0.406	0.129	0.260	26.9	0.96
38	F	44.7	191	76.0	1.72	0.410	0.401	0.112	0.282	25.7	0.98
39	F	24.1	193	55.2	1.56	0.337	0.363	0.111	0.240	22.7	1.08

used in subsequent analyses. The difference between the measured $\dot{V}O_2$ from minutes 3 and 4 and stRMR was calculated and these values were then used to develop a subject-specific, linear equation that predicted $net\dot{V}O_2$ (in $mlO2/min$) from velocity (all p's <0.001 and $r^2 = 0.68$–0.99). This equation was used to determine $net\dot{V}O_2$ for the appropriate motion analysis trial velocity (described below). The measured velocity of each trial was matched to the individual's velocity-$\dot{V}O_2$ curve and this metabolic value was used in subsequent analyses.

Motion and force data collection and analysis

Motion and ground reaction force profiles of the subjects were assessed in a human motion analysis laboratory, which is equipped with a 6-camera Qualysis (Gothenburg, Sweden) infrared system to capture 3-dimensional motion and an embedded force plate to measure ground reaction force. Data were collected at 120 Hz and stored for later analyses. Calibration of the motion capture volume occurred immediately before each subject's test in accordance with the manufacturer's instructions and marker positions were determined to be within 2 mm of their known position. A standard marker set was attached to the following landmarks of each subject: left and right acromion, anterior superior iliac spine, greater trochanter, superior patella, lateral knee, tibial tuberosity, lateral malleolus, posterior heel, and the space between the second and third metatarsal heads and the superior sacral border. Subjects wore athletic shoes with socks that exposed the malleoli, spandex shorts, and sleeveless shirts during the walking trials. Sacral, ASIS, and trochanteric markers were placed over the landmarks on the shorts; heel and metatarsal head markers were placed on the shoes. Other markers were attached directly to the skin. Once placed, these markers remained in place for all trials. Additional markers on the left and right medial knee and medial malleolus were used to determine joint widths in an initial standing trial and then removed.

Subjects walked at their self-selected slow, normal and fast velocities 10 times across the force plate (5 trials each with left and right foot contact with the force plate), which resulted in 30 walking trials for each subject. Subjects were instructed to watch a point on the laboratory wall and maintain a smooth motion. Trials in which the appropriate foot did not fully contact the force plate or which had excessive gaps in marker data (which can occur when the arm does not swing enough to reveal the trochanteric marker to the cameras) were redone.

After post-processing using standard Qualysis software, analyses were conducted with custom-developed LabView (National Instruments Corporation, Austin TX) programs to determine 1) peak hip range of motion for each trial to be used in the Matlab simulation described below; 2) external work using the sacral marker motion, ground reaction forces, and force production methods; and 3) total work from joint moments.

Matlab model

We developed a mechanical model using SimMechanics, the mechanical simulation module of Matlab (R2010a, The Math Works, Natick, MA). The model included rigid bodies representing the left and right thigh, calf and foot segments and a pelvis/trunk which linked the two legs. Motion of the knee and ankle joints was restricted to the para-sagittal plane while that of the hip joints was allowed in all three planes. Two groups of inputs were required by the SimMechanics model: limb segment parameters and angular displacements.

Thigh, calf and foot segmental variables include segment length and proximal and distal circumferences. Segment lengths and joint widths were determined from the initial standing trial of the

motion analysis using the distance between appropriate markers. Knee and ankle circumferences were derived assuming that the joint widths were diameters. Thigh circumference was calculated from a linear regression equation relating thigh circumference to knee circumference, developed from the data contained in the 1988 US Army Anthropometric Survey [61]. Mass moments of inertia and segment masses were calculated assuming that the thigh and calf were idealized truncated cones of circular cross-section, while the foot was assumed to be a rectangular block. All segments were assumed to be of homogenous density. These shapes are similar to those recommended by others [62]. For the thigh segment, the thigh circumference was used as the proximal diameter of the truncated cone and the knee circumference as the distal diameter. For the calf segment, the knee circumference was the proximal diameter and the ankle circumference the distal one.

Typical hip angular displacement profiles were obtained for average adult humans walking at slow, normal and fast velocities [63] and have been used previously in a similar model [31]. These general profiles were modified to reflect the maximum hip excursion of each subject for each trial. Knee and ankle angular velocities were not subject-specific.

Linear velocities of the centers of gravity and angular velocity for the segments were output from the SimMechanics model (which used an inverse dynamic solution) and were reported for each limb segment for temporal increments from 0–50% of stride cycle. These were used to calculate internal work at each temporal increment from the standard equations, similar to the procedure of Cavagna and Kaneko [34]. Full (100%) energy transfer was allowed between the thigh, calf and foot of the same limb, but not between a limb and the body, as has been done previously [31,64]. Intra-limb energy transfers are feasible because the accelerations and masses and, consequently, forces, are similar, but this is not the case between the body and the limbs [64].

The internal energy of a limb at one temporal increment was compared to that of the next temporal increment. If the energy of a later increment was greater than that of the previous increment, extra energy was added to the system to create motion. If a subsequent increment had a lower energy than the previous, this energy was not stored for later use and was set to zero. This approach is similar to previous work [31,64]. The extra energy required for each interval was summed across the step for left and right legs. Internal work for that iteration was the sum of the extra energy required by the left and right legs. External work was calculated from the change in position of the body's center of gravity.

Every trial for each subject from the motion analysis was evaluated separately using the SimMechanics model.

Mechanical calculations

The individual data described above were used to calculate mechanical energy using several methods as detailed in Table 1. These approaches can be grouped into those that calculate external work (EXT-xx), internal work (INT-xx) or the combination of internal and external work (COMB-xx). External work was calculated using contact time via force production (EXT-FP), ground reaction forces (EXT-GRF), and sacral motion (measured by a sacral marker (EXT-SAC) and determined by the Matlab model (EXT-MAT). Internal work was calculated via the Matlab model (INT-MAT). Combined work was determined from joint moments (COMB-JM) and the sum of internal and external work via the Matlab model (COMB-MAT).

Statistical analysis

The pairwise correlation coefficients between metabolic and mechanical energy approaches were calculated to see if the methods varied together. Then, each method of predicting energy expenditure was regressed against $net\dot{V}O_2$ (except for ACSM which was regressed against $\dot{V}O_2$) to see whether or not it accurately reflected the change in $net\dot{V}O_2$ with increasing intensity. Both ordinary least squares (OLS) and maximum likelihood estimation (MLE) statistical techniques were used. As detailed below, OLS analysis allows for many of the relationships to be examined using familiar statistical criteria such as coefficients of determination, but some relationships are more complex and a formulation to evaluate them exists only for MLE. We chose to do both to allow readers who are less familiar with MLE to access the analysis from a familiar perspective. The anthropometric variables listed in Table 2 were also included in a stepwise OLS regression.

Because previous work [65] indicated that considerable between individual variability exists in walking $\dot{V}O_2$ and that at least some of this variability is due to physiological factors for which we are not currently able to control, we wanted to distinguish variability that exists within an individual from that which exists between individuals. This is important because it provides information regarding the degree to which the method accounts for these two sources of variation (within and between individuals). The goal of collecting this kind of information is to begin to discern where the methods are weak and need more sophisticated approaches.

To accomplish this goal, we used hierarchical linear modeling to examine the relationship between our dependent variable, $\dot{V}O_2$ (metabolic energy), and the potential independent variables, i.e., the various approaches to calculating of mechanical energy. This type of statistical procedure provides two advantages over non-hierarchical techniques. First, because each subject was measured during multiple trials, data points within a subject are not independent and clustering is required to account for the non-independence of the repeated measures. Second, measured metabolic energy can be explained by both variance within an individual subject and variance that exists between subjects. Hierarchical linear modeling partitions the variance of the independent variable and determines the separate and combined contributions to predicting the dependent variable.

In the first analysis, subjects were considered clusters of data points (an individual subject measured during multiple trials of walking). In this analysis, all subjects are constrained to have the same slope (termed "fixed slope") relating $measured\dot{V}O_2$ to the predicted metabolic or mechanical energy, but each subject is permitted to have a different intercept (termed "random intercept"). Using OLS, these analyses result in three coefficients of determination: one for the within subject variance, one for the between subject variance, and one using the total combined variance. Coefficients of determination are an absolute measure of the degree to which a statistical model incorporating independent variables explains the variability of the dependent variable. The fixed slope-random intercept analyses were repeated using MLE.

In the second set of analyses, both the intercept and the slope were allowed to vary between subjects (termed random slope-random intercept) using MLE. (This analysis was not done using OLS because the formulation does not exist [66].) The MLE results were interpreted using the Akaike information criterion (AIC) and the Bayesian information criterion (BIC). Information criteria are relative (i.e., they are not equivalent to coefficients of determination) and are used to select among potential models. Models with lower information criteria have a better balance between accuracy of prediction and the number of independent variables included.

All statistical analyses were accomplished in StataSE (Version 9, Stata Corporation, College Station, TX). Where appropriate, statistical significance was set at an alpha of $p \leq 0.05$.

Results

All methods of predicting $net\dot{V}O_2$ were correlated with each other (Table 3), with correlation coefficients ranging from 0.42–0.99.

Using OLS and requiring a fixed slope for all subjects but allowing a random intercept for each (fixed slope-random intercept), the coefficients of determination were calculated for all predictive methods relative to $net\dot{V}O_2$ (Table 4). All methods predict $net\dot{V}O_2$, explaining 38–76% of the overall variation. The ACSM method, which is the representative metabolic energy approach, explains more of the variation in $\dot{V}O_2$ than do the mechanical energy methods. Among the mechanical energy methods, the method using sacral motion was the poorest predictor, explaining 38% of the variation in $net\dot{V}O_2$. All methods were good at predicting within subject variation, but only the ACSM, force production, and joint moment methods were able to account for between subject variation.

To try to understand why the predictions are less effective at accounting for differences between people than they are within a person, we used our subject-specific variables (Table 2) in a stepwise regression to determine a best-fit equation via OLS assuming a fixed slope-random intercept for each method. The predictive ability of all methods improved with the addition of either crural index (ACSM and ground reaction force methods) or mass (all other methods). Overall predictive ability improved to 52–83% with the addition of a subject specific variable (Table 4).

We further tested the efficacy of the predictive methods by employing MLE. We repeated the fixed slope-random intercept analysis that was completed using OLS and added another analysis, where we allowed the intercept and the slope to vary among subjects (random slope-random intercept). As with the OLS results, the MLE results (Table 5) indicate that all methods produce predictions of similar usefulness and all methods, except the ACSM equation, exhibit better fits with random slope-random intercept than fixed slope-random intercept. The Matlab model and the force production methods produce the best results, while the joint moments and sacral motion the worst.

Discussion

We had two goals at the onset of this research. The first was to establish the degree to which the various methods of calculating mechanical energy are related. The second was to characterize the relationship of the predictive methods with measured energy expenditure.

Relating mechanical energy approaches

We found that all mechanical energy approaches produced predictions that are significantly correlated. The sacral motion method consistently produces the lowest correlation coefficients, although the relationship between joint moment method and the Matlab simulations are also relatively low (but still >0.5). We anticipated that the methods would be correlated, because all approaches are different mathematical descriptions of the same biological phenomenon.

Of the four ways to calculate external work (i.e., the mechanical energy required to move the whole body), all are correlated, but the method that uses measured sacral motion stands out as having lower correlation coefficients (0.42-0.55) with the others than the others have with themselves (0.83-0.94). The differences in correlation between the prediction methods reflect the difficulty in obtaining the inputs for the calculations. As mentioned previously, all of the methods require assumptions about inputs

Table 3. Correlation coefficients of metabolic and mechanical energy approaches.

Variable name	ACSM	EXT-FP	EXT-GRF	EXT-MAT	EXT-SAC	INT-MAT	COMB-JM	COMB-MAT
ACSM	1							
EXT-FP	0.91	1						
EXT-GRF	0.90	0.83	1					
EXT-MAT	0.90	0.87	0.94	1				
EXT-SAC	0.69	0.55	0.42	0.47	1			
INT-MAT	0.90	0.87	0.89	0.96	0.48	1		
COMB-JM	0.70	0.70	0.52	0.56	0.71	0.62	1	
COMB-MAT	0.90	0.87	0.93	0.99	0.47	0.97	0.57	1

needed to calculate energy. The variables of body mass, segment lengths, and velocity are relatively simple to measure accurately. The values that are used for the movement of an anatomical landmark, however, have error associated with measuring the marker's position (that can be assessed rigorously and is less than 2 mm) plus error from any movement that occurs between the marker and the landmark (that is of unknown magnitude). For instance, we believe that the cause of the sacral motion discrepancy is that the sacral marker must be placed on the subject's clothing that, even though tightly fitting spandex, does not adhere to the skin as closely in this area as it does at ASIS or greater trochanter. Consequently, our sacral markers may have tended to vibrate or wiggle more than do more closely adhering markers. This observation is based solely on visual assessment and we present it only as a suggested explanation for the discrepancy. Nonetheless, movement in location can become a spike when position is differentiated with respect to time to obtain velocity. Even though smoothing techniques are used, velocity spikes cause anomalous spikes in the energy expenditure calculation. Measuring sacral motion with a marker attached to shorts, then, seems to be the least attractive method to calculate external work.

Some variables, like mass moment of inertia, are impossible to measure in living creatures and have to be estimated. In our case, we assumed that the thigh and calf could be idealized as truncated cones of homogenous density and circular cross-section. We further assumed that the thigh circumference could be estimated from knee circumference. Inaccuracies in the estimation of segmental inertias would affect the Matlab model, but it does not appear to be substantially different from the other methods.

Characterizing the relationship between predicted and measured energy expenditure

The second of our goals was to characterize the relationship of the predictive methods with measured energy expenditure. We did this using both OLS and MLE statistical techniques. Using OLS, as expected, the ACSM method predicts $\dot{V}O_2$ well, explaining 76% of the overall variation in $\dot{V}O_2$, while the force production method explains 73% of the overall variation in net$\dot{V}O_2$. Both of these methods rely on body mass and a measure of intensity (in the form of velocity or ground contact time) to determine energy expenditure.

Mass and intensity variables have been shown to be particularly relevant to locomotor energy expenditure both using metabolic and mechanical energy approaches in all species studied [24]. It seems, therefore, fundamental at this point that any method to predict energy expenditure must incorporate the effect of these two quantities. Body mass and intensity do not, however, explain all the variation in energy expenditure and any possible effects of shape differences within the body cannot be explored by using only these two variables. The other predictive methods, however,

Table 4. Coefficients of determination (r^2) between energy prediction methods and net$\dot{V}O_2$, including within a subject, between subjects and overall effects using OLS and requiring fixed slopes but allowing random intercepts.

Variable name	net$\dot{V}O_2$			net$\dot{V}O_2$ and mass or crural index**		
	Within a subject r^2	Between subjects r^2	Overall r^2	Within a subject r^2	Between subjects r^2	Overall r^2
ACSM*	0.91	0.74	0.76	0.91	0.76	0.79
EXT-FP	0.83	0.85	0.73	0.83	0.85	0.83
EXT-GRF	0.82	0.14	0.45	0.82	0.46	0.61
EXT-MAT	0.88	0.14	0.48	0.88	0.65	0.72
EXT-SAC	0.67	0.31	0.38	0.67	0.55	0.52
INT-MAT	0.86	0.17	0.45	0.86	0.61	0.68
COMB-JM	0.50	0.63	0.55	0.50	0.86	0.68
COMB-MAT	0.87	0.17	0.46	0.86	0.62	0.69

*ACSM regression statistics are for gross $\dot{V}O_2$.
**ACSM and EXT-GRF are crural index; all other variables methods are mass.

Table 5. Information criteria for MLE for three sets of assumptions: fixed slope-fixed intercept, fixed slope-random intercept, and random slope-random intercept.

Method	Variable name	Fixed slope-fixed intercept		Fixed slope-random intercept		Random slope-random intercept	
		AIC	BIC	AIC	BIC	AIC	BIC
ACSM-walk*	ACSM	2601	2608	2268	2281	**	**
Force production	EXT-FP	2642	2648	2255	2268	1959	1978
CoM-GRF	EXT-GRF	2650	2657	2321	2335	2089	2108
CoM-sacrum-model	EXT-MAT	2664	2671	2292	2304	2018	2038
CoM- sacrum-measured	EXT-SAC	2771	2778	2546	2559	2508	2527
Internal work	INT-MAT	2656	2663	2256	2269	1965	1985
Joint moments	COMB-JM	2708	2714	2603	2616	2554	2574
Model (int + ext work)	COMB-MAT	2662	2669	2283	2296	2002	2022

*ACSM regression statistics are for gross $\dot{V}O_2$.
**random slope-random intercept model not different from fixed slope-random intercept model.

produced lower coefficients of determination than either ACSM or force production methods, but this overall lower explanatory ability was due to particularly low between subjects predictive ability. The within subjects r^2 for all the other methods (except sacral motion and joint moments) was similar to that of ACSM and force production.

To explore this further, we included the subject-specific anthropomorphic variables in a stepwise OLS regression with a fixed slope and random intercept to see if one of the variables would improve the between subjects predictive ability. Although adding a subject-specific variable improved the between subjects fit for all methods, the improvement was marginal for either the ACSM or joint moment method. The other methods saw more improvement. Mass and crural index emerged as the most significant additional predictor and both were independently and positively predictive of measured net$\dot{V}O_2$ in the presence of each other and the predicted metabolic or mechanical energy. We did not, however, have sufficient participants to include more than one subject-specific variable in the OLS regressions. Given that mass is already accounted in all predictive methods, it seems likely that it is acting as a proxy for another subject-specific variable, perhaps a physiological one, that we did not assess. We could speculate that a likely candidate for this is some measure of "physical fitness," but we have no data to address the subject. Another possibility is that body mass is acting as a proxy for activated muscle volume [44] or the muscular energy used in joint stabilization. Dynamic models that incorporate muscles and allow these muscles to drive the simulation [32,41,42,43] are one way to test this possibility and we look forward to the further development of the methods and the opportunity to test this possibility with them.

It is also unclear how crural index is functioning. Other work has indicated that calf length is negatively associated with energy expenditure [67], but whether or not it is functioning as a causal or proxy agent is unclear. It is also possible that crural index (or body mass) is acting as a proxy for effective limb length (the distance between the hip and the center of rotation of the hip during stance) [68], but it is unclear why a length variable would not have been a more predictive proxy. More data is needed to explore these relationships.

Using MLE, we repeated the fixed slope-random intercept analysis which we completed using OLS and were able to extend the analysis to a random slope-random intercept statistical model. All mechanical energy approaches benefited from inclusion of a random slope. Using either the Akaike or Bayesian information criteria, the predictive methods, with the exception of measured sacral motion, have similar likelihoods of representing the measured data appropriately. The MLE regressions, therefore, mirror those obtained using OLS.

Within a subject, the metabolic and mechanical methods produce excellent agreement with measured net$\dot{V}O_2$, but between subjects the methods are less effective. We propose that the explanatory ability of a method within an individual reflects directly on those factors that vary among trials (e.g. velocity, hip angular excursion), while that among individuals reflects the factors that vary among trials *and* among individuals (e.g. velocity, anthropometrics, physiological factors). Consequently, in the within subject statistics, which are most-easily appreciated by examination of the coefficients of determination shown in Table 4, each person is compared only to themselves. Thus, the fit of that part of the statistical model is due to the amalgamation of the predictive ability of the method within a person across all people. This approach has been useful in evaluating growth curves where similar patterns are present among individuals in the presence of substantial intra-individual variation (Rabe-Hesketh and Skrondal 2005).

Summary

The general picture that emerges from these analyses is that all mechanical approaches are predictive of $\dot{V}O_2$ with approximately the same explanatory ability and they are all correlated with each other. This result was expected. Although within subject variation (i.e., the variation introduced solely by intensity) was well-matched, the more unexpected result here is that variation among individuals was not particularly well-predicted with any method except joint moments, which was less able to replicate intra-individual variation.

The chief limitation of this work is the small sample size, especially given that it includes women and men with different physical activity levels and of different ages. The reason to sample broadly was to be able to generalize, but that choice may have limited our ability to detect subtle differences. Nonetheless, we believe that the results of our analyses demonstrate that the choice of methodology should be dependent on the question(s) being asked and not on any perceived theoretical superiority of the method. Inherent in this analysis is our assumption that the principles of Newtonian mechanics and the methods that flow from it are important to the calculation of locomotor energy expenditure and are sensitive to variability in the variables of both large (interspecific) and small scale (intraspecific) analyses. Body mass and velocity are significant predictors of metabolic function in empirical studies of humans (e.g. [16,19,20]) and of diverse groups of animal (e.g. [24]). These same variables are also critical components in the mechanical formulations, suggesting causality to us. When the value of body mass and/or velocity span orders of magnitude, their effect may well overwhelm any other more subtle effects (e.g. kinematic differences or segment inertias), but within species, body mass and velocity vary much less and subtle effects may contribute more to the observed variation in energy expenditure. While the major drivers of energy expenditure (mass and intensity) are accounted in all the methods, more subtle potential contributors can only be addressed by methods that incorporate their effect.

In a general example, changes in shape, like variations in crural index, can be addressed by the forward and inverse dynamics methods, because they incorporate a linked-segment model which has individual limb segment lengths, but not by the force production method. This is not to say that there is anything wrong with the force production method, just that it does not include the level of detail that is needed to explore the specific question of the influence of crural index on energy expenditure.

Specific examples can be easily found in the current anthropological literature. On the one hand, Jungers and colleagues [69] suggest that kinematic differences from modern humans existed in the gait of *Homo floresiensis*, because the foot of *H. floresiensis* is proportionately longer than that of modern humans. This long foot requires that the knee be more flexed at mid-swing, so that the toes can clear the ground. This change in angles potentially changes energy expenditure, but it can only be evaluated with the inverse dynamics approach and not the other mechanical methods, because only inverse dynamics addresses kinematic variability. In this case, a mechanical model is the only choice for the analysis. A metabolic approach for this problem is less-easily implemented or interpreted. One could artificially increase the foot length in an experimental group of humans (by, for instance, requiring them to wear shoes with exaggerated toe boxes), but it is difficult to know if any difference in energetics

between the long-foot and normal-foot groups that might be found is due to foot length or to the inexperience of the subjects in dealing with long feet.

On the other hand, determining the energetic expenditure of pursuit hunting in *Homo* [70] would probably be best done with a metabolic approach using empirically-determined equations. The principle reason is that modern humans are available for study so little extrapolation is required. Human data can be directly used to evaluate the question of interest.

Although we have drawn our examples here from the locomotion of modern humans and their extinct ancestors and relatives, the ideas are applicable to other groups as well. The ability to choose analysis method based on the type of information available should be useful in general to biologists, particularly given that extant nonhuman species are often more difficult to study than humans. Although we acknowledge that this work should be extended to other species, we are encouraged that the methods, when applied to humans, produce consistent results.

Conclusion

Our critical points are that the choice of method is dependent on the question of interest and that no method is intrinsically better or worse than another. The study of locomotion, whether in creatures from the deep past or modern people, benefits from multiple lines of inquiry from diverse perspectives. The performance of any simulation of reality is dependent on the quality of the data available as inputs, the assumptions made to allow the calculations to proceed, and the question of interest.

Acknowledgments

The authors thank Robert Price for his invaluable help in developing the LabView post-processing software and overseeing the motion analysis data collection. Three reviewers provided invaluable help in clarifying our ideas and to them we are indebted.

Author Contributions

Conceived and designed the experiments: PAK ADS. Performed the experiments: PAK ADS. Analyzed the data: PAK ADS. Wrote the paper: PAK ADS.

References

1. Zuntz N, Geppert G (1886) Ueber die Natur der normalen Athemreize und den Ort ihrer Wirkung. Eur J Appl Physiol 38: 337–338.
2. Smith E, Winterhalder B (1984) Natural Selection and Decision Making: Some Fundamental Principles. In: Smith E, Winterhalder B, eds. Evolutionary Ecology and Human Behavior. New York: Aldine de Gruyter. pp 25–60.
3. Kaplan H (1996) A theory of fertility and parental investment in traditional and modern societies Ybk Phys Anthropol 39: 91–135.
4. Tracer DP (1996) Lactation, nutrition, and postpartum amenorrhea in lowland Papua New Guinea. Hum Biol 68: 277–292.
5. Jones JH, Wilson ML, Murray C, Pusey A (2010) Phenotypic quality influences fertility in Gombe chimpanzees. J Anim Ecol 79: 1262–1269.
6. Valeggia C, Ellison PT (2009) Interactions between metabolic and reproductive functions in the resumption of postpartum fecundity. Am J Hum Biol 21: 559–566.
7. Valeggia C, Ellison PT (2004) Lactational amenorrhoea in well-nourished Toba women of Formosa, Argentina. J Biosoc Sci 36: 573–595.
8. Jasienska G, Ellison PT (1998) Physical work causes suppression of ovarian function in women. Proc Biol Sci 265: 1847–1851.
9. Richard AF, Dewar RE, Schwartz M, Ratsirarson J (2000) Mass change, environmental variability and female fertility in wild Propithecus verreauxi. J Hum Evol 39: 381–391.
10. Tardif S, Power M, Layne D, Smucny D, Ziegler T (2004) Energy restriction initiated at different gestational ages has varying effects on maternal weight gain and pregnancy outcome in common marmoset monkeys (Callithrix jacchus). Br J Nutr 92: 841–849.
11. Ellison P (2008) Energetics, Reproductive Ecology and Human Evolution. PaleoAnthropology. pp 172–200.
12. Starr C (2006) Biology A Human Emphasis. BelmontCA: Thomson Brooks/ Cole.
13. Taylor CR (1994) Relating mechanics and energetics during exercise. Adv Vet Sci Comp Med 38A: 181–215.
14. Zelik KE, Kuo AD (2010) Human walking isn't all hard work: evidence of soft tissue contributions to energy dissipation and return. The Journal of experimental biology 213: 4257–4264.
15. Marsh RL, Ellerby DJ, Carr JA, Henry HT, Buchanan CI (2004) Partitioning the energetics of walking and running: swinging the limbs is expensive. Science 303: 80–83.
16. Pimental NA, Pandolf KB (1979) Energy expenditure while standing or walking slowly uphill or downhill with loads. Ergonomics 22: 963–973.
17. Taylor CR, Heglund NC (1982) Energetics and mechanics of terrestrial locomotion. Annu Rev Physiol 44: 97–107.
18. Sarton-Miller I (2006) Noninvasive assessment of energy expenditure in children. Am J Hum Biol 18: 600–609.
19. Steudel-Numbers KL, Tilkens MJ (2004) The effect of lower limb length on the energetic cost of locomotion: implications for fossil hominins. J Hum Evol 47: 95–109.
20. Glass S, Dwyer G (2007) ACSM's Metabolic Calculations Handbook. Philadelphia: Lippencott Williams & wilkins.
21. Dawson TJ, Taylor CR (1973) Energetic cost of locomotion in kangaroos. Nature 246: 313–314.
22. Farley CT, Taylor CR (1991) A mechanical trigger for the trot-gallop transition in horses. Science 253: 306–308.
23. Langman VA, Roberts TJ, Black J, Maloiy GM, Heglund NC, et al. (1995) Moving cheaply: energetics of walking in the African elephant. J Exp Biol 198: 629–632.
24. Taylor CR, Heglund NC, Maloiy GM (1982) Energetics and mechanics of terrestrial locomotion. I. Metabolic energy consumption as a function of speed and body size in birds and mammals. J Exp Biol 97: 1–21.

25. Taylor CR, Schmidt-Nielsen K, Raab JL (1970) Scaling of energetic cost of running to body size in mammals. Am J Physiol 219: 1104–1107.

26. Alexander RM, Jayes AS (1983) A dynamic similarity hypothesis for the gaits of quadrupedal mammals. J Zool Lond 201: 135–152.

27. Kramer P, Sarton-Miller I (2008) The energetics of human walking: Is Froude number (Fr) useful for metabolic comparisons? Gait and Posture 27: 209–215.

28. FAO/WHO/UNU (1985) Energy and Protein Requirements; Technical report Series n, editor. Geneva: World Health Organization.

29. Crompton RH, Yu L, Weijie W, Gunther M, Savage R (1998) The mechanical effectiveness of erect and "bent-hip, bent-knee" bipedal walking in Australopithecus afarensis. J Hum Evol 35: 55–74.

30. Kramer P (1998) Locomotor energetics and leg length in hominid evolution. Seattle: PhD dissertation, University of Washington.

31. Kramer PA (1999) Modelling the locomotor energetics of extinct hominids. J Exp Biol 202: 2807–2818.

32. Sellers WI, Dennis LA, Crompton RH (2003) Predicting the metabolic energy costs of bipedalism using evolutionary robotics. J Exp Biol 206: 1127–1136.

33. Cavagna GA, Margaria R (1966) Mechanics of walking. J Appl Physiol 21: 271–278.

34. Cavagna GA, Kaneko M (1977) Mechanical work and efficiency in level walking and running. J Physiol 268: 467–481.

35. Cavagna GA (1975) Force platforms as ergometers. J Appl Physiol 39: 174–179.

36. Umberger B, Martin P (2007) Mechanical power and efficiency of level walking with different stride rates. J Exp Biol 210: 3255–3265.

37. Cavagna GA, Thys H, Zamboni A (1976) The sources of external work in level walking and running. J Physiol 262: 639–657.

38. Yamazaki N, Ishida H, Kimura T, Okada M (1979) Biomechanical Analysis of Primate Bipedal Walking by Computer Simulation. J Hum Evol 8: 337–349.

39. Kram R, Taylor CR (1990) Energetics of running: a new perspective. Nature 346: 265–267.

40. Pontzer H (2005) A new model predicting locomotor cost from limb length via force production. J Exp Biol 208: 1513–1524.

41. Nagano A, Umberger BR, Marzke MW, Gerritsen KG (2005) Neuromusculoskeletal computer modeling and simulation of upright, straight-legged, bipedal locomotion of Australopithecus afarensis (A.L. 288-1). Am J Phys Anthropol 126: 2–13.

42. Sellers WI, Cain GM, Wang W, Crompton RH (2005) Stride lengths, speed and energy costs in walking of Australopithecus afarensis: using evolutionary robotics to predict locomotion of early human ancestors. J R Soc Interface 2: 431–441.

43. Sellers WI, Dennis LA, W JW, Crompton RH (2004) Evaluating alternative gait strategies using evolutionary robotics. J Anat 204: 343–351.

44. Pontzer H, Raichlen DA, Sockol MD (2009) The metabolic cost of walking in humans, chimpanzees, and early hominins. J Hum Evol 56: 43–54.

45. Crompton RH, Sellers WI, Thorpe SK (2010) Arboreality, terrestriality and bipedalism. Philos Trans R Soc Lond B Biol Sci 365: 3301–3314.

46. Chumanov ES, Wall-Scheffler C, Heiderscheit BC (2008) Gender differences in walking and running on level and inclined surfaces. Clin Biomech (Bristol, Avon) 23: 1260–1268.

47. Wall-Scheffler CM, Chumanov E, Steudel-Numbers K, Heiderscheit B (2010) Electromyography activity across gait and incline: The impact of muscular activity on human morphology. Am J Phys Anthropol.

48. Bertram JE, Chang YH (2001) Mechanical energy oscillations of two brachiation gaits: measurement and simulation. Am J Phys Anthropol 115: 319–326.

49. Nakatsukasa M, Hirasaki E, Ogihara A, Hamada Y (2002) Energetics of bipedal and quadrupedal walking in Japanese macaques. Am J Phys Anth Suppl 34: 117.

50. Nakatsukasa M, Ogihara N, Hamada Y, Goto Y, Yamada M, et al. (2004) Energetic costs of bipedal and quadrupedal walking in Japanese macaques. Am J Phys Anthropol 124: 248–256.

51. Griffin TM, Kram R, Wickler SJ, Hoyt DF (2004) Biomechanical and energetic determinants of the walk-trot transition in horses. J Exp Biol 207: 4215–4223.

52. Pfau T, Witte TH, Wilson AM (2006) Centre of mass movement and mechanical energy fluctuation during gallop locomotion in the Thoroughbred racehorse. J Exp Biol 209: 3742–3757.

53. Full RJ, Tu MS (1991) Mechanics of a rapid running insect: two-, four- and six-legged locomotion. J Exp Biol 156: 215–231.

54. Reilly SM, McElroy EJ, Andrew Odum R, Hornyak VA (2006) Tuataras and salamanders show that walking and running mechanics are ancient features of tetrapod locomotion. Proc Biol Sci 273: 1563–1568.

55. Sellers WI, Manning P (2007) Estimating dinosaur maximum running speeds using evolutionary robotics. Proc Roy Soc B-Biol Sci 274: 2711–2716.

56. Steudel-Numbers KL (2006) Energetics in Homo erectus and other early hominins: the consequences of increased lower-limb length. J Hum Evol 51: 445–453.

57. Weaver T, Steudel-Numbers KL (2005) Does Cimate or Mobility Explain the Differences in Body Proportions between Neandertals and their Upper Paleolithic Successors? Evol Anthro 14: 218–223.

58. Lovejoy CO, Latimer B, Suwa G, Asfaw B, White TD (2009) Combining prehension and propulsion: the foot of Ardipithecus ramidus. Science 326: 72e71–78.

59. Lovejoy CO, McCollum MA (2011) Spinopelvic pathways to bipedality: why no hominids ever relied on a bent-hip-bent-knee gait. Philos Trans R Soc Lond B Biol Sci 365: 3289–3299.

60. Lovejoy CO, Suwa G, Simpson SW, Matternes JH, White TD (2009) The great divides: Ardipithecus ramidus reveals the postcrania of our last common ancestors with African apes. Science 326: 100–106.

61. Gordon C, Bradtmiller B, Churchill T, Clauser C, McConville J, et al. (1988) 1988 Anthropometric Survey of US Army Personnel: Methods and Summary Statistics.

62. Hanavan EP, Jr. (1964) A Mathematical Model of the Human Body. Amrl-Tr-64-102. AMRL TR. pp 1–149.

63. Winter DA (1987) The Biomechanics and Motor Control of Human Gait. Ontario: University of Waterloo press.

64. Willems PA, Cavagna GA, Heglund NC (1995) External, internal and total work in human locomotion. J Exp Biol 198: 379–393.

65. Kramer PA (2010) The effect on energy expenditure of walking on gradients or carrying burdens. Am J Hum Biol 22: 497–507.

66. Rabe-Hesketh S, Skrondal A (2005) Multilevel and Longitudinal Modeling using Stata. College Station: Stata Press.

67. Bereket S (2005) Effects of anthropometric parameters and stride frequency on estimation of energy cost of walking. J Sports Med Phys Fitness 45: 152–161.

68. Pontzer H (2007) Effective limb length and the scaling of locomotor cost in terrestrial animals. J Exp Biol 210: 1752–1761.

69. Jungers WL, Harcourt-Smith WE, Wunderlich RE, Tocheri MW, Larson SG, et al. (2009) The foot of Homo floresiensis. Nature 459: 81–84.

70. Steudel-Numbers KL, Wall-Scheffler CM (2009) Optimal running speed and the evolution of hominin hunting strategies. J Hum Evol 56: 355–360.

5

Influence of Passive Muscle Tension on Electromechanical Delay in Humans

Lilian Lacourpaille, François Hug*, Antoine Nordez

University of Nantes, Laboratory "Motricité, Interactions, Performance" (EA 4334), Nantes, France

Abstract

Background: Electromechanical delay is the time lag between onsets of muscle activation and muscle force production and reflects both electro-chemical processes and mechanical processes. The aims of the present study were two-fold: to experimentally determine the slack length of each head of the biceps brachii using elastography and to determine the influence of the length of biceps brachii on electromechanical delay and its electro-chemical/mechanical processes using very high frame rate ultrasound.

Methods/Results: First, 12 participants performed two passive stretches to evaluate the change in passive tension for each head of the biceps brachii. Then, they underwent two electrically evoked contractions from 120 to 20° of elbow flexion (0°: full extension), with the echographic probe maintained over the muscle belly and the myotendinous junction of biceps brachii. The slack length was found to occur at 95.5 ± 6.3° and 95.3 ± 8.2° of the elbow joint angle for the long and short heads of the biceps brachii, respectively. The electromechanical delay was significantly longer at 120° (16.9 ± 3.1 ms; p<0.001), 110° (15.0 ± 3.1 ms; p<0.001) and 100° (12.7 ± 2.5 ms; p = 0.01) of elbow joint angle compared to 90° (11.1 ± 1.7 ms). However, the delay between the onset of electrical stimulation and the onset of both muscle fascicles (3.9 ± 0.2 ms) and myotendinous junction (3.7 ± 0.3 ms) motion was not significantly affected by the joint angle (p>0.95).

Conclusion: In contrast to previous observations on gastrocnemius medialis, the onset of muscle motion and the onset of myotendinous junction motion occurred simultaneously regardless of the length of the biceps brachii. That suggests that the between-muscles differences reported in the literature cannot be explained by different muscle passive tension but instead may be attributable to muscle architectural differences.

Editor: Christof Markus Aegerter, University of Zurich, Switzerland

Funding: This study was supported by grants from the European Regional Development Fund (ERDF, number 37400), the Association Française contre les Myopathie (AFM number 14597) and the Region des Pays de la Loire. The funders had no role in study design, data collection and analysis, decision to publish, or preparation of the manuscript.

Competing Interests: The authors have declared that no competing interests exist.

* E-mail: francois.hug@univ-nantes.fr

Introduction

Electromechanical delay (EMD) is the time lag between onsets of muscle activation and muscle force production. It reflects both electro-chemical processes (i.e., synaptic transmission, propagation of the action potential, excitation-contraction coupling) as well as mechanical processes (i.e., force transmission along the active and the passive part of the series elastic component, SEC) [1]. The relative contributions of both electro-chemical and mechanical processes involved in EMD has recently been characterized on gastrocnemius medialis [2] and biceps brachii [3,4] using very high frame rate ultrasound. More precisely, the delay between the muscle electrical stimulation and the onset of muscle fascicles motion has been mainly attributed to electro-chemical processes and the delay between the onset of fascicles motion and the onset of both the myotendinous junction motion and the force production has been attributed to mechanical processes [2,3,4]. While the study of gastrocnemius medialis reported a delay of about 2.4 ms between the onset of muscle fascicles motion and the onset of myotendinous junction motion (i.e., the delay to transmit force along the aponeurosis) [2], fascicles and myotendinous

junction motion occurred concomitantly in biceps brachii [3,4]. As proposed by Hug et al. [3], this discrepancy could be explained by architectural differences between these two muscles (pennate vs. fusiform, [5]) and/or different levels of passive tension induced by the experimental setup. Indeed, the ankle joint angle (10° in plantar flexion) used in the study of Nordez et al. [2] induces slight passive muscle tension [6,7,8,9]. In contrast, in the study of Hug et al. [3] the biceps brachii muscle-tendon unit was likely to be slack (elbow joint = 90°) and thus did not produced any passive tension. In this latter case, one would expect a rigid body motion inducing a simultaneous displacement onset of the fascicles and myotendinous junction.

Some studies have reported significant changes in EMD through experimental manipulation of tension in the SEC [6,10,11]. More precisely, they showed that EMD is influenced by the time to stretch the SEC when the muscle-tendon unit length is shorter than the estimated slack length (defined here as the length from which the muscle begins to develop passive elastic force). In contrast, these earlier studies also showed that EMD is independent of the passive tension when the muscle-tendon unit is longer than the slack length. One of the main limitations of these studies is that they arbitrarily determined the slack length (i.e., at 90° of elbow angle) [11], or determined it to be at the angle at which no passive joint moment was produced [6]. The utility of this last method is questionable, because the passive joint moment is associated with all structures that cross the joint (i.e., muscles, tendons, skin, articular structures) [12] whereas EMD is only associated with the muscle-tendon unit. Furthermore, none of these studies simultaneously recorded the onset of motion of muscle fascicles and myotendinous junction making them unable to attribute changes to electro-chemical and/or mechanical process. Thus, due to shortcomings in experimental techniques, the relationship between muscle passive tension and the mechanisms involved in EMD has never been investigated.

The aims of the present study were two-fold. First, we experimentally determined the slack length of each head of the biceps brachii using an ultrasound shear wave elastographic technique named supersonic shear imaging (SSI). The main advantage of this technique is that it can be used to accurately estimate passive tension and slack length of an individual muscle [8]. For instance, as biceps brachii is composed of two heads with different proximal insertions one would expect different passive tension within each head at a given joint angle. Secondly, we determined the influence of biceps brachii length on EMD and its mechanisms. We hypothesized that for a muscle-tendon unit length shorter than the measured slack length the onset of fascicle motion would not be different to the onset of myotendinous junction motion (i.e., transmission force as rigid body motion) [3]. For a muscle-tendon unit length longer than the slack length, we hypothesized that a significant delay should exist between the onset of fascicles motion and the onset of myotendinous junction motion, attributed to the time to transmit force along the aponeurosis, as previously shown in gastrocnemius medialis [2].

Materials and Methods

Participants

Twelve males volunteered to participate in the present study (age: 21.8 ± 2.3 years; height: 180.5 ± 3.6 cm, body mass: 76.0 ± 6.1 kg). Participants were informed of the purpose of the study and methods used before providing written consent. The experimental design of the study was approved by the Ethical Committee of Nantes Ouest IV and was conducted in accordance with the Declaration of Helsinki (last modified in 2004).

Instrumentation

Ergometer. Participants sat on an isokinetic dynamometer (Biodex System 3 Research, Biodex Medical, Shirley, USA) with their right shoulder abducted at 90° and with their wrist in a neutral position as described previously [4] (Fig. 1). The torso was strapped to the dynamometer chair to ensure that the participant's shoulder/trunk position did not change throughout the experiment.

Due to the lack of sensitivity of the isokinetic ergometer to precisely detect the onset of elbow flexion force, a force transducer (SML-50, range: 0–50 Ibf, sensibility: 2 mV/V, Interface, Arizona, USA) was incorporated in the ergometer and connected with Velcro straps to the wrist to ensure constant contact (Fig. 1). Elbow flexion force was digitized at a sampling rate of 5 kHz (MP36, BIOPAC, Goleta, California, USA).

Elastography. During the first part of the protocol (i.e., passive stretching cycles), an Aixplorer ultrasound scanner (version 4.2; Supersonic Imagine, Aix-en-Provence, France), coupled with a linear transducer array (4–15 MHz, SuperLinear 15-4, Vermon, Tours, France) was used in SSI mode (musculo-skeletal preset) as

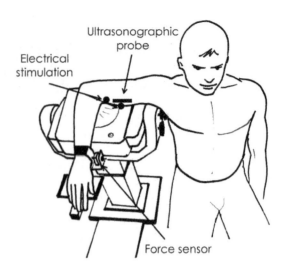

Figure 1. Schematic representation of the experimental setup. Positioning of the subject with shoulder abducted at 90 degrees and forearm placed in a 90 flexed position. The wrist was directly in contact with a force sensor and velcro straps ensured constant contact. Adapted from Lacourpaille et al. (in press) with permission from Elsevier.

previously described [13,14]. Assuming a linear elastic behavior, the muscle shear elastic modulus was calculated as follow:

$$\mu = \rho V s^2$$

Where ρ is the muscle mass density (1000 kg.m^3) and Vs is the shear wave speed. As discussed previously [15,16], the hypothesis of linear material is well accepted in muscle elastographic studies, for both transient elastography [13,17] and magnetic resonance elastography [18,19]. Maps of the shear elastic modulus were obtained at 1 Hz with a spatial resolution of 1×1 mm (Fig. 2).

Surface EMG activity. Surface EMG electrodes (Delsys DE 2.1, Delsys Inc., Boston, MA, USA; 1 cm interelectrode distance) were placed on the muscle belly biceps brachii and long head of triceps brachii. EMG signals were amplified (ξ1000) and digitized (6–400 Hz bandwidth) at a sampling rate of 1 kHz (Bagnoli 16, Delsys, Inc. Boston, USA). EMG was monitored during the passive stretching cycles, and trials with EMG greater than 1% of maximal voluntary contraction were discarded [9,20,21].

Electrical stimulation. During the second part of the protocol (i.e., electromechanical delay), elbow flexion was initiated by means of percutaneous electrical stimulation over the biceps brachii. A constant current stimulator (Digitimer DS7A, Digitimer, Letchworth Garden City, UK) delivered a single electrical pulse (pulse duration = 500 μs, 400 V) through two electrodes (2×1.5 cm, Compex, Annecy-le-vieux, France) placed on the main motor point and on the distal portion of biceps brachii [3,4]. The motor point was determined by detecting the location that induced the strongest muscle twitch with the lowest electrical stimulation intensity. To determine the minimal stimulation intensity required to induce the maximal muscle torque (107 ± 24 mA), the output current was incrementally increased (from 0 mA, with an incremental step of 5 mA) until a maximum torque output was reached.

Ultrasonography. To assess the electromechanical delay, a very high frame rate ultrasound scanner (Aixplorer, version 4.2, Supersonic Imagine, Aix en Provence, France) coupled with

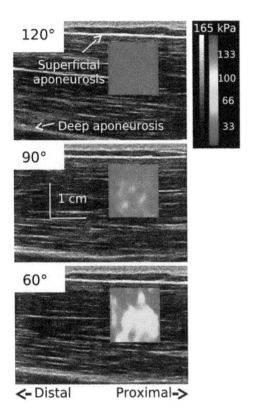

Figure 2. Typical example of shear elastic modulus measurement at different elbow angles. Typical example of shear elastic modulus of the long head of biceps brachii at 120°, 90°, and 20° of elbow joint angle. The colored region represents the map of shear elastic modulus values.

a linear transducer array (4–15 MHz, SuperLinear 15-4, Vermon, Tours, France) was used in « research » mode to acquire raw radio frequency (RF) signals at 4 kHz. At the start of each ultrasound acquisition, the scanner sent a transistor-transistor logic (TTL) pulse to a train/delay generator (DS7A, Digitimer Ltd, Welwyn Garden City, UK) that generated a TTL pulse to the electrical stimulator with a 48.00-ms delay to have a sufficient baseline to detect the onset of tissue motion. To check the consistency of synchronization throughout the experiments, TTL pulses from both the ultrasound scanner and the train/delay generator were recorded using the same device that recorded the force signal (MP36, Biopac, Goleta, California, USA).

Protocol

Passive tension. To account for a possible effect of conditioning, participants first performed five slow (10°/s) passive loading/unloading cycles between 120° and 20° of elbow flexion (0° represents full extension) that were not analyzed [22]. Immediately after, the ultrasound probe was placed on either head of the biceps brachii (in random order) and participant's biceps brachii was passively stretched through 2 very slow (2°/s) loading/unloading cycles over the same range of motion. The shear elastic modulus of each head of the biceps brachii was measured during the extension phase. Online EMG feedback was provided to the participants and the examiner. Participants were asked to stay as relaxed as possible throughout the loading/unloading cycles. If EMG activity was observed during the trial, recording ceased, and another trial initiated. However, this did not occur.

Electromechanical delay. Immediately after completion of the first part of the protocol, EMD was evaluated at a range of elbow flexion angles. First, five slow (10°/s) passive loading/unloading cycles were performed to account for a possible effect of conditioning (no data were recorded during these cycles). Then, two electrically evoked contractions of biceps brachii (designated as muscle trials and tendon trials, when the ultrasound probe was positioned above the muscle and tendon, respectively) were performed at 11 angles, i.e., in 10° increments from 20° to 120° of elbow flexion, in a randomized order, with one minute of rest between each contraction. Participants were instructed to be fully relaxed prior to each stimulation. During the muscle and tendon trials, the echographic probe was maintained parallel to the muscle fascicles and on the previously localized distal myotendinous junction of the biceps brachii, respectively. Because it was not possible to selectively stimulate one head of biceps brachii by percutaneous electromyostimulation without stimulating the other head, we were not able to determine a specific EMD for each head. Thus, the measured EMD corresponded to the EMD of the whole muscle [3,4].

Data Processing

All the data were processed using custom Matlab scripts (The Mathworks, Nathick, USA).

SSI recordings were exported from software (Version 4.2, Supersonic Imagine, Aix en Provence, France) in "mp4" format and sequenced in "jpeg". Image processing was performed to convert the colored map into shear elastic modulus values. The average value of shear elastic modulus over the largest muscular region was calculated for each image. The slack length was visually determined by an experienced examiner for both the short and long head [4].

Ultrasonic raw data (i.e., RF signals) obtained using the very high frame rate ultrasound device were used to create echographic images by applying a conventional beam formation, i.e., applying a time-delay operation to compensate for the travel time differences. These ultrasound images were used to determine the region of interest (ROI; see Fig. 3 of ref [4]) for each contraction, i.e., between the two aponeuroses of the biceps brachii muscle for muscle trials and on the biceps brachii myotendinous junction for tendon trials. Using a one-dimensional cross correlation of windows of consecutive RF signals, the displacements along the ultrasound beam axis (y-axis) were calculated [23,24,25]. Thus, the tissue motion between the two consecutive images (i.e., particle velocity) was measured with a micrometric precision. Displacements were then averaged over the previously determined ROI, and these averaged signals were used to detect the onset of motion. The onset of tissue motion (for the muscle fascicles and myotendinous junction) and the onset of force production were detected visually [4]. The time (delay) between the electrical stimulation (i.e., beginning of stimulation artefact) and the onset of muscle fascicles motion (Dm), myotendinous junction motion (Dt), and force production (EMD) were calculated for each elbow angle.

Statistical Analysis

Normality testing (Kolmogorov-Smirnov) was consistently passed and thus values are reported as mean ± standard deviation. A paired t-test was used to compare the slack length of the two heads of biceps brachii. The effect of probe location [i.e., 4 locations (Dm and EMD for muscle trials and Dt and EMD for tendon trials)] and elbow joint angle [i.e., 11 elbow angles (20, 30, 40, 50, 60, 70, 80, 90, 100, 110, and 120°)] was tested using a two-way repeated measures ANOVA. Post-hoc analyses were

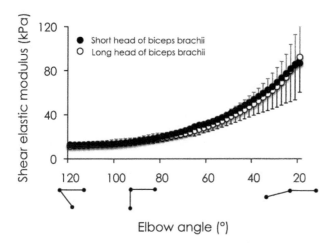

Figure 3. Relationship between shear elastic modulus and elbow joint angle for both heads of biceps brachii. Shear elastic modulus (kPa) was obtained for all participants using supersonic shear imaging during passive loading cycles performed between 20° and 120° of elbow flexion (0° represents full extension). The change of shear elastic modulus for both the short head (mean values in black circles and standard deviation in black lines) and the long head (mean values in open circles and standard deviation in gray) of biceps brachii is represented.

performed when appropriated using Scheffe's method. The statistical significance was set at p<0.05.

Results

Due to technical problems in the export of high frame rate ultrasound data and amplification of force signals during the experimentation, two participants were not included in the analysis. Results are therefore presented from 10 participants.

Relationship between Muscle Shear Elastic Modulus and Elbow Joint Angle

Fig. 3 depicts the relationship between shear elastic modulus and elbow joint angle for each head of the biceps brachii. In accordance with previous literature [8], the change in muscles stiffness during the passive stretching was exponential. The smallest elbow flexion angle at which the shear elastic modulus increased (the slack length) was similar between the two heads of the biceps brachii (95.5 ± 6.3° and 95.3 ± 8.2° for the long and short head of the biceps brachii, respectively) (p = 0.99).

Effect of Elbow Joint Angle on EMD, Dm and Dt

The influence of the elbow joint angle on EMD and its mechanisms (Dm and Dt) is depicted in Fig. 4. ANOVA revealed a significant main effect of location (p<0.001). More precisely, Dm was significantly shorter than EMD for muscle trials (3.9 ± 0.2 ms vs. 11.8 ± 2.3 ms; p<0.001), and Dt was significantly shorter than EMD for tendon trials (3.7 ± 0.3 ms vs. 11.8 ± 2.2 ms; p<0.001). No significant difference was found between Dm and Dt (p = 0.96) or between EMD measured during muscle trials and tendon trials (p = 0.99).

A main effect of elbow joint angle on the delays was found (p<0.001) corresponding to an overall decrease when the elbow joint was extended. In addition, a significant interaction location x elbow joint angles was found (p<0.001), indicating that Dm, Dt, and EMD were not similarly altered by the elbow joint angle. More precisely, 120°, 110° and 100° of the elbow joint angle

induced a significantly longer EMD compared to 90° (i.e., p<0.001, p<0.001, and p = 0.01, respectively). However, there were no significant changes in Dm and Dt across elbow angles (p>0.95 for all the paired comparisons).

Discussion

The aim of the present work was to determine the slack length of each head of the biceps brachii muscle, and to evaluate the influence of muscle length (relative to this slack length) on the electro-chemical and mechanical processes involved in the electromechanical delay. The results demonstrate that the slack length of both heads of biceps brachii occur at the same elbow angle (≈95°). EMD was significantly longer for the most flexed elbow angles (100°, 110°, and 120°) compared to 90°, and it was not significantly changed for more extended angles, i.e when muscle-tendon length was longer than the slack length. The onset of muscle motion and the onset of myotendinous junction motion occurred simultaneously regardless of the muscle length.

A passive torque-angle curve is classically used to study the behaviour of the muscle-tendon unit *in vivo* [9,21,22,26,27]. However, this curve is a composite of several structures including agonist and antagonist muscles, tendons, skin, ligaments, joint capsule, etc. [12]. Consequently, it cannot be used to directly estimate the slack length of a given muscle-tendon unit. Maisetti et al. [8] recently showed that the shear elastic modulus of the gastrocnemius medialis can be reliably measured using SSI during the loading phase of passive stretches providing a direct estimation of passive muscle-tendon tension and slack length. Using the same experimental technique, we determined the slack length of the biceps brachii in the present study at about 95°, corresponding to a muscle-tendon length of about 35.1 cm (calculating using the model proposed by Martin et al. [28] and Valour and Pousson, [29]). The main advantage of the elastographic method used in the present study is that it can be easily used to individualize neuromusculoskeletal models. As the muscle-tendon slack length is one of the parameters in Hill-type muscle models [30,31] this individualization is of great interest. Despite the differences in proximal insertion between the two heads of the biceps brachii and the potential "pre-tension" of the short head of biceps brachii induced by the experimental setup (i.e., shoulder abducted 90°), the slack length of both heads occurred at the same joint angle. Mechanical interactions between muscles have been shown in animals [32,33] and humans [34]. As the two heads of the biceps brachii are connected by the bicipital aponeurosis and their common distal tendon, it is possible that intermuscular force transmission occurred between the two heads. In other words, passive tension within one head could have been transmitted to the other one, explaining that the slack length occurred at the same angle for each of them.

We report EMD values ranging from 10.2 ± 1.4 ms to 17.2 ± 3.4 ms for 50° and 120° of elbow flexion, respectively. These values are close to those reported in the literature during electrically evoked contractions and confirm that EMD is affected by the muscle-tendon unit length [2,3,4,10,11,35]. More precisely, for muscle-tendon unit lengths shorter than the measured slack length (i.e., 95° of elbow flexion), the EMD decreased with increase in elbow joint angle (Fig. 4) until a plateau of 90° of elbow flexion, after which EMD remained stable. As previously suggested by Sasaki et al. [11], the increase in EMD at short muscle lengths (i.e., shorter than the slack length) is likely to be explained by the time required for the muscle to take up the slack within the muscle-tendon unit.

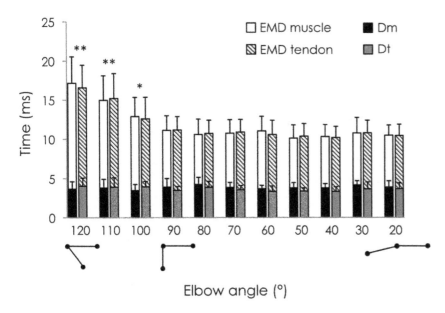

Figure 4. Effect of elbow joint angle on EMD, Dm, and Dt. For each angle, electromechanical delay (EMD), the onset of muscle fascicle motion (Dm) and the onset of myotendinous junction motion (Dt) were determined during an electrically evoked contraction. Two histograms are depicted for each angle (for muscle trials and for tendon trials). EMD for muscle and tendon trials is represented by the addition of filled and open bars (muscle trials) and filled and hatched bars (tendon trials). Dm and Dt are symbolized by the filled bars in black and grey, respectively. *: $p < 0.05$ and **: $p < 0.001$: Significant difference in EMD from the elbow joint angle of $90°$.

To our knowledge, only Sasaki et al. [11] previously studied the influence of joint angle on electrochemical processes of EMD, which was determined as the delay between the onset of stimulation and the onset of muscle contraction (assessed by accelerometers placed on the skin). They showed that this delay was not influenced by elbow joint angle. However, no study has evaluated the relationship between elbow joint angle and the force transmission between muscle fascicles and myotendinous junction during EMD. The results of the present study demonstrate that Dm and Dt were not significantly altered by the elbow joint angle and occurred concomitantly regardless of the muscle length. Therefore, the discrepancy in the force transmission in EMD between gastrocnemius medialis [2] and biceps brachii [3] previously reported in the literature cannot be due to differences in muscle passive tension induced by the experimental setup. The architectural differences between these two muscles (pennate vs. fusiform) are likely to explain the differences in muscle force transmission suggested by Dm, Dt and EMD measurements.

Conclusion

This study shows that the slack length determined by SSI does not differ between the two heads of the biceps brachii. Our results also show that the discrepancy in electro-chemical and mechanical processes of EMD between gastrocnemius medialis [2] and biceps brachii [3] is likely due to muscle architecture rather than a difference in passive tension. Both the determination of the slack length by SSI and EMD could be useful to follow changes in mechanical and contractile properties of target muscles particularly affected by neuromuscular disorders or involved in rehabilitation/training programs.

Acknowledgments

The authors thank Dr Kylie TUCKER (The University of Queensland, Australia) for editing the manuscript and Jean HUG for drawing Fig. 1.

Author Contributions

Conceived and designed the experiments: LL FH AN. Performed the experiments: LL. Analyzed the data: LL. Contributed reagents/materials/analysis tools: LL FH AN. Wrote the paper: LL FH AN.

References

1. Cavanagh PR, Komi PV (1979) Electromechanical delay in human skeletal muscle under concentric and eccentric contractions. Eur J Appl Physiol 42: 159–163.
2. Nordez A, Gallot T, Catheline S, Guevel A, Cornu C, et al. (2009) Electromechanical delay revisited using very high frame rate ultrasound. J Appl Physiol 106: 1970–1975.
3. Hug F, Gallot T, Catheline S, Nordez A (2011) Electromechanical delay in biceps brachii assessed by ultrafast ultrasonography. Muscle Nerve 43: 441–443.
4. Lacourpaille L, Nordez A, Hug F Influence of stimulus intensity on electromechanical delay and its mechanisms. J Electromyogr Kinesiol. In press.
5. Murray WM, Buchanan TS, Delp SL (2000) The isometric functional capacity of muscles that cross the elbow. J biomech 33: 943–952.
6. Muraoka T (2004) Influence of tendon slack on electromechanical delay in the human medial gastrocnemius in vivo. J Appl Physiol 96: 540–544.
7. Hoang PD, Gorman RB, Todd G, Gandevia SC, Herbert RD (2005) A new method for measuring passive length-tension properties of human gastrocnemius muscle in vivo. J Biomech 38: 1333–1341.
8. Maïsetti O, Hug F, Bouillard K, Nordez A (2012) Characterization of passive elastic properties of the human medial gastrocnemius muscle belly using supersonic shear imaging. J Biomech 45: 978–984.
9. Nordez A, Gennisson JL, Casari P, Catheline S, Cornu C (2008) Characterization of muscle belly elastic properties during passive stretching using transient elastography. J Biomech 41: 2305–2311.
10. Muro A, Nagata A (1985) The effects on electromechanical delay of muscle stretch of the human triceps surae. In: Biomechanics IX-A, edited by Winter DA, Norman RW, Wells R P, Hayes KC, Patla A E Champaign, IL: Human Kinetics (1985) 86–90.
11. Sasaki K, Sasaki T, Ishii N (2011) Acceleration and force reveal different mechanisms of electromechanical delay. Med Sci Sports Exerc 43: 1200–1206.

12. Riemann BL, DeMont RG, Ryu K, Lephart SM (2001) The effects of sex, joint angle, and the gastrocnemius muscle on passive ankle joint complex stiffness. J Athl Train 36: 369–375.

13. Bercoff J, Tanter M, Fink M (2004) Supersonic shear imaging: a new technique for soft tissue elasticity mapping. IEEE Trans Ultrason Ferroelectrics Freq Contr 51: 396–409.

14. Tanter M, Bercoff J, Sinkus R, Deffieux T, Gennisson JL, et al. (2008) Quantitative assessment of breast lesion viscoelasticity: initial clinical results using supersonic shear imaging. Ultrasound Med Biol 34: 1373–1386.

15. Nordez A, Hug F (2010) Muscle shear elastic modulus measured using supersonic shear imaging is highly related to muscle activity level. J Appl Physiol 108: 1389–1394.

16. Lacourpaille L, Hug F, Bouillard K, Hogrel JY, Nordez A (2012) Supersonic shear imaging provides a reliable measurement of resting muscle shear elastic modulus. Physiol Meas 33: 19–28.

17. Catheline S, Gennisson JL, Delon G, Fink M, Sinkus R, et al. (2004) Measuring of viscoelastic properties of homogeneous soft solid using transient elastography: an inverse problem approach. J. Acoust Soc Am 116: 3734–3741.

18. Dresner MA, Rose GH, Rossman PJ, Muthupillai R, Manduca A, et al. (2001) Magnetic resonance elastography of skeletal muscle. J Magn Reson Imaging 13: 269–276.

19. Debernard L, Robert L, Charleux F, Bensamoun SF (2011) Analysis of thigh stiffness from childhood to adulthood using magnetic resonance elastography (MRE) technique. Clin Biomech 26: 836–840.

20. McNair PJ, Dombroski EW, Hewson DJ, Stanley SN (2001) Stretching at the ankle joint: viscoelastic responses to holds and continuous passive motion. Med Sci Sports Exerc. 33: 354–358.

21. McNair PJ, Hewson DJ, Dombroski E, Stanley SN (2002) Stiffness and passive peak force changes at the ankle joint: the effect of different joint angular velocities. Clin Biomech (Bristol, Avon) 17: 536–540.

22. Nordez A, McNair PJ, Casari P, Cornu C (2008) Acute changes in hamstrings musculo-articular dissipative properties induced by cyclic and static stretching. Int J Sports Med 29: 414–418.

23. Catheline S, Wu F, Fink M. (1999) A solution to diffraction biases in sonoelasticity: the acoustic impulse technique. J Acoust Soc Am 105: 2941–2950.

24. Deffieux T, Gennisson JL, Tanter M, Fink M, Nordez A (2006) Ultrafast imaging of in vivo muscle contraction using ultrasound. Appl Phys Lett 89: 184107–184111.

25. Deffieux T, Gennisson JL, Tanter M, Fink M (2008) Assessment of the mechanical properties of the musculoskeletal system using 2-D and 3-D very high frame rate ultrasound. IEEE Trans Ultrason Ferroelectrics Freq Contr 55: 2177–2190.

26. Magnusson SP (1998) Passive properties of human skeletal muscle during stretch maneuvers. A review. Scand J Med Sci Sports 8: 65–77.

27. Gajdosik RL (2001) Passive extensibility of skeletal muscle: review of the literature with clinical implications. Clin Biomech 16: 87–101.

28. Martin A, Morlon B, Pousson M, Van Hoecke J (1996) Viscosity of the elbow flexor muscles during maximal eccentric and concentric actions. Eur J Appl Physiol 73: 157–162.

29. Valour D, Pousson M (2003) Compliance changes of the series elastic component of elbow flexor muscles with age in humans. Pflügers Arch 445: 721–727.

30. De Groote F, Van Campen A, Jonkers I, De Schutter J (2010) Sensitivity of dynamic simulations of gait and dynamometer experiments to hill muscle model parameters of knee flexors and extensors. J Biomech 43: 1876–1883.

31. Ackland DC, Lin YC, Pandy MG (2012) Sensitivity of model predictions of muscle function to changes in moment arms and muscle–tendon properties: A Monte-Carlo analysis. J Biomech 45: 1463–1471.

32. Maas H, Sandercock TG (2008) Are skeletal muscles independent actuators? Force transmission from soleus muscle in the cat. J Appl Physiol 104: 1557–1567.

33. Maas H, Baan GC, Huijing PA (2001) Intermuscular interaction via myofascial force transmission: effects of tibialis anterior and extensor hallucis longus length on force transmission from rat extensor digitorum longus muscle. J Appl Physiol 34: 927–940.

34. Tian M, Herbert RD, Hoang P, Gandevia SC, Bilston LE Myofascial force transmission between the human soleus and gastrocnemius muscles during passive knee motion. J Appl Physiol. In press.

35. Moritani T, Berry MJ, Bacharach DW, Nakamura E (1987) Gas exchange parameters, muscle blood flow and electromechanical properties of the plantar flexors. Eur J Appl Physiol 56: 30–37.

6

Increased Residual Force Enhancement in Older Adults Is Associated with a Maintenance of Eccentric Strength

Geoffrey A. Power[1]*, **Charles L. Rice**[1,2], **Anthony A. Vandervoort**[1,3]

1 Canadian Centre for Activity and Aging, School of Kinesiology, Faculty of Health Sciences, The University of Western Ontario, London, Ontario, Canada, **2** Department of Anatomy and Cell Biology, The University of Western Ontario, London, Ontario, Canada, **3** School of Physical Therapy, Faculty of Health Sciences, The University of Western Ontario, London, Ontario, Canada

Abstract

Despite an age-related loss of voluntary isometric and concentric strength, muscle strength is well maintained during lengthening muscle actions (i.e., eccentric strength) in old age. Additionally, in younger adults during lengthening of an activated skeletal muscle, the force level observed following the stretch is greater than the isometric force at the same muscle length. This feature is termed residual force enhancement (RFE) and is believed to be a combination of active and passive components of the contractile apparatus. The purpose of this study was to provide an initial assessment of RFE in older adults and utilize aging as a muscle model to explore RFE in a system in which isometric force production is compromised, but structural mechanisms of eccentric strength are well-maintained. Therefore, we hypothesised that older adults will experience greater RFE compared with young adults. Following a reference maximal voluntary isometric contraction (MVC) of the dorsiflexors in 10 young (26.1 ± 2.7y) and 10 old (76.0 ± 6.5y) men, an active stretch was performed at $15°$/s over a $30°$ ankle joint excursion ending at the same muscle length as the reference MVCs ($40°$ of plantar flexion). Any additional torque compared with the reference MVC therefore represented RFE. In older men RFE was ~2.5 times greater compared to young. The passive component of force enhancement contributed ~37% and ~20% to total force enhancement, in old and young respectively. The positive association ($R^2 = 0.57$) between maintained eccentric strength in old age and RFE indicates age-related mechanisms responsible for the maintenance of eccentric strength likely contributed to the observed elevated RFE. Additionally, as indicated by the greater passive force enhancement, these mechanisms may be related to increased muscle series elastic stiffness in old age.

Editor: Kelvin E. Jones, University of Alberta, Canada

Funding: This research is supported by funding from The Natural Sciences and Engineering Research Council of Canada (NSERC) (http://www.nserc-crsng.gc.ca/index_eng.asp). G.A. Power is supported by The Queen Elizabeth II Graduate Scholarship in Science and Technology. The funders had no role in study design, data collection and analysis, decision to publish, or preparation of the manuscript.

Competing Interests: The authors have declared that no competing interests exist.

* E-mail: gpower@uwo.ca

Introduction

Impaired force generating capacity is a consequence of natural adult aging resulting from many factors [1] including: the loss of contractile muscle mass [2,3], decreased neural activation [4,5], changes in muscle architecture [2] and excitation-contraction uncoupling [6]. Despite the age-related loss of isometric strength, during active lengthening (i.e., eccentric; ECC) of muscle, strength is well-maintained [7,8]. Muscular force is dependent highly upon contractile history, such that isometric force of activated skeletal muscles following active stretch is greater than isometric force produced at the same muscle length prior to the stretch [9,10]. This muscle property is termed residual force enhancement (RFE). Currently, it is unknown whether RFE is present in older adults and if the maintenance of ECC strength in old age contributes to RFE.

Age-related reductions in muscle contractile capacity are disparate when considered in terms of contractile mode [3]. The initial observation of Vandervoort et al. [8] reported older women had well-maintained knee extensor ECC strength compared with young [8]. This finding was later confirmed in older men [11] and other muscles [12,13]. The maintenance of ECC strength with

aging could relate to neural and mechanically mediated mechanisms. Neural factors could include: reduced agonist and increased antagonist activation during concentric actions thus reducing concentric strength, however older adults, if well practiced and accustomed with the task can fully activate their muscles, and antagonist coactivation is often not altered with aging [14,15,16,17]. Therefore, the mechanism is likely related to the non-contractile and structural properties of the muscle tissue. Thus, an increase in muscle series elastic stiffness [18,19] in older adults may yield greater passive resistance during muscle lengthening [11]. The elevated passive stiffness of muscle in old age could increase the effective 'storage' of elastic energy to optimise force production. Support of an intrinsic muscle property leading to maintained eccentric strength in older adults is the elevated tension (i.e. force) following a quick active stretch in single muscle fibers of older adults [20]. Elevated force could be related to increased force produced by individual cross-bridges during lengthening muscle actions. As well, the increased instantaneous stiffness in single muscle fibers from older adults observed by Ochala et al. [20] provides evidence of altered elastic, or structural properties of the muscle, independent of cross-bridge cycling responsible for the maintenance of ECC strength.

Residual force enhancement is evident in various muscle [10,21,22,23,24,25] and human [26,27,28,29,30] preparations with active and passive properties of muscle force generating and transmitting structures suggested to contribute to RFE (for review see [31,32,33]). Mechanisms include: an increased proportion of strongly bound cross-bridges [34], increased average force produced by each cross-bridge [26] and the engagement of passive force (PFE) transmitting elements following stretch [35,36] effectively 'stiffening' the contracting agonist thereby providing increased resistance to stretch. As well, RFE appears to be related, in part to the level of active muscle stiffness [37]. Noteworthy, the mechanisms of RFE following stretch appear to be similar to those responsible for maintenance of ECC strength in old age. Therefore, it is reasonable to propose RFE in older adults would be elevated compared with younger adults.

The purpose of this study is to utilize the aged muscle model to further explore RFE in a system in which isometric strength is compromised, but ECC strength is well-maintained. This study aims to determine whether RFE exists for the dorsiflexor muscles in older adults and to what extent as compared with young adults. We hypothesised steady-state isometric torque after active muscle stretch will be greater than the reference isometric steady state torque, in both absolute and relative terms, when compared with their younger counterparts. Thus, older adults will have greater RFE than young adults. As well, due to the age-related increase in muscle series elastic stiffness, passive force enhancement will be greater in older than younger adults following stretch.

Materials and Methods

Participants

All young (n = 10, 26.1±2.7y, 178.5±4.4 cm, 82.9±8.7 kg) and old men (n = 10, 76.0±6.5y, 174.4±5.9 cm, 82.8±10.4 kg) were asked to refrain from unaccustomed and strenuous exercise prior to testing and not to consume caffeine within 2 h prior to testing. All participants were recreationally active with no known neurological or musculoskeletal conditions. The young adults were recruited from the university population and the older adults were recruited from a local senior's fitness group which includes walking, light stretching and calisthenics 3 times per week. This study was approved by The University of Western Ontario Health Science Research Ethics Board for Research Involving Human Subjects and conformed to the Declaration of Helsinki. Informed verbal and written consent was obtained from all participants prior to testing.

Experimental arrangement

All testing was conducted on a HUMAC NORM dynamometer (CSMi Medical Solutions, Stoughton, MA). The left foot was fastened tightly to the ankle attachment footplate with inelastic straps, aligning the lateral malleolus with the rotational axis of the dynamometer. Extraneous movements were minimized using non-elastic shoulder, waist and thigh straps. Participants sat in a slightly reclined position with the hip, and knee angles set at ~110°, and ~140° (180°; straight), respectively. All voluntary and evoked isometric dorsiflexion contractions were performed at an ankle joint angle of 40° of plantar flexion (PF). The ankle angle of 40° of PF was chosen to maximize the stretch of the dorsiflexor muscles during active lengthening. Lengthening contractions began at 10° PF until 40° of PF, and thus moved through a 30° joint excursion.

Electromyography (EMG)

Electromyography signals were collected using self-adhering Ag-AgCl surface electrodes (1.5×1 cm; Kendall, Mansfield, MA).

Prior to electrode placement, the skin was cleaned with pre-soaked alcohol swabs. The electrode configuration involved the active electrode positioned over the proximal portion of the tibialis anterior at the innervation zone (7 cm distal to the tibial tuberosity and 2 cm lateral to the tibial anterior border) [38] and a reference surface electrode was placed over the distal tendinous portion of the tibialis anterior just proximal to the level of the malleoli. The surface active electrode for the soleus was positioned 2 cm distal to the lower border of the medial head of the gastrocnemius and a reference was placed over the calcaneal tendon. The ground electrode was positioned over the patella. These electrode configurations were chosen to allow for a more global recording area.

Experimental procedures

Stimulated contractions of the dorsiflexors were evoked electrically with two round carbon rubber electrodes (Empi, St. Paul, Minnesota, USA), coated in conductive gel positioned to maximize the twitch torque response, and secured with tape. The anode was positioned anterior and the cathode posterior to the fibular head over the deep branch of the common fibular nerve. A computer-triggered stimulator (model DS7AH, Digitimer, Welwyn Garden City, Hertfordshire, UK) set at 400V provided the electrical stimulation using a pulse width of 100 µs. Peak twitch torque (P_t) was determined by increasing the current until a plateau in dorsiflexor P_t and tibialis anterior compound muscle action potential (M-wave) peak to peak amplitude were reached, and then the current was further increased by at least 15% to ensure activation of all motor axons via supramaximal stimulation. This stimulation intensity was used for the evoked doublet (P_d) (two pulses at a 10 ms interpulse interval) to assess voluntary activation. Finally, a 10 and 50 Hz stimulus was delivered to assess low frequency torque depression and peak tetanic torque. For tetanic stimulation the current was increased until there was a plateau in evoked 50 Hz torque.

A 3–5s duration isometric dorsiflexor baseline MVC was performed to ensure there was sufficient time for subjects to reach peak MVC torque. During all MVCs, participants were provided visual feedback of the torque tracing on a computer monitor, and were exhorted verbally. Voluntary activation was assessed using the modified interpolated twitch technique [39]. The amplitude of the interpolated torque evoked during the peak plateau of the MVC was compared with a resting P_d evoked 1s following the MVC when the muscles were relaxed fully. Percent voluntary activation was calculated as voluntary activation (%) = [1-interpolated P_d/resting P_d] ×100%. Values from the MVC with the highest peak torque were recorded. Contractile speeds were analyzed for twitch and 50 Hz tetanus, and time to peak twitch (TPT) was determined as the time for baseline torque to reach peak twitch torque. Half relaxation time of the twitch (HRT) and 50 Hz tetanus were determined as the time from peak torque amplitude to when half of the peak torque amplitude was reached. The protocol used to determine residual force enhancement (Figure 1) involved a 10 s isometric reference MVC at 40° of PF followed by 3 min of rest. The dorsiflexors were activated maximally for 10s, consisting of a 1s isometric contraction at the shortened muscle length (10° PF), followed by a 2 s lengthening stretch at 15°/s, and ending with a 7 s isometric MVC at the same ankle angle as the 10 s reference MVC (40° PF) (Figure 1). This sequence was repeated 2 times with the greater RFE value reported. Passive force enhancement (PFE) was calculated as the difference between resting torque after stretch and resting torque after a reference MVC (Figure 1). To compare the maximal strength of young and old during differing contraction types,

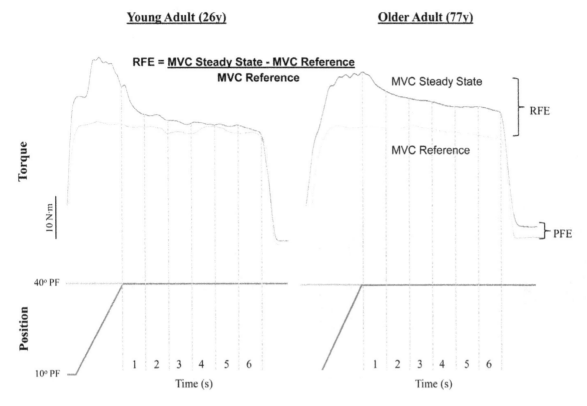

Figure 1. Raw data depicting the determination of residual force enhancement (RFE) in older and young men. Passive force enhancement (PFE) was determined as elevated force above rested baseline upon relaxation after stretch.

eccentric strength (ECC) was determined as the maximum torque amplitude during stretch. After 3 min rest, a maximal voluntary shortening dorsiflexor contraction (15°/s) was performed to determine concentric (CON) strength.

Data reduction and analysis

Torque and position data were sampled by the dynamometer at a rate of 500Hz. All data were converted to digital format using a 12-bit analog-to-digital converter (model 1401 Power, Cambridge Electronic Design, Cambridge, UK). Residual force enhancement was calculated by determining the mean torque value over 1s epochs during the last 6s of the 10s of the contractions. The values for the reference MVC, were divided into the mean torque value for each of the 6 1s epoch during the steady state MVC following the end of stretch, corresponding to the same time as the reference MVC (Figure 1). Steady state was defined as when the torque value following stretch reached a statistically significant difference from the first time epoch and force transients were no longer present. Residual force enhancement during steady state was defined as the percent increase in isometric torque following stretch, relative to the reference MVC.

Surface EMG signals were pre-amplified (×100), amplified (×2), band-pass filtered (10–1,000 Hz), and sampled online at 2500 Hz using Spike 2 software (version 7.07, Cambridge Electronic Design Ltd). The EMG signals for the tibialis anterior and soleus muscles were recorded during the dorsiflexor MVCs and expressed as a root mean square (RMS) value over each 1s epoch. Following stretch, EMG was analysed over each of the 6 1s epochs. Soleus EMG recorded during those periods was used to estimate antagonist coactivation as a soleus:tibialis anterior EMG ratio ×100%. All RMS values of EMG recorded from the tibialis anterior and soleus

muscles for both the reference and steady state 10s contractions were normalized to the tibialis anterior and soleus EMG RMS values for the baseline agonist MVC. EMG from the trial which yielded the greater RFE was used for analysis. Post-activation potentiation was determined by calculating the ratio between the amplitude of the peak twitch torque recorded before and following the baseline isometric MVC. Spike 2 software (Version 7.07) was used off line to determine torque values of all contractions.

Statistical analysis

Using SPSS software (version 16, SPSS Inc. Chicago, IL) a one way analysis of variance (ANOVA) was performed to assess baseline neuromuscular function of the young and old adults. A two way ANOVA was performed to assess RFE between young and old over time. When significance was observed a *post hoc* analysis using unpaired t-tests was performed with a Bonferroni correction factor to determine where significant differences existed in RFE over time during the steady state. Voluntary activation values were not normally distributed, and thus a Mann-Whitney U-test was employed for this particular variable. The level of significance for all tests was set at $P<0.05$. A power calculation was determined to ensure there was sufficient power $(1–\beta = 0.98–0.99)$ to detect significant differences. The tables are presented as means $\pm$ standard deviations (SD), and figure 2 as means $\pm$ standard error (SE). A Pearson correlation coefficient (r) and a linear regression analysis (R^2) were performed to evaluate the relationship and shared variance between the ratio of eccentric to concentric strength and residual force enhancement.

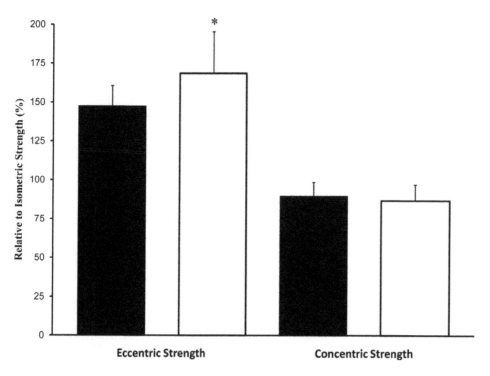

Figure 2. Eccentric and concentric strength in old (open bars) and young men (closed bars) relative to isometric strength. Values are Means ± standard error.

Results

As shown in Table 1, older adults had a 26% lower twitch torque ($P<0.05$) compared to young, but both groups had similar evoked 10 Hz and 50 Hz torques ($P>0.05$). Contractile speeds for Pt and 50 Hz were 20–30% slower in the older adults compared with young. As well, the older adults had a 10% reduced capacity for potentiation compared to the young ($P<0.05$). During voluntary efforts, the old men were 13% weaker for isometric MVC torque ($P<0.05$) compared with the young men despite similar and equal high voluntary activations (~98%, $P>0.05$) and similar levels of muscle co-activation ($P>0.05$) in both groups. Furthermore, concentric strength was 16% lower in older adults ($P<0.05$) compared to young. However, eccentric strength was well-maintained in the older men relative to isometric and concentric strength ($P<0.05$) and was not different to that reported for young ($P>0.05$) (Figure 2; Figure 3).

Residual force enhancement

Peak eccentric torque values during active stretch were 70% and 50% greater than torque values reached during baseline isometric contractions in old and young ($P<0.05$), respectively (Table 2). Torque values were consistently higher in the steady state (isometric) phase following stretch for both old and young compared to the reference isometric MVC (Table 3; $P<0.05$). The steady state mean RFE for young and old was 8.4±5.0 and 21.7±13.5, respectively. Root mean square amplitudes of EMG for the tibialis anterior and co-activation of the soleus were similar for the isometric reference MVC and the steady state isometric phase following stretch in both old and young ($P>0.05$). Residual force enhancement was ~2.5 times greater in the older adults compared to young ($P<0.05$) during the steady state isometric phase following stretch (Table 3). Both old and young adults experienced the typical exponential decay of torque to steady state following stretch (Figure 1); however the old

had a longer time to steady state torque (2s) compared to young (1 s) ($P<0.05$). Passive force enhancement (PFE) (Table 2) was greater in older adults and contributed 37% and 20% to total RFE in old and young, respectively.

Regression analysis

There was a positive association ($r=0.75$, $P<0.05$) between the ratio of eccentric to concentric strength compared with RFE with a significant linear regression [RFE (%) $=0.286\times$ Ecc:Con strength -36.78, $R^2=0.57$, $P<0.05$] (Figure 3A). Furthermore, there was a similar association ($r=0.71$, $P<0.05$) between the ratio of eccentric to concentric strength compared with PFE with a significant linear regression [PFE (Nm) $=0.034\times$ Ecc:Con strength -4.48, $R^2=0.51$, $P<0.05$] (Figure 3B). Additionally, there was another positive association ($r=0.84$, $P<0.05$) between PFE and RFE with a significant linear regression [RFE (%) $=6.68\times$ PFE (Nm) $+4.19$, $R^2=0.70$, $P<0.05$] (Figure 3C). These relationships suggest that the muscle stiffness of older men leading to the maintenance of ECC strength in old age is paramount in explaining the elevated RFE in older compared to young adults.

Discussion

We investigated the effects of natural adult aging on residual force enhancement (RFE) in a cross-sectional comparison of young and older men. Older men were weaker and slower for electrically evoked twitch properties, had blunted potentiation capacity and were weaker for isometric and concentric strength compared to young. However, despite impairments in these neuromuscular measures, eccentric strength was well-maintained in older adults and not different from the young. Residual force enhancement was calculated as the increase in torque during the isometric steady state following stretch compared to a reference MVC performed prior to stretch. In line with our hypothesis, older men had on

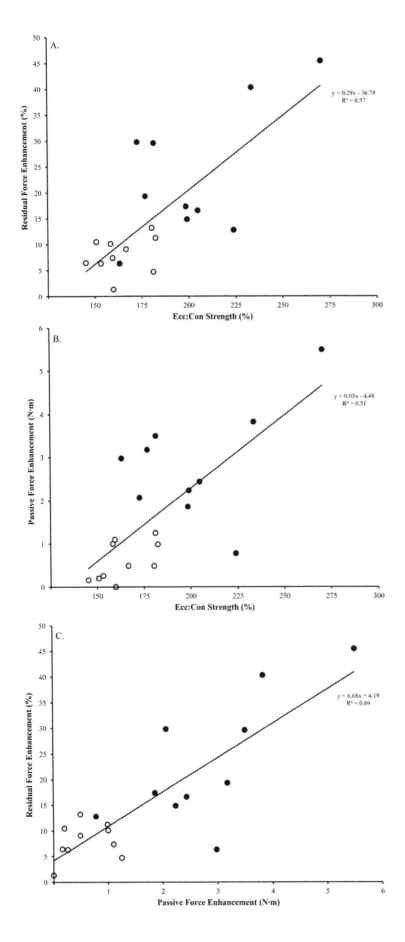

Figure 3. Relationship between the ratio of eccentric strength to concentric strength (Ecc:Con) and residual force enhancement (RFE) for old (closed circle) and young (open circle) (A.). Relationship between the ratio of eccentric strength to concentric strength (Ecc:Con) and passive force enhancement (PFE) for old (closed circle) and young (open circle) (B.). Relationship between the passive force enhancement (PFE) residual force enhancement (RFE) for old (closed circle) and young (open circle) (C.).

average ~2.5 times greater RFE during the isometric steady state following stretch compared to their younger counterparts, and passive force enhancement (PFE) contributed ~37% and ~20% to RFE for old and young, respectively. The impetus behind elevated RFE in older men appears to be related partly to the mechanisms responsible for the age-related maintenance of eccentric strength (Figure 3 A, B).

Comparison with previous investigations of RFE in humans

Residual force enhancement was present in all young and older participants (Table 3). Force enhancement in the young (7–11%) was similar to values reported previously for voluntary contractions of the adductor pollicis 14% [26], plantar flexors 7–13% [27], and dorsiflexors 6–19% [27,28,30]. The present study is the first reported to investigate RFE in older adults and we found values ranging from 7–30%, with a mean of ~25%. This level of RFE is considerably more than that reported for investigations on younger adults, with the exception of one study following exercise induced muscle damage in which RFE was elevated 150% above baseline values [30]. In older men, PFE contributed ~17% more to RFE compared with young (Table 2), and thus PFE appears to be a key component of the overall increase in force production observed following active stretch, particularly in older adults (Figure 3C). After stretch, old and young followed the typical exponential decline in torque [32], but more time was required for the older men to reach a steady state torque level compared to young (Table 3). This longer time to steady state and elevated PFE indicates structural elastic mechanisms may have a disproportionately greater contribution to force enhancement in old age. Residual force enhancement in the present study is likely more related to mechanical factors compared to neural influences. Central activation (agonist; RMS EMG) levels were similar for the reference isometric MVC and steady-state MVC following stretch and differed minimally between young and older men. As well, antagonist coactivation was not significantly different between young and old, which is similar to previous findings for dorsiflexion contractions (14). Additionally, voluntary activation as assessed using the interpolated twitch technique [39] was near maximal and was similar for young and old. Thus, any confounding influence of age-related reductions in neuromuscular

activation was avoided in the determination of RFE and the enhancement in older men likely can be attributed to age-related alterations within the muscle's structure.

For the determination of RFE, active stretch was initiated at $10°$ plantar flexion, which falls presumably on the ascending limb of the whole muscle force-length relationship for the dorsiflexors [40]. Stretch then continued to $40°$ of plantar flexion and at this muscle length most of the active sarcomeres would be operating near the plateau region of their length-tension relationship [40]. Residual force enhancement can be observed during stretch over the ascending limb of the force-length relationship [36], whereas PFE appears to be more dependent on activation over the descending limb in isolated preparations [36,41] and humans [29]. Therefore, based upon the greater amount of PFE in old compared to young the force-length relationship may be different between young and older men. Passive force enhancement following muscle stretch after relaxation was present (Table 2) in every older participant (1.9–5.5 Nm) whereas the young participants displayed minimal passive force enhancement (0–1.3 Nm) upon relaxation. Because PFE is highly dependent upon stretch amplitude, the tibialis anterior of older men may lie further along the sarcomere length-tension curve. Thus, muscle of older men likely experienced greater stretch amplitude, which contributed to the greater RFE. However, this suggestion needs further investigation.

Age-related maintenance of eccentric strength and elevated residual force enhancement

Mechanisms responsible for the age-related reduction in isometric strength, other than neural factors, can be attributed to intrinsic changes at the cellular and whole muscle level. Reduced force production of single muscle fibers with adult aging is likely related to the decrease in the number of viable cross-bridges and amount of force generated by each cross-bridge [42]. As well, excitation-contraction uncoupling contributes to impairments in force production [6] through failure to activate intact force generators. Following muscle stretch (i.e., isometric steady state) age-related decrements in cross-bridge function may be modified temporarily to improve isometric force generation which would contribute to elevated RFE compared to the young. With active stretch, there is potential for greater availability of actomyosin binding sites, allowing for the recruitment of weakly

Table 1. Electrically evoked neuromuscular properties of the dorsiflexors.

Neuromuscular Properties of the Dorsiflexors

Group (n = 10)	P_t (N·m)	TPT (ms)	HRT (ms)	Twitch Potentiation	10Hz (N·m)	50Hz (N·m)	50Hz$_{HRT}$ (ms)	10:50Hz (%)
		Electrically Evoked Isometric Properties						
Young	5.3±1.2	110.7±15.7	109.5±22.7	119.8±15.6	14.8±3.1	21.5±5.1	138.2±26.7	0.69±0.11
Old	3.9±1.2*	133.3±9.1*	146.0±23.9*	108.1±12.5*	14.5±3.2	20.0±5.3	173.2±19.0*	0.73±0.11

Old men had lower absolute evoked peak twitch torque (P_t), twitch potentiation (%), time to peak twitch (TPT), half-relaxation time (HRT) and 50Hz$_{HRT}$ compared with young men. The 10Hz peak torque, 50Hz peak torque and 10:50Hz ratio were not different between age groups. Values are means ± standard deviation. * Denotes significant age difference.

Table 2. Voluntary evoked neuromuscular properties of the dorsiflexors.

Neuromuscular Properties of the Dorsiflexors

Group (n = 10)	Voluntary Activation (%)	Voluntary Contractile Properties					MVC	
		Isometric Strength (N·m)	Concentric Strength (N·m)	Eccentric Strength (N·m)	Ecc:Iso (%)	Ecc:Con (%)	Co- Act (%)	PFE (N·m)
Young	99.6±1.3	33.2±6.4	29.9±4.7	48.5±7.3	147.8±12.9	162.9±13.1	22.6±6.5	0.59±0.45
Old	97.9±2.1	28.8±3.7*	25.0±4.6*	48.2±6.4	168.6±26.9*	199.2±32.8*	20.2±4.5	2.84±1.29*

Old men had lower maximal voluntary isometric contraction (MVC) strength and concentric strength. Voluntary activation and antagonist coactivation (MVC Co-act) was not significantly different between groups. Eccentric strength was well maintained in old men relative to young and other contraction modes (ratio of eccentric to isometric strength; Ecc:Iso, ratio of eccentric to concentric strength; Ecc:Con). Passive force enhancement (PFE) was greater in old than young. Values are means ± standard deviation. * Denotes significant age difference.

bound cross-bridges into a strongly bound cross-bridge state [20]. Therefore, the age-related decline in cross-bridge function could have been modified by stretch to increase the average force per cross bridge [43] contributing to RFE. Additionally, increased series elastic stiffness of the muscles of older adults, suggested to be an intrinsic muscle property leading to maintained eccentric strength in older adults [20], could also contribute to increased RFE in older men. Following a quick stretch the elevated tension (i.e. force) of fibers from older men may be related to increased force produced by individual cross-bridges during lengthening muscle actions [20], thereby increasing steady state force following stretch relative to reference MVC.

At the whole muscle level, age-related changes in muscle architecture contribute to force loss owing to shorter fascicle lengths and a less pennate fascicle organization, as well as increased tendon compliance (i.e. less stiff) [2,44]. These changes in muscle architecture have functional implications on the overall musculotendinous unit. For example, during isometric contractions the greater tendon compliance in older men causes sarcomeres to shorten more compared to young, thus impairing their working length and force production by creating a state of less optimal myofilament overlap [45]. Hence, during isometric contractions the force generators work over a less optimal operational sarcomere length-tension range, impairing force production. Therefore, during the MVC steady state phase following stretch, the muscle from an older adult would potentially benefit from "taking up the slack" of the musculotendinous unit to optimize sarcomeric force production and effectively stiffening the

series elastic complex for greater force transmission attenuating some of the age-related reduction in isometric force production. Furthermore, increased joint stiffness in old age [46,47] and increased series elastic stiffness [18,19] may have provided higher passive resistance during muscle lengthening [11] to optimise force production during the isometric steady state following stretch. Therefore, the engagement of passive series elastic structures in the muscle of older adults could contribute to greater overall force production as evident by the increased PFE in older compared to younger adults.

It seems in the present study that the passive component of force enhancement (i.e., PFE) contributed greatly to elevated force enhancement in older adults. Therefore, it appears that a system with compromised isometric force production such as natural aging, may share some similarities to lengthening-induced muscle damage model [30] in which the contribution of PFE to overall total force enhancement is markedly increased. The increased instantaneous stiffness following stretch in old muscle fibers observed by Ochala et al. [20] which contributes to the age-related maintenance of eccentric strength, contributes to elevated RFE in older adults. These findings support the role of an elastic structural mechanism of the muscle cell, independent of cross-bridge cycling contributing to RFE. Force enhancement following stretch has been attributed to the involvement of a passive structural element [25,48] such as titin whose stiffness is increased by Ca^{2+} influx during force development in active muscle [24,25]. In light of this, the greater PFE in older adults could be related to a potential age-related modification to titin, but this remains to be explored.

Table 3. Residual force enhancement (RFE).

Time Following Stretch (s)	Absolute Residual Force Enhancement (N·m)		Relative Residual Force Enhancement (%)	
	Young	Old	Young	Old
1	5.0±1.4	9.5±3.7*	17.1±4.4	37.8±15.6*
2	3.2±1.1†	7.7±3.6*	11.2±4.6†	30.9±15.4*
3	2.8±1.2†	5.7±3.2*†	8.6±5.3†	22.7±13.1*†
4	2.3±0.9†	5.2±3.3*†	7.1±4.7†	20.9±14.3*†
5	1.7±0.9†	5.1±2.9*†	6.4±4.9†	20.7±12.8*†
6	1.9±1.2†	5.3±3.2*†	6.9±3.9†	22.4±14.0*†

Old men reached a steady state torque profile later than young men succeeding stretch and benefited from greater force enhancement in absolute and relative terms. Values are means ± standard deviation. * Denotes significant age difference. † Denotes steady state torque level.

To explore possible mechanisms of residual force enhancement we utilized a model of natural human aging, in which age-related changes to the neuromuscular system yield impaired isometric strength while strength during lengthening actions is well maintained. Residual force enhancement is regarded as a fundamental property of muscle unaccounted for by the current swinging cross-bridge and sliding filament theory of muscle contraction. In the aged system, following stretch, RFE was elevated compared to young, possibly owing to increased cross-bridge function and the engagement of passive elements following stretch. Although the exact mechanisms cannot be elucidated at this time, stretch appeared to attenuate detrimental effects of aging on subsequent torque production and provided a mechanical strategy for enhanced muscle function over isometric actions.

Acknowledgments

We would like to thank all those who participated in the study.

Author Contributions

Conceived and designed the experiments: GAP CLR AAV. Performed the experiments: GAP CLR AAV. Analyzed the data: GAP CLR AAV. Contributed reagents/materials/analysis tools: GAP CLR AAV. Wrote the paper: GAP CLR AAV.

References

1. Russ DW, Gregg-Cornell K, Conaway MJ, Clark BC (2012) Evolving concepts on the age-related changes in "muscle quality". J Cachexia Sarcopenia Muscle 3: 95–109.
2. Narici MV, Maffulli N (2010) Sarcopenia: characteristics, mechanisms and functional significance. Br Med Bull 95: 139–159.
3. Vandervoort AA (2002) Aging of the human neuromuscular system. Muscle Nerve 25: 17–25.
4. Aagaard P, Suetta C, Caserotti P, Magnusson SP, Kjaer M (2010) Role of the nervous system in sarcopenia and muscle atrophy with aging: strength training as a countermeasure. Scand J Med Sci Sports 20: 49–64.
5. Roos MR, Rice CL, Vandervoort AA (1997) Age-related changes in motor unit function. Muscle Nerve 20: 679–690.
6. Payne AM, Delbono O (2004) Neurogenesis of excitation-contraction uncoupling in aging skeletal muscle. Exerc Sport Sci Rev 32: 36–40.
7. Roig M, Macintyre DL, Eng JJ, Narici MV, Maganaris CN, et al. (2010) Preservation of eccentric strength in older adults: Evidence, mechanisms and implications for training and rehabilitation. Exp Gerontol 45: 400–409.
8. Vandervoort AA, Kramer JF, Wharram ER (1990) Eccentric knee strength of elderly females. J Gerontol 45: B125–128.
9. Abbott BC, Aubert XM (1952) The force exerted by active striated muscle during and after change of length. J Physiol 117: 77–86.
10. Rassier DE, Herzog W, Wakeling J, Syme DA (2003) Stretch-induced, steady-state force enhancement in single skeletal muscle fibers exceeds the isometric force at optimum fiber length. J Biomech 36: 1309–1316.
11. Hortobagyi T, Zheng D, Weidner M, Lambert NJ, Westbrook S, et al. (1995) The influence of aging on muscle strength and muscle fiber characteristics with special reference to eccentric strength. J Gerontol A Biol Sci Med Sci 50: B399–406.
12. Porter MM, Vandervoort AA, Kramer JF (1997) Eccentric peak torque of the plantar and dorsiflexors is maintained in older women. J Gerontol A Biol Sci Med Sci 52: B125–131.
13. Poulin MJ, Vandervoort AA, Paterson DH, Kramer JF, Cunningham DA (1992) Eccentric and concentric torques of knee and elbow extension in young and older men. Can J Sport Sci 17: 3–7.
14. Jakobi JM, Rice CL (2002) Voluntary muscle activation varies with age and muscle group. J Appl Physiol 93: 457–462.
15. Klass M, Baudry S, Duchateau J (2005) Aging does not affect voluntary activation of the ankle dorsiflexors during isometric, concentric, and eccentric contractions. J Appl Physiol 99: 31–38.
16. Roos MR, Rice CL, Connelly DM, Vandervoort AA (1999) Quadriceps muscle strength, contractile properties, and motor unit firing rates in young and old men. Muscle Nerve 22: 1094–1103.
17. Power GA, Dalton BH, Rice CL, Vandervoort AA (2011) Power loss is greater following lengthening contractions in old versus young women. Age (Dordr). 2012 Jun; 34(3): 737-50. Available: http://www.ncbi.nlm.nih.gov/pubmed/21559865.
18. Ochala J, Frontera WR, Dorer DJ, Van Hoecke J, Krivickas LS (2007) Single skeletal muscle fiber elastic and contractile characteristics in young and older men. J Gerontol A Biol Sci Med Sci 62: 375–381.
19. Hasson CJ, Miller RH, Caldwell GE (2011) Contractile and elastic ankle joint muscular properties in young and older adults. PLoS One 6: e15953.
20. Ochala J, Dorer DJ, Frontera WR, Krivickas LS (2006) Single skeletal muscle fiber behavior after a quick stretch in young and older men: a possible explanation of the relative preservation of eccentric force in old age. Pflugers Arch 452: 464–470.
21. Julian FJ, Morgan DL (1979) The effect on tension of non-uniform distribution of length changes applied to frog muscle fibres. J Physiol 293: 379–392.
22. Telley IA, Stehle R, Ranatunga KW, Pfitzer G, Stussi E, et al. (2006) Dynamic behaviour of half-sarcomeres during and after stretch in activated rabbit psoas myofibrils: sarcomere asymmetry but no 'sarcomere popping'. J Physiol 573: 173–185.
23. Rassier DE, Pavlov I (2012) Force produced by isolated sarcomeres and half-sarcomeres after an imposed stretch. Am J Physiol Cell Physiol 302: C240–248.
24. Joumaa V, Leonard TR, Herzog W (2008) Residual force enhancement in myofibrils and sarcomeres. Proc Biol Sci 275: 1411–1419.
25. Leonard TR, DuVall M, Herzog W (2010) Force enhancement following stretch in a single sarcomere. Am J Physiol Cell Physiol 299: C1398–1401.
26. Lee HD, Herzog W (2002) Force enhancement following muscle stretch of electrically stimulated and voluntarily activated human adductor pollicis. J Physiol 545: 321–330.
27. Pinniger GJ, Cresswell AG (2007) Residual force enhancement after lengthening is present during submaximal plantar flexion and dorsiflexion actions in humans. Journal of applied physiology 102: 18–25.
28. Tilp M, Steib S, Herzog W (2009) Force-time history effects in voluntary contractions of human tibialis anterior. Eur J Appl Physiol 106: 159–166.
29. Shim J, Garner B (2012) Residual force enhancement during voluntary contractions of knee extensors and flexors at short and long muscle lengths. J Biomech 45: 913–918.
30. Power GA, Rice CL, Vandervoort AA (2012) Residual force enhancement following eccentric induced muscle damage. J Biomech 45: 1835–1841.
31. Campbell SG, Campbell KS (2011) Mechanisms Of Residual Force Enhancement In Skeletal Muscle: Insights From Experiments And Mathematical Models. Biophys Rev 3: 199–207.
32. Edman KA (2012) Residual force enhancement after stretch in striated muscle. A consequence of increased myofilament overlap? J Physiol 590: 1339–1345.
33. Rassier DE (2012) The mechanisms of the residual force enhancement after stretch of skeletal muscle: non-uniformity in half-sarcomeres and stiffness of titin. Proc Biol Sci 279: 2705–2713.
34. Rassier DE, Herzog W (2004) Considerations on the history dependence of muscle contraction. Journal of applied physiology 96: 419–427.
35. Edman KA, Elzinga G, Noble MI (1982) Residual force enhancement after stretch of contracting frog single muscle fibers. J Gen Physiol 80: 769–784.
36. Herzog W, Leonard TR (2002) Force enhancement following stretching of skeletal muscle: a new mechanism. J Exp Biol 205: 1275–1283.
37. Rassier DE, Herzog W (2005) Relationship between force and stiffness in muscle fibers after stretch. J Appl Physiol 99: 1769–1775.
38. Botter A, Oprandi G, Lanfranco F, Allasia S, Maffiuletti NA, et al. (2011) Atlas of the muscle motor points for the lower limb: implications for electrical stimulation procedures and electrode positioning. Eur J Appl Physiol 111: 2461–2471.
39. Gandevia SC (2001) Spinal and supraspinal factors in human muscle fatigue. Physiol Rev 81: 1725–1789.
40. Maganaris CN (2001) Force-length characteristics of in vivo human skeletal muscle. Acta Physiol Scand 172: 279–285.
41. Herzog W, Leonard TR (2005) The role of passive structures in force enhancement of skeletal muscles following active stretch. J Biomech 38: 409–415.
42. D'Antona G, Pellegrino MA, Adami R, Rossi R, Carlizzi CN, et al. (2003) The effect of ageing and immobilization on structure and function of human skeletal muscle fibres. J Physiol 552: 499–511.
43. Mehta A, Herzog W (2008) Cross-bridge induced force enhancement? J Biomech 41: 1611–1615.
44. Narici MV, Maganaris CN, Reeves ND, Capodaglio P (2003) Effect of aging on human muscle architecture. J Appl Physiol 95: 2229–2234.
45. Narici MV, Maffulli N, Maganaris CN (2008) Ageing of human muscles and tendons. Disabil Rehabil 30: 1548–1554.
46. Vandervoort AA, Chesworth BM, Cunningham DA, Paterson DH, Rechnitzer PA, et al. (1992) Age and sex effects on mobility of the human ankle. J Gerontol 47: M17–21.
47. Winegard KJ, Hicks AL, Sale DG, Vandervoort AA (1996) A 12-year follow-up study of ankle muscle function in older adults. J Gerontol A Biol Sci Med Sci 51: B202–207.
48. Herzog W, Duvall M, Leonard TR (2012) Molecular mechanisms of muscle force regulation: a role for titin? Exerc Sport Sci Rev 40: 50–57.

7

Dystrophin Deficiency Compromises Force Production of the Extensor Carpi Ulnaris Muscle in the Canine Model of Duchenne Muscular Dystrophy

Hsiao T. Yang[1,⑨], Jin-Hong Shin[2,⑨,¤], Chady H. Hakim[2], Xiufang Pan[2], Ronald L. Terjung[1], Dongsheng Duan[2]*

1 Department of Biomedical Sciences, College of Veterinary Medicine, The University of Missouri, Columbia, Missouri, United States of America, 2 Department of Molecular Microbiology and Immunology, School of Medicine, The University of Missouri, Columbia, Missouri, United States of America

Abstract

Loss of muscle force is a salient feature of Duchenne muscular dystrophy (DMD), a fatal disease caused by dystrophin deficiency. Assessment of force production from a single intact muscle has been considered as the gold standard for studying physiological consequences in murine models of DMD. Unfortunately, equivalent assays have not been established in dystrophic dogs. To fill the gap, we developed a novel *in situ* protocol to measure force generated by the extensor carpi ulnaris (ECU) muscle of a dog. We also determined the muscle length to fiber length ratio and the pennation angle of the ECU muscle. Muscle pathology and contractility were compared between normal and affected dogs. Absence of dystrophin resulted in marked histological damage in the ECU muscle of affected dogs. Central nucleation was significantly increased and myofiber size distribution was altered in the dystrophic ECU muscle. Muscle weight and physiological cross sectional area (PCSA) showed a trend of reduction in affected dogs although the difference did not reach statistical significance. Force measurement revealed a significant decrease of absolute force, and the PCSA or muscle weight normalized specific forces. To further characterize the physiological defect in affected dog muscle, we conducted eccentric contraction. Dystrophin-null dogs showed a significantly greater force loss following eccentric contraction damage. To our knowledge, this is the first convincing demonstration of force deficit in a single intact muscle in the canine DMD model. The method described here will be of great value to study physiological outcomes following innovative gene and/or cell therapies.

Editor: James M. Ervasti, University of Minnesota, United States of America

Funding: This work was supported by grants from the National Institutes of Health AR-49419, Jesse's Journey-The Foundation for Gene and Cell Therapy, and the Muscular Dystrophy Association (DD). The funders had no role in study design, data collection and analysis, decision to publish, or preparation of the manuscript.

Competing Interests: The authors have declared that no competing interests exist.

* E-mail: duand@missouri.edu

¤ Current address: Pusan National University Yangsan Hospital, Yangsan, Republic of Korea

⑨ These authors contributed equally to this work.

Introduction

The absence of dystrophin leads to Duchenne muscular dystrophy (DMD), an incurable lethal muscle disease that affects approximately 1 to 3 boys per every 10,000 male births [1,2,3]. The dystrophin gene was discovered in 1987 by Kunkel and colleagues [4,5]. It was soon determined that dystrophin scaffolds a series of cytosolic and trans-membrane proteins into the dystrophin-associated glycoprotein complex (DGC). A major cellular function of the DGC is to crosslink the cytoskeleton with the extra cellular matrix and protects the sarcolemma from mechanical injuries generated during muscle contraction.

With the knowledge of the dystrophin gene, two naturally occurring dystrophin-null animals were soon identified. These are mdx mice and golden retriever muscular dystrophy (GRMD) dogs [6,7,8,9]. Dystrophin expression is abolished in these animals due to point mutations in the dystrophin gene. Both mdx mice and GRMD dogs show characteristic muscle pathology including degeneration/regeneration, necrosis, fibrosis and inflammation. Interestingly, young adult mdx mice appear quite healthy and they

manifest minimal dystrophic symptoms. In striking contrast, young adult dogs are clinically crippled and display apparent muscle wasting and loss of mobility.

The phenotypic resemblance between dystrophic dogs and human patients suggests that dystrophin-null dogs may serve as a more relevant preclinical model [10,11,12,13,14]. Further, the body size similarity between dogs and affected children may offer additional advantages in translation. Unfortunately, few studies have been performed in the canine model [14]. A factor that has limited the use of the dog model is the lack of robust outcome measurements. In particular, no assay has been established to allow reliable determination of force changes in a single intact muscle in dystrophic dogs. Studying effect in a single intact muscle represents a logical approach at the early stage of new therapy development. As a matter of fact, the proof-of-principle for essentially every ongoing genetic therapy was originally demonstrated in a single intact muscle in mdx mice. Some of these examples include adeno-associated virus (AAV) mediated micro/mini-dystrophin gene replacement therapy and anti-sense oligonucleotides mediated exon skipping. Corroboration of promising murine results in the dog model has now become a rate-limiting factor in the development of novel DMD therapies. So far, the contractile profile of dystrophic dogs has only been studied using whole hind limb preparation which measures force generated from a group of muscles rather than a single discrete muscle [15]. Attempts to delineate contraction deficiency in a single intact muscle in dystrophic dogs have not been very successful [16]. Kornegay and colleagues measured force in the peroneus longus muscle of GRMD dogs. Characteristic dystrophic muscle pathology was observed. However, the authors did not detect a significant difference in muscle weight normalized forces between normal and affected dogs, nor was a cardinal feature of muscle deficit, susceptibility to eccentric contraction examined [16].

To meet the need of preclinical translational studies, here we explored whether a robust and sensitive physiology assay can be developed to faithfully study contraction defects in a single intact muscle in dystrophic dogs. *In vitro* force measurement in the extensor digitorum longus (EDL) muscle and *in situ* force assay in the tibialis anterior (TA) muscle are two most frequently used methods in murine studies [17]. Considering the size of the muscle (a large muscle cannot be fully oxygenated *in vitro*) and the accessibility for therapeutic agent delivery (e.g. gene or cell transfer), we decided to focus on the extensor carpi ulnaris (ECU) muscle and an *in situ* force measurement approach. We examined dystrophin expression, histopathology, tetanic muscle force, fatigue and eccentric contraction profiles in seven normal and seven affected dogs. Characteristic pathological lesions were observed in dystrophin-deficient ECU muscles. Compared to that of wild type controls, dystrophic dogs showed a significant reduction in both absolute and specific tetanic forces. During isometric contractions there was no difference in the fatigue profile between two groups. Importantly, however, affected dogs showed a much larger force decline upon repeated cycles of eccentric contraction challenge.

Materials and Methods

Animals

All animal experiments were approved by the Animal Care and Use Committee of the University of Missouri (# 6739) and were performed in accordance with NIH guidelines. Experimental dogs were produced at the University of Missouri by artificial insemination. These dogs were on a mixed genetic background of golden retriever, labrador retriever, welsh corgi and beagle. Affected dogs were initially diagnosed by elevated creatine kinase levels and PCR genotyping using our published protocols [18,19]. The diagnosis was further confirmed by dystrophin immunofluorescence staining (see below) (Figure 1). Age and body weight of experimental dogs are shown in Table 1.

Morphology Studies

General muscle histopathology was revealed with haematoxylin and eosin (HE) staining. Muscle fibrosis was evaluated by immunofluorescence staining with the wheat germ agglutinin (WGA)-Oregon Green conjugate (Molecular Probes, W6748; 5 µg/mL PBS). Fibrotic tissues stain in green color. Dystrophin was examined by immunofluorescence staining with a monoclonal antibody against the dystrophin C-terminal domain (Dys-2, 1:30 dilution, Novocastra, Newcastle, UK). Immunofluorescence staining was performed according to our previously published protocol [20,21]. The percentage of centrally nucleated myofibers were quantified in HE stained muscle cross-sections as we described before [18]. The cross-sectional area of individual myofiber was determined from the digitized images using the quantitative image

analysis module of the extended version of the Photoshop CS5.5 software (Photoshop version CS5.5 extended, Adobe Systems Incorporated, San Jose, CA). Photomicrographs were taken with a Qimage Retiga 1300 camera using a Nikon E800 fluorescence microscope.

Muscle Function Evaluation

Surgical preparation. The experimental subject was sedated with ketamine (15 mg/kg body weight) and acepromazine (0.12 mg/kg body weight). Anesthesia was induced with 4% isoflurane. The subject was then intubated with an endotracheal tube connected to a mechanical ventilator (Ohmeda 7000, Ohmeda, Madison, WI). The breath rate was set at 15–18 per min and the tidal volume was set at 10 ml/min/kg body weight. During the experiment, anesthesia was maintained with 2% isoflurane and 98% oxygen.

Body hair in the surgical area was shaved. The right carotid artery and jugular vein were surgically exposed. A catheter was inserted into the carotid artery and advanced to the thoracic aorta for blood pressure monitoring. Another catheter was inserted into the jugular vein for intravenously lactated saline infusion. Core body temperature (rectal temperature), blood pressure and electrocardiograph (including the heart rate) were monitored throughout the experiment.

The dog was placed in a supine position on a force transducer plate that was specially designed for *in situ* muscle function assay. A 3 cm incision was made at the medial side of the upper forelimb. The brachial artery was exposed and a 3P transonic flow probe was put around the brachial artery for blood flow measurement (Module TS 420, Transonic Systems, Ithaca, NY). Another incision was made on the lateral side of the forearm to expose the entire ECU muscle. The length of the entire ECU preparation (muscle plus tendon) was measured as the distance from the proximal tendon insertion at the medial epicondyle of the humerus to the distal tendon insertion at the carpus. The length of the tendons (proximal and distal) accounts for 16% of the length of a complete ECU preparation (muscle plus tendon) (Yang, Shin, Terjung and Duan, unpublished observation). The length of the experimental ECU muscle was calculated by subtracting the tendon length (16% of the total length) from the total measured length (Table 1). The distal ECU tendon was cut at the insertion on the carpus. The free end of the distal tendon of ECU muscle was then sewn on a metal washer (5/16 size) with #2 surgical silk. The washer was tightly held by two metal blocks each with a U shaped groove in the middle to let the muscle tendon pass through. The metal block was fastened with two screws onto the force transducer (SM-250–38, Interface, Scottsdale, AZ). The forearm was subsequently fixed with two bone pins to allow the ECU muscle in line with the muscle force transducer. One stainless steel bone pin was placed on the olecranon and the other was placed on the radius about 3 cm away from its distal end. The radial nerve was located at the lateral side of the distal humerus bone. To expose the radial nerve for electric stimulation, the forearm incision was slightly extended proximately until the nerve was clearly visible. The radial nerve was carefully dissected and tied. The nerve was then cut and its distal end was mounted on a bipolar electrode for triggering muscle contraction. Radial nerve stimulation resulted in contraction of the whole extensor muscle groups. However, since the force transducer was only connected to the ECU muscle tendon, only the force produced by the ECU muscle was recorded. It should be pointed out that since the forelimb was tightly held by two strong bone pins (one on the olecranon and the other on the radius), radial nerve stimulation did not cause any movement of the forelimb except for foot kicking

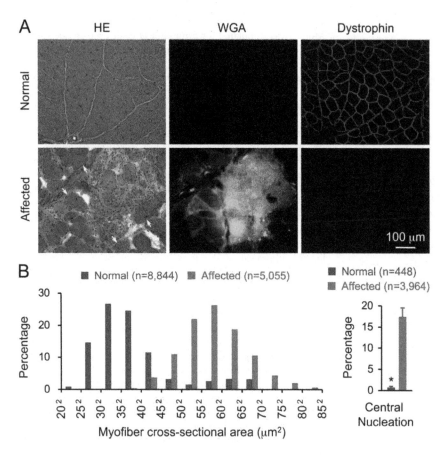

Figure 1. Dystrophin deficiency leads to severe muscle damage in the extensor carpi ulnaris muscle in affected dogs. A, Haematoxylin and eosin (HE) staining (left panel), wheat germ agglutinin (WGA) staining (middle panel) and dystrophin immunofluoresence staining (right panel) of the extensor carpi ulnaris muscle from a normal dog (top panel) and an affected dog (bottom panel). WGA staining reveals tissue fibrosis. Arrow, regenerative myofibers with centrally located nuclei. **B,** Morphometric quantification of the myofiber size (left panel) and central nucleation in normal and affected ECU muscles. The myofiber size is expressed according to the distribution of the cross-sectional area of individual myofibers. Results for the normal ECU muscle was from 8,844 myofibers of five normal dogs. Results for the dystrophic ECU muscle was from 5,055 myofibers of four affected dogs. The central nucleation is expressed as the percentage of myofiber with centrally localized nuclei among all myofibers counted. Results for the normal ECU muscle was from 9,467 myofibers of five normal dogs. Results for the dystrophic ECU muscle was from 3,964 myofibers of four affected dogs. Asterisk, significantly different (p = 0.0001).

due to extensor muscle contraction. To determine whether foot kicking affected tension measurement, we compared the results with or without foot fixation. We did not see any difference in the recorded tension. The exposed ECU muscle and tendon were moistened with warm (37°C) saline gauze. The temperature of the ECU muscle surface was maintained at 37°C with a surgical lamp. After the preparation was done, the subject was allowed to stabilize for 10 minutes before force measurement. In some subjects, the same experiment was conducted on both sides of the forelimb. At the end of study, the subject was euthanized and necropsied.

Force measurements. For all experiments, electric stimulation was set at 8 volts and 0.2 ms pulse duration (Grass S48 Stimulator, Grass Instruments, Quincy, MA). Muscle force, brachial arterial blood flow and aorta blood pressure were recorded with Powerlab (AD Instruments, Castle Hill, Australia) interfaced with a Mac power PC computer. The optimal muscle length was determined using single twitch stimulation. Briefly, twitch stimulation was applied while the muscle was hold at different lengths. The muscle length which yielded the highest twitch force was defined as the optimal muscle length (Lo). At the optimal muscle length, the force-frequency relationship was

determined by applying 200 ms tetanic stimulation at various stimulation frequencies (Figure 2A). The frequency that yielded the highest force (usually 90 to 100 Hz) was defined as the optimal stimulation frequency. The optimal muscle length (Lo) and optimal stimulation frequency were used in all subsequent force measurements. The peak tetanic force was determined as the highest force produced during 100 to 200 ms tetanic stimulation (Table 1).

Determination of the fiber length (Lf) to optimal muscle length ratio (Lf/Lo) in the ECU muscle. The freshly isolated ECU muscle was pinned at Lo with two 22G 1.5-inch needles on a piece of 4-inch thick Styrofoam board. The blood was rinsed off the muscle with the Ringer's buffer. The muscle was then sutured to a piece of wood stick using 1–0 suture to fix it at the Lo. After 3 to 4 days' fixation in 10% formaldehyde, the muscle was macerated in 15% nitric acid (HNO_3) for five days. After 5 days of maceration in 15% nitric acid, the muscle was then transferred to 30% nitric acid for ~30 min until the myofiber bundles became loosely attached to the muscle. The muscle was carefully rinsed with 50% glycerol several times and then stored in 50% glycerol. Approximately 10 to 20 myofiber bundles (~5 to 10 intact myofibers per bundle) were gently teased from the proximal,

Table 1. Animal information and muscle data.

	Normal	n	Affected	n	P value
Age (year)	1.64±0.30	7	1.61±0.30	7	0.944
Body weight (Kg)	20.34±2.76	7	16.57±1.55	7	0.256
ECU muscle					
Muscle weight (g)	8.37±1.83	7	6.08±0.93	7	0.287
Weight ratio (g/kg body weight)	0.39±0.04	7	0.36±0.03	7	0.604
Muscle length (cm)	14.48±1.40	7	16.04±0.81	7	0.354
Fiber length (cm)	0.65±0.06	7	0.72±0.04	7	0.354
PCSA (cm^2)	11.37±1.70	7	7.68±0.82	7	0.074
Tetanic force					
Absolute (N)	97.15±16.40	7	54.94±7.07	7	0.034
Specific, per muscle weight (N/g)	12.45±0.82	7	9.21±0.54	7	0.006
Specific, per PCSA (N/cm^2)	8.38±0.41	7	7.04±0.36	7	0.031
Eccentric contraction parameters					
Maximal tension (N)	282.76±22.68	3	204.84±59.21	4	0.332
% Length stretched	5.00±0.00	3	4.97±0.02	7	0.360
Stretch rate (mm/s)	7.90±1.15	3	7.14±0.65	7	0.500

ECU, extensor carpi ulnaris muscle.
n, number of dogs studied.
N, Newton.
PCSA, physiological cross-sectional area.
P value obtained from unpaired Student T test.

middle and distal portions of the muscle under a dissection microscope. Individual intact myofiber was carefully separated from the bundle and digital images were taken under 2x magnification. The myofiber length was then measured with the Photoshop CS5.5 software. The fiber length of approximately 100 myofibers was measured for each ECU muscle from three normal dogs (16.22±4.32 month-old, mean ± sem) using the length measurement function of the NIH image J software (version 1.45h). The Lf/Lo ratio was 0.0448±0.0025 (mean ± sem). The value 0.0448 was used as the average Lf/Lo ratio for physiological cross-sectional area (PCSA) calculation.

Determination of the PCSA of the ECU muscle. The ECU muscle is a bi-pennate muscle. Its PCSA is proportional to the cosine of the pennation angle [22,23,24]. We first measured the pennation angle from the ECU muscles of three normal dogs (the same dogs used for Lf/Lo ratio determination) [25]. The pennation angle was 10.03±0.80 (mean ± sem). The value 10.03 was used as the average pennation angle for PCSA calculation. The PCSA (cm^2) of each muscle was calculated according to the equation PCSA = (muscle weight in gram x cos10.03)/(1.056 g/cm^3 x optimal fiber length in cm). 1.0597 g/cm^3 is the muscle density [26]. The optimal fiber length was determined by multiplying the measured Lo of the muscle by the Lf/Lo ratio of 0.0448.

Determination of the specific muscle force. The specific muscle force was calculated by normalizing the tetanic muscle force by the PCSA. For comparison, we also determined the muscle weight normalized muscle force (Table 1).

Fatigue protocol. Muscle was rested for 1 min. Resistance to fatigue was then tested by applying trains of repeated 200 ms tetanic stimulation at gradually increasing train frequencies of 4, 8,

12, 16, 20, 25, 30, 45, 60, 75, and 90 tetani per min (TPM). Muscle was stimulated for 5 minutes at each train frequency and immediately shifted to a higher train frequency without interruption.

Eccentric contraction protocol. After the fatigue protocol, the ECU muscle was rested for 20 min. The peak force was recovered by 95±10.6% in normal dogs, and 90±4.6% in affected dogs. The ECU muscle was then subjected to eccentric contraction. The stimulation parameters were the same as described above (8 volts, 0.2 ms pulse duration, optimal muscle length and optimal stimulation frequency). In each cycle of eccentric contraction, the ECU muscle was stimulated for a total of 1200 msec. No stretch was performed during the first 100 msec to allow collection of the tetanic force data. In subsequent 1100 msec, the ECU muscle was stretched manually by ~ 5% of its original length. Briefly, muscle stretch was established manually by uniform rotation of a large screw-thread-knob to achieve a linear withdrawal of the force transducer, with the force and length recorded over time (Powerlab). This record was used to calculate the actual stretch length (mm/ECU muscle length) and uniform stretch rate (mm/sec). The details of the stretching parameters are listed in Table 1. After a 2 min rest, a second cycle of eccentric contraction was applied. A total of ten cycles of eccentric contraction were conducted in each ECU muscle. The tetanic force generated at the beginning of the first cycle eccentric contraction was defined as 100%. The tetanic forces obtained in each subsequent cycle were used to calculate force drop induced by eccentric contraction. The percentage of force drop was determined according to the formula, force drop % = 100×(T1–Tn)/T1, where T1 stood for the tetanic force obtained during the first cycle and Tn represented the tetanic force obtained during the nth cycle.

Blood Flow

Blood flow rate (ml/min) in the brachial artery and aortic blood pressure were recorded throughout the entire experiment. To more accurately reflect blood flow change during repeated tetanic contraction, we calculated blood flow conductance using the formula, conductance = blood flow rate (ml/min)/blood pressure (mmHg).

Statistical Analysis

Data are presented as mean ± standard error of mean. For comparison of two groups, unpaired Student t test was applied. For muscle performance, blood pressure and blood flow data, repeated measures one way analysis of variance was applied. This analysis allowed determination of the effect of muscle disease (muscular dystrophy) and muscle contraction as well as the interaction between muscle disease and muscle contraction. Tukey's test was used for *post hoc* analysis. P<0.05 was considered statistically significant.

Results

A total of seven normal and seven affected dogs were studied. There was no statistically significant difference in body weight and age between normal and affected dogs (Table 1). Normal dog ECU muscle showed characteristic sarcolemmal dystrophin expression (Figure 1). As expected, dystrophin was not detected in the ECU muscles obtained from affected dogs (Figure 1). ECU muscle pathology was examined by HE staining. Normal dog muscle had uniform fiber size, peripherally located myonuclei and there was minimal inflammatory cell infiltration. Affected dogs showed prominent muscle degeneration, necrosis, myofiber size

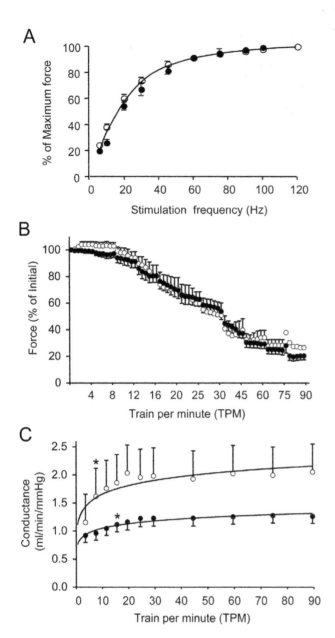

Figure 2. Force-frequency relationship in the ECU muscle and impact of repetitive tetanic contraction on muscle force and blood flow. A, Force-frequency relationship in the ECU muscle of normal and dystrophin-null dogs. Single tetanic force at different stimulation frequency was recorded under optimal muscle length (L_0). After normalizing to muscle weight, relative tetanic force at each stimulation frequency was calculated as the percentage of the maximal single tetanic force (Table 1). Relative tetanic force was then graphed against stimulation frequency. Data are presented as mean ± standard error of mean. Open circle, normal dogs (n = 4). Closed circle, dystrophic dogs (n = 7). B, Force profile during continuous tetanic stimulation. Uninterrupted stimulation was started at a train frequency of 4 TPM. The train frequency increased every 5 min to 8, 12, 16, 20, 25, 30, 45, 60, 75 and finally 90 TPM. Muscle force was recorded every minute. The tetanic force prior to the start of train stimulation was defined as 100%. Subsequent force change was compared accordingly and expressed as the percent of the starting tetanic force. Open circle, normal dogs (n = 4). Closed circle, dystrophic dogs (n = 7). C, Forearm blood flow conductance (ml/min per mmHg) during continuous tetanic stimulation. Logarithm trend lines are depicted for both normal and affected dogs. Open circle, normal dogs (n = 4). Closed circle, dystrophic dogs (n = 7). Asterisk, significantly different from that of pre-contraction (0 TPM) in the same group. No statistically significant difference was

noted between normal and affected dogs by repeated measures analysis of variance ($0.1 > p > 0.05$).

variation and inflammation (Figure 1). More then 15% of myofibers contained centrally localized nuclei in affected dogs while it was only less than 1% in normal dogs (Figure 1). The distribution of the cross-sectional area of individual myofibers was also altered in dystrophic dogs (Figure 1). To evaluate muscle fibrosis, we performed WGA immunostaining. Only affected dog ECU muscle showed pronounced fibrosis (Figure 1).

Force from ten normal and eight affected ECU muscles was examined. These include ten ECU muscles from seven normal dogs and eight ECU muscles from seven affected dogs. In four normal dogs, force was measured from only one ECU muscle. In the other three normal dogs, force was measured from both sides. In six affected dogs, force was measured from only one ECU muscle. In one affected dog, force was measured from both sides) (Table 1). In cases where both side ECU muscles were studied, force from the left and right ECU muscles were combined as the data from one dog for statistical comparisons. There was no significant difference in body weight, muscle weight, muscle length, fiber length and PCSA between normal and affected dogs (Table 1). Force-frequency relationship was not altered by dystrophin deficiency (Figure 2A). The half relaxation time was 29.7 ± 1.68 ms in normal group and 29.2 ± 0.92 ms in affected group. There was no significant difference between normal and affected dogs ($p > 0.05$). Absolute muscle force and specific tetanic force (normalized either by muscle weight or PCSA) were significantly reduced in affected dogs (Table 1).

To evaluate muscle fatigue, we applied continuous tetanic contractions at the rate of 4 to 90 TPM (Figure 2B). A similar pattern was observed in both normal and affected dogs. No loss of initial tension was observed up to 16 TPM. At the end of 90 TPM contractions, ~25% of initial force was still retained in both groups (Figure 2B).

We also measured the change of brachial blood flow during repeated tetanic contraction (Figure 2C). Blood flow increased as the frequency of the train stimulation increased from 4 to 30 TPM. Statistic analysis by ANOVA suggests that there is a strong correlation between contraction and blood flow increase ($p < 0.001$). Interestingly, the rate of conductance increase in normal dogs was 67% higher than that of affected dogs. For normal dogs, the slope before reaching plateau was 0.10 ± 0.04. For affected dogs, the slop was 0.06 ± 0.02 ($p < 0.1$) (Figure 2C). After 30 TPM, blood flow reached plateau and no further increase was noted.

To characterize contraction-induced muscle damage, we challenged the ECU muscle with 10 cycles of eccentric contraction (Figure 3, Table 1). The ECU muscle was stretched while it underwent tetanic contraction. Similar stretch parameters (maximal tension, percentage of length stretched and the stretch rate) were applied to normal and affected dogs (Table 1). In normal dogs, no significant force reduction was observed until the sixth cycle of eccentric contraction. Even after all 10 cycles of eccentric contraction, the normal ECU muscle still maintained ~64% of the initial force (Figure 3). In sharp contrast, a dramatic force drop was observed even after the first cycle of eccentric contraction in affected dogs ($p < 0.01$). By the end of the 10th cycle of eccentric contraction, tetanic force reduced to only ~12% of the initial force in the dystrophic ECU muscle (Figure 3). Statistic analysis by ANOVA showed a strong interaction ($p < 0.01$) of dystrophin deficiency and eccentric contraction in force decline. Blood pressure and brachial blood flow showed no statistical difference

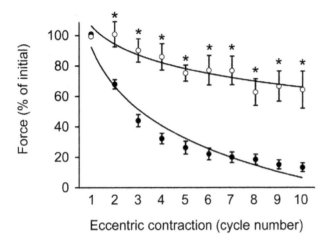

Figure 3. The ECU muscle of affected dogs was more vulnerable to eccentric contraction induced damage. Relative changes of the tetanic force before the start of eccentric contraction and after each cycle during 10 cycles of eccentric contraction. The force at the beginning of the first cycle of eccentric contraction was designated as 100%. Logarithm trend lines are depicted for both normal and affected dogs. Open circle, normal dogs (n = 3). Closed circle, dystrophic dogs (n = 7). Asterisk, significantly different from that of affected dogs.

(either within the same group or between groups) during eccentric contraction.

Discussion

A bottleneck in the development of DMD gene and/or cell therapy is the dog study. Despite consensus agreement on the importance and relevance of the canine model, it remains a great challenge to convincingly demonstrate physiological benefits of treatment in dystrophic dogs. Studies conducted so far have been mainly focused on dystrophin expression and morphological amelioration [27,28,29]. Definitive force improvement data that are essential to buttress the microscopic findings are missing [14]. Even worse, a solid protocol has not been developed to demonstrate force deficiency in a single intact muscle in dystrophin-deficient dogs, not to mention quantifying variable levels of (potentially subtle) improvements incurred by experimental therapy. A major goal of the current study is to fill this knowledge gap and establish a rigorous and sensitive assay to evaluate contractility of a single intact dog muscle. This platform can then be used to test functional outcome of any gene/cell therapy strategies in the canine model.

We first determined which muscle to use. We considered the following factors in decision making. These are (1) whether the muscle can be readily approached and fully saturated by local injection, (2) whether the muscle have defined anatomic structure (such as a long slender tendon) for *in situ* mounting on the force transducer plate and (3) muscle pathology. A preliminary study was performed on the gastrocnemius, extensor carpi radialis and ECU muscles (data not shown). The results suggest that the ECU muscle is an ideal target muscle for our purpose. The ECU muscle can be easily identified based on the surface marks. Saturated delivery can be achieved in the ECU muscle via surgical or percutaneous injection (data not shown) [28]. This muscle also showed characteristic muscle pathology and yielded consistent force data in dogs of different size and breeds (Figure 1).

The following major findings were made. First, we observed a significant reduction of tetanic force in affected dogs (Table 1). In contrast to what have been reported for the peroneus longus muscle [16], the ECU muscle of dystrophin-deficient dogs uniformly showed a significantly reduced specific isometric tetanic muscle force (either normalized by muscle weight or PCSA) (Table 1). As a consequence of muscle degeneration and necrosis, a loss of specific isometric force is expected in dystrophin-deficient muscle. However, this has only been shown in mdx mice. Our results here provide direct evidence that specific force reduction also presents in large mammals that carry a null mutation in the dystrophin gene.

The second major finding is on eccentric contraction. We observed a much greater force decline in affected ECU muscles. A statistically significant difference was obtained even after one cycle of eccentric contraction (Figure 3). A major function of dystrophin is to protect muscle cells from contraction-induced injury. Forcibly lengthening of an actively contracted muscle is one of the most sensitive and stringent physiological tests of muscle integrity [30]. The degree of immediate force drop after eccentric contraction is now a widely accepted index for evaluating the therapeutic efficacy of an experimental DMD therapy in the murine model. Immediate force changes after eccentric contraction have not been evaluated in the DMD dog model until recently [31]. Tegeler et al tested the effect of eccentric contraction using a tibiotarsal joint preparation. This preparation measures the collective effect from all muscles in the cranial tibial compartment. After 30 cycles of eccentric contraction, normal and affected dogs lost 8% and 63% of their initial torque, respectively [31]. The authors concluded that the flexor muscles of dystrophic dogs induced a greater force drop than that of normal dogs [31]. Our results here have confirmed and extended the study by Tegeler et al and suggest that the extensor muscle is also quite sensitive to lengthening contraction injury in dystrophic dogs. It is worth to point out that the method reported by Tegeler et al measures cumulative responses from many muscles and it cannot distinct the contribution of individual muscle. The ability to measure force alteration in a single dog muscle has significant advantages in translational studies. It provides a convenient avenue to compare different therapeutic strategies before launching much more expensive whole limb or whole body therapy. This is especially relevant in the case of AAV micro-dystrophin vectors. More than a dozen different constructs have been described (reviewed in [14,32,33]). A side-by-side comparison in a single dog muscle will be cost-effective to prioritize these microgene vectors. Another advantage of the single muscle approach is the possibility of correlating transduction efficiency and force improvement in the same muscle. It is currently not clear what percentage of myofibers should be transduced in order to see a physiological improvement in dystrophin-null large mammals. The single muscle assay platform described here may allow investigators to achieve this goal by titrating vector dose, viral serotype and injection protocol (such as the volume and speed etc).

Besides specific tetanic force and eccentric contraction, we also examined the fatigue profile and blood perfusion during tetanic muscle contraction. Similar to what have been reported in the limb muscle of mdx mice [34,35], the ECU muscle from normal and affected dogs showed the same fatigue profile (Figure 2B). An important role of dystrophin is to anchor neuronal nitric oxide synthase (nNOS) to the sarcolemma [36]. Nitric oxide produced by membrane-associated nNOS counteracts sympathetic vasoconstriction in contracting muscle. In the absence of dystrophin, this protective mechanism is compromised [37,38]. The resulting functional ischemia is now considered as a crucial pathogenic mechanism for DMD. In agreement with this theory, we indeed found a blunted (though not statistically significant) blood flow in affected dogs when the ECU muscle was subject to continuous tetanic stimulation (Figure 2C). Future studies are needed to further corroborate this exciting preliminary observation.

The reduction of specific muscle force and the increase of susceptibility to eccentric contraction injury are the most consistent findings in the murine DMD model (reviewed in [39]). Our results demonstrated for the first time that a single intact muscle from dystrophin-null dogs share the same features. A straining issue in the use of the dog model is the lack of rigorous physiological methods to objectively evaluate the outcome. The *in situ* protocol described here, though a terminal assay, may therefore serve as a highly informative endpoint to accurately measure muscle force improvement in dog studies in the future.

Acknowledgments

The authors thank Drs Bruce Smith, Dietrich Volkmann, Dawna L. Voelkl, Scott Korte, Lonny Dixon and Mr. Clayton Douglas, Ms Yongping Yue and Keqing Zhang for technical help with dog breeding and colony maintenance.

Author Contributions

Conceived and designed the experiments: DD RLT. Performed the experiments: CHH HTY JS XP. Analyzed the data: CHH DD HTY JS RLT. Contributed reagents/materials/analysis tools: CHH DD HTY JS RLT. Wrote the paper: DD HTY.

References

1. Emery AEH, Muntoni F (2003) Duchenne muscular dystrophy. Oxford; New York: Oxford University Press. x, 270 p.
2. Romitti P, Mathews K, Zamba G, Andrews J, Druschel C, et al. (2009) Prevalence of Duchenne/Becker muscular dystrophy among males aged 5–24 years - four states, 2007. MMWR Morb Mortal Wkly Rep 58: 1119–1122.
3. Dooley J, Gordon KE, Dodds L, MacSween J (2010) Duchenne muscular dystrophy: a 30-year population-based incidence study. Clin Pediatr (Phila) 49: 177–179.
4. Koenig M, Hoffman EP, Bertelson CJ, Monaco AP, Feener C, et al. (1987) Complete cloning of the Duchenne muscular dystrophy (DMD) cDNA and preliminary genomic organization of the DMD gene in normal and affected individuals. Cell 50: 509–517.
5. Hoffman EP, Brown RH Jr, Kunkel LM (1987) Dystrophin: the protein product of the Duchenne muscular dystrophy locus. Cell 51: 919–928.
6. Cooper BJ, Winand NJ, Stedman H, Valentine BA, Hoffman EP, et al. (1988) The homologue of the Duchenne locus is defective in X-linked muscular dystrophy of dogs. Nature 334: 154–156.
7. Sicinski P, Geng Y, Ryder-Cook AS, Barnard EA, Darlison MG, et al. (1989) The molecular basis of muscular dystrophy in the mdx mouse: a point mutation. Science 244: 1578–1580.
8. Bulfield G, Siller WG, Wight PA, Moore KJ (1984) X chromosome-linked muscular dystrophy (mdx) in the mouse. Proc Natl Acad Sci U S A 81: 1189–1192.
9. Kornegay JN, Tuler SM, Miller DM, Levesque DC (1988) Muscular dystrophy in a litter of golden retriever dogs. Muscle Nerve 11: 1056–1064.
10. Wells DJ, Wells KE (2005) What do animal models have to tell us regarding Duchenne muscular dystrophy? Acta Myol 24: 172–180.
11. Shelton GD, Engvall E (2005) Canine and feline models of human inherited muscle diseases. Neuromuscul Disord 15: 127–138.
12. Howell JM, Fletcher S, Kakulas BA, O'Hara M, Lochmuller H, et al. (1997) Use of the dog model for Duchenne muscular dystrophy in gene therapy trials. Neuromuscul Disord 7: 325–328.
13. Smith BF, Wrighten R (2010) Animal models for inherited muscle diseases. In: Duan D, editor. Muscle gene therapy. New York: Springer Science + Business Media, LLC. 1–21.
14. Duan D (2011) Duchenne muscular dystrophy gene therapy: lost in translation? Resarch and Report in Biology 2: 31–42.
15. Childers MK, Grange RW, Kornegay JN (2011) In vivo canine muscle function assay. J Vis Exp: pii 2623.
16. Kornegay JN, Sharp NJ, Bogan DJ, Van Camp SD, Metcalf JR, et al. (1994) Contraction tension and kinetics of the peroneus longus muscle in golden retriever muscular dystrophy. J Neurol Sci 123: 100–107.
17. Hakim CH, Li D, Duan D (2011) Monitoring murine skeletal muscle function for muscle gene therapy. Methods Mol Biol 709: 75–89.
18. Smith BF, Yue Y, Woods PR, Kornegay JN, Shin JH, et al. (2011) An intronic LINE-1 element insertion in the dystrophin gene aborts dystrophin expression and results in Duchenne-like muscular dystrophy in the corgi breed. Lab Invest 91: 216–231.
19. Fine DM, Shin JH, Yue Y, Volkmann D, Leach SB, et al. (2011) Age-matched comparison reveals early electrocardiography and echocardiography changes in dystrophin-deficient dogs. Neuromuscul Disord 21: 453–461.
20. Yue Y, Li Z, Harper SQ, Davisson RL, Chamberlain JS, et al. (2003) Microdystrophin Gene Therapy of Cardiomyopathy Restores Dystrophin-Glycoprotein Complex and Improves Sarcolemma Integrity in the Mdx Mouse Heart. Circulation 108: 1626–1632.
21. Yue Y, Liu M, Duan D (2006) C-terminal truncated microdystrophin recruits dystrobrevin and syntrophin to the dystrophin-associated glycoprotein complex

and reduces muscular dystrophy in symptomatic utrophin/dystrophin double knock-out mice. Mol Ther 14: 79–87.
22. Sacks RD, Roy RR (1982) Architecture of the hind limb muscles of cats: functional significance. J Morphol 173: 185–195.
23. Ward SR, Kim CW, Eng CM, Gottschalk LJ, Tomiya A, et al. (2009) Architectural analysis and intraoperative measurements demonstrate the unique design of the multifidus muscle for lumbar spine stability. J Bone Joint Surg Am 91: 176–185.
24. Fukunaga T, Roy RR, Shellock FG, Hodgson JA, Day MK, et al. (1992) Physiological cross-sectional area of human leg muscles based on magnetic resonance imaging. J Orthop Res 10: 928–934.
25. Maxwell LC, Faulkner JA, Hyatt GJ (1974) Estimation of number of fibers in guinea pig skeletal muscles. J Appl Physiol 37: 259–264.
26. Mendez J, Keys A (1960) Density and composition of mammalian muscle. Metabolism 9: 184–188.
27. Wang Z, Kuhr CS, Allen JM, Blankinship M, Gregorevic P, et al. (2007) Sustained AAV-mediated Dystrophin Expression in a Canine Model of Duchenne Muscular Dystrophy with a Brief Course of Immunosuppression. Mol Ther 15: 1160–1166.
28. Shin JH, Yue Y, Srivastava A, Smith B, Lai Y, et al. (2012) A simplified immune suppression scheme leads to persistent micro-dystrophin expression in duchenne muscular dystrophy dogs. Hum Gene Ther 23: 202–209.
29. Yokota T, Lu QL, Partridge T, Kobayashi M, Nakamura A, et al. (2009) Efficacy of systemic morpholino exon-skipping in duchenne dystrophy dogs. Ann Neurol 65: 667–676.
30. Proske U, Morgan DL (2001) Muscle damage from eccentric exercise: mechanism, mechanical signs, adaptation and clinical applications. J Physiol 537: 333–345.
31. Tegeler CJ, Grange RW, Bogan DJ, Markert CD, Case D, et al. (2010) Eccentric contractions induce rapid isometric torque drop in dystrophin-deficient dogs. Muscle Nerve 42: 130–132.
32. Athanasopoulos T, Graham IR, Foster H, Dickson G (2004) Recombinant adeno-associated viral (rAAV) vectors as therapeutic tools for Duchenne muscular dystrophy (DMD). Gene Ther 11 Suppl 1: S109–121.
33. Blankinship MJ, Gregorevic P, Chamberlain JS (2006) Gene therapy strategies for Duchenne muscular dystrophy utilizing recombinant adeno-associated viral vectors. Mol Ther 13: 241–249.
34. Gregorevic P, Plant DR, Lynch GS (2004) Administration of insulin-like growth factor-I improves fatigue resistance of skeletal muscles from dystrophic mdx mice. Muscle Nerve 30: 295–304.
35. Harcourt LJ, Schertzer JD, Ryall JG, Lynch GS (2007) Low dose formoterol administration improves muscle function in dystrophic mdx mice without increasing fatigue. Neuromuscul Disord 17: 47–55.
36. Lai Y, Thomas GD, Yue Y, Yang HT, Li D, et al. (2009) Dystrophins carrying spectrin-like repeats 16 and 17 anchor nNOS to the sarcolemma and enhance exercise performance in a mouse model of muscular dystrophy. J Clin Invest 119: 624–635.
37. Thomas GD, Sander M, Lau KS, Huang PL, Stull JT, et al. (1998) Impaired metabolic modulation of alpha-adrenergic vasoconstriction in dystrophin-deficient skeletal muscle. Proc Natl Acad Sci U S A 95: 15090–15095.
38. Sander M, Chavoshan B, Harris SA, Iannaccone ST, Stull JT, et al. (2000) Functional muscle ischemia in neuronal nitric oxide synthase-deficient skeletal muscle of children with Duchenne muscular dystrophy. Proc Natl Acad Sci U S A 97: 13818–13823.
39. Watchko JF, O'Day TL, Hoffman EP (2002) Functional characteristics of dystrophic skeletal muscle: insights from animal models. J Appl Physiol 93: 407–417.

8

Subject-Specific Tendon-Aponeurosis Definition in Hill-Type Model Predicts Higher Muscle Forces in Dynamic Tasks

Pauline Gerus[1]*, Guillaume Rao[2], Eric Berton[2]

1 Centre for Musculoskeletal Research, Griffith Health Institute, Griffith University, Gold Coast, Australia, **2** Institute of Movement Sciences E-J Marey, Aix-Marseille Université, Marseille, France

Abstract

Neuromusculoskeletal models are a common method to estimate muscle forces. Developing accurate neuromusculoskeletal models is a challenging task due to the complexity of the system and large inter-subject variability. The estimation of muscles force is based on the mechanical properties of tendon-aponeurosis complex. Most neuromusculoskeletal models use a generic definition of the tendon-aponeurosis complex based on *in vitro* test, perhaps limiting their validity. Ultrasonography allows subject-specific estimates of the tendon-aponeurosis complex's mechanical properties. The aim of this study was to investigate the influence of subject-specific mechanical properties of the tendon-aponeurosis complex on a neuromusculoskeletal model of the ankle joint. Seven subjects performed isometric contractions from which the tendon-aponeurosis force-strain relationship was estimated. Hopping and running tasks were performed and muscle forces were estimated using subject-specific tendon-aponeurosis and generic tendon properties. Two ultrasound probes positioned over the muscle-tendon junction and the mid-belly were combined with motion capture to estimate the *in vivo* tendon and aponeurosis strain of the *medial head of gastrocnemius muscle*. The tendon-aponeurosis force-strain relationship was scaled for the other ankle muscles based on tendon and aponeurosis length of each muscle measured by ultrasonography. The EMG-driven model was calibrated twice - using the generic tendon definition and a subject-specific tendon-aponeurosis force-strain definition. The use of subject-specific tendon-aponeurosis definition leads to a higher muscle force estimate for the soleus muscle and the plantar-flexor group, and to a better model prediction of the ankle joint moment compared to the model estimate which used a generic definition. Furthermore, the subject-specific tendon-aponeurosis definition leads to a decoupling behaviour between the muscle fibre and muscle-tendon unit in agreement with previous experiments using ultrasonography. These results indicate the use of subject-specific tendon-aponeurosis definitions in a neuromusculoskeletal model produce better agreement with measured external loads and more physiological model behaviour.

Editor: Hani A. Awad, University of Rochester, United States of America

Funding: These authors have no support or funding to report.

Competing Interests: The authors have declared that no competing interests exist.

* E-mail: pauline@gerus.fr

Introduction

The force produced by the muscle fibres is transmitted to the bones via the aponeurosis and tendon. The aponeurosis and the tendon are not rigid and therefore their lengths change in some proportion to applied loading. This elasticity of the aponeurosis and tendon is important in transmitting force from muscles to bone. For example, during an isometric contraction when the overall muscle-tendon unit length remains constant muscle force production results from the shortening of muscle fascicles while the tendon-aponeurosis complex stretches [1]. During a dynamic task such as walking, Ishikawa and al. [2] have used ultrasonography to quantify the in vivo behaviour of the muscle fibre with respect to the muscle-tendon unit length change. The muscle-tendon unit undergoes a stretching followed by a shortening, while the muscle fibre behaviour may be different. The muscle fibre could shorten or remain constant during the stretching of the muscle-tendon unit. The independent behaviour of the muscle fibre and muscle-tendon unit, called decoupling, is a result of the compliance of the

aponeurosis-tendon unit. Decoupling reduces the muscle fibre velocity and thus directly affects the production of muscle fibre force. Furthermore, the decoupling within the muscle-tendon unit could be influenced by the intensity of tasks, with a decrease in decoupling related to an increase in task intensity [3], [4]. The tendon and the aponeurosis thus are important to the decoupling between the muscle fibre and the muscle-tendon unit, and to muscle force production during either static or dynamic tasks.

Neuromusculoskeletal (NMS) models are developed to estimate muscle forces important to the investigation of motor control and neuromusculoskeletal disorders. Developing accurate models is a challenging task because of system complexity and the presence of high inter-subject variability in many of the system components. The interaction between the muscle fibre and the tendon-aponeurosis complex is usually represented in a NMS model with a Hill-type muscle model. In a Hill-type muscle model, an elastic element (Series Elastic Element: SEE) representing the tendon-aponeurosis complex is in series with two parallel elements representing the muscle fibre. The series elastic element is usually defined by a generic force-strain relationship based on *in vitro* tests on tendon. [5]. The use of this generic definition is questionable for several reasons. First, the mechanical properties were measured in cadaveric specimens and do not reflect human *in vivo* behaviour [6]. Second, the generic definition is applied to models regardless of the nature of the task and the subject. Recent studies have shown a large variability in tendon mechanical properties depending on the sex [7], the type exercise [8], the age [9], and the loading rate (rate of force application to the tissue) [10], [11]. Finally, the generic definition is used to represent both the tendon and aponeurosis mechanical properties assuming their respective mechanical properties are equivalent. Given the recent advances in tendon characterization and the inter-subject variability, it is necessary to properly define the SEE in a NMS model in order to accurately estimate muscle forces.

The mechanical properties of the tendon and aponeurosis have previously been estimated for different muscles using ultrasonography during isometric contractions. Previous studies have found a similar strain of the tendon and aponeurosis [12], [13], and both a higher strain for the aponeurosis [14], [15] and tendon [16], [17]. The lack of consistent results may be explained by experiments being conducted on various muscles, with different methods, or by the large variability in muscle-tendon mechanics between individuals. Due to the variability in tendon and aponeurosis mechanical properties, it is necessary to represent the tendon and aponeurosis as two separate elements within a Hill-type muscle model. Lieber et al [18] developed a Hill-type muscle model which modelled the tendon and aponeurosis as two elements in series with the muscle fibre. The force-strain relationship of the tendon and aponeurosis was estimated from experiments on frog muscle. Importantly, the simulation of fixed-end contraction has shown that the mechanical definition of the SEE influenced the model outputs [18]. The attempt by Lieber et al. [18] to separate the tendon and aponeurosis was promising, but limited to animal experimentation and during fixed-end contraction.

The aim of this study was to investigate the influence of the tendon and aponeurosis considered as two separate elements in Hill-type muscle model defined by subject-specific mechanical properties on EMG-driven model outputs such as the muscle force estimations and muscle fibre behaviours during highly dynamic tasks. By using a simulation, Bobbert [19] has found that a Series Elastic Element more compliant increases the maximal squat jump height. Thus our hypothesis was that the use of a subject-specific tendon-aponeurosis force-strain relationship in a Hill-type muscle model will lead to higher estimates of muscle forces compared to the model estimates using a generic tendon force-strain relationship.

Materials and Methods

Experimental Design

Seven healthy males (age 25.9 ± 1.6 years, body mass 72.7 ± 9.8 kg, height 1.77 ± 0.05 m) participated in this study. All participants gave informed written consent. The study was approved by the Ethical Committee of Aix-Marseille University and was conducted in accordance with the Declaration of Helsinki. Subjects performed two types of tasks to investigate the influence of subject-specific definition of the SEE on muscle forces and estimated fibre behaviours: (i) Isometric contractions to estimate the *in vivo* tendon-aponeurosis force-strain relationships, and (ii) running and hopping tasks.

For the isometric contractions, subjects were seated on the bench of a custom ergometer with the knee fully extended and the ankle joint at $0°$ dorsiflexion. This ankle angle was chosen to minimize effects from the passive joint moment and obtain large forces from the medial head of the gastrocnemius (GM) muscle. The right foot was set in a rigid shoe fixed to a plate with both joint and static torquemeter (CS3, Meiri, France) axis aligned. Subjects performed three 3-second maximal voluntary isometric plantar-flexion contractions (MVIC) with verbal encouragement and on-screen joint moment feedback. Then subjects performed ramp-up contractions (from rest to 100% MVIC) in minimal time with on-screen feedback. (Two trials were recorded for each condition with a resting time of 2 min. The contraction duration was chosen to be close to loading rates encompassed during running and hopping tasks.

During isometric contractions, the ankle joint net moment was recorded by the static torquemeter at 2000 Hz. Kinematic data were recorded synchronously at 125 Hz by a six-camera VICON system (Vicon Motion System, Lake Forest, CA). Three retrore-flective markers were attached to an ultrasound probe located over the muscle-tendon junction (MTJ) in order to create a probe reference frame parallel to the image plane and further used to estimate the tendon length [11]. Additional markers were attached to the Achilles' tendon insertion over the calcaneus, the first metatarsal head of the foot, the lateral and medial malleoli of the ankle, and the fibula head. The first 50 mm linear array ultrasound probe (BK-Med Pro-Focus) was positioned over the MTJ of the GM muscle, while a second 40 mm linear array ultrasound probe (BK-Med Ultra-view) was fixed over the mid-belly of GM muscle (Fig. 1) at the level of 30% of the lower leg length (i.e. from the popliteal crease to the centre of the lateral malleolus) and aligned approximately in the same plane as the muscle line action [20]. The probes were carefully attached to the leg using foam fixation and secured with elastic bandage. Images were recorded synchronously at 30 Hz with two image acquisition boards (National Instrument, PCI 1410). The synchronization of the ultrasound video acquisition with Vicon motion capture system was triggered by an analog signal (0–5V). In rest position, a single ultrasound probe was used to measure the tendon length, the fascicle length and the pennation angle for the *lateral head of the gastrocnemius* (GL), *medial head of the gastrocnemius* (GM), and *soleus* (SOL).

For the dynamic contractions, subjects performed hopping and running tasks. They performed two series of 15 continuous hops on the right leg over a force plate (Kistler, USA) at an approximate frequency of 2 Hz [21]. They were asked to hop in-place without shoes and with their hands on their hips. Then, subjects performed two running trials at a self-selected speed with their right foot landing on the force plate. Markers were attached over the insertion of the Achilles' tendon on the calcaneus, the fifth and first metatarsal heads of the foot, the lateral and medial malleoli of the ankle, the fibula head, the lateral and medial condyles of the femur, the great trochanter for both legs, and the right and left anterior superior iliac spines. The coordinates of each marker was recorded at 125 Hz. EMG signals were recorded at 2000 Hz (Trigno Wireless, Delsys, USA) using surface electrodes placed over the muscles according to recommendations of the SENIAM group. Muscle activity for the GL, GM, SOL and tibialis anterior (TA) were recorded.

Estimation of the Tendon and Aponeurosis Force-strain Relationships for the GM Muscle

Ultrasound images from the first probe were used to track the MTJ defined as the intersection between the GM muscle fascicles and the GM tendon. Raw images were processed by adjusting the contrast and then binarized using a graythreshold

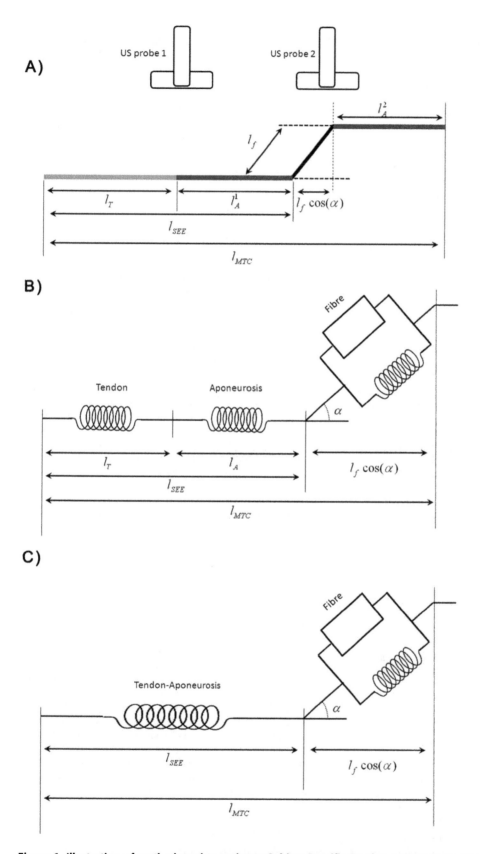

Figure 1. Illustration of method used to estimate Subject-Specific Tendon-Aponeurosis. (A) Geometric model of the muscle-tendon-aponeurosis complex that includes fascicle, tendon, and aponeurosis adapted from Fukashiro et al. [23]. The aponeurosis length is: $l_A = l_A^1 + l_A^2$. Hill-type muscle model with the tendon and the aponeurosis in series (B) and a resulting Tendon-Aponeurosis element representing the tendon and aponeurosis in series (C).

value. The MTJ displacements were tracked using the method presented by Korstanje et al. [22] with manual adjustment when necessary. All possible pixel displacements within the search region were evaluated with normalized cross-correlation, with the higher value used to determine the MTJ position on the next frame. For each frame, the tendon length was computed as the distance between the markers placed on calcaneus and the MTJ position in the global coordinate system using the probe reference frame [11].

The tendon strain of the GM muscle (ε_T) was defined as:

$$\varepsilon_T = \frac{\Delta l_T}{l_T^0} \tag{1}$$

Where l_T^0 is the initial tendon length computed in the rest position and Δl_T is the elongation of tendon.

The aponeurosis length was computed based on the geometric model (Fig. 1) presented by Fukashiro et al. [23] with muscle fascicle length, pennation angle, tendon length and muscle-tendon length as input at each time step. First, the muscle fascicle length (Lf) and the pennation angle (α) of GM muscle were computed using ultrasound data obtained from the second probe. The muscle fascicle length was defined as the distance between the intersection of the fascicle with the superficial and deeper aponeurosis. The proximal and distal ends of both superficial and deep aponeurosis were tracked automatically for each frame [22] (Fig. 2). Each aponeurosis was defined by linear interpolation between the proximal and distal end. This process directly accounts for changes in position of the aponeurosis during contraction and indirectly took into account the effect of the internal pressure of the muscle. Proximal and distal ends of each fascicle were tracked automatically for each following frame using the method presented by Korstanje et al. [22]. The entire muscle fascicle could not be seen on the US image, thus the missing part of fascicle was estimated by linear extrapolation of both aponeurosis and fascicle [24] (Fig. 2). The pennation angle was defined as the angle between the deeper aponeurosis and the muscle fascicle. The curvature of the fascicle was not taken into account. The possible error of this assumption is less than 6% [25]. The fascicle length and pennation angle were estimated for two fascicles and averaged at each time instance with the US probe placed over the mid-belly of GM muscle to account for variability amongst the fascicles. The averaged data were used to represent the entire muscle fibre. Shin et al. [26] have shown by using MRI data that there is no difference in muscle fascicle length along the GM muscle but that the pennation angle could change from the distal to the proximal region of GM muscle. The value of the pennation angle for the middle part of the GM muscle is the average of the distal and proximal regions. Sampling the mid-part of the GM muscle appears a reasonable way to represent the entire muscle.

To estimate the aponeurosis length, we hypothesized that the muscle fibre lengths and pennation angles estimated using ultrasonography in the muscle mid-belly were representative of the entire muscle behaviour [27].

The muscle-tendon length was computed from Opensim by using kinematic data of the isometric task. First, a geometric musculoskeletal model was scaled for each subject by using a static upright trial. Then, the markers positions obtained at each time during contraction were used in Opensim to estimate joint angles with the Inverse Kinematic Tool. Finally, the muscle-tendon length was computed at each time for all subjects and all trials [28].

The aponeurosis length was computed at each time using:

$$l_A(t) = l_{MTC}(t) - l_f(t)\cos(\alpha(t)) - l_T(t) \tag{2}$$

Where $l_{MTC}(t)$ is the muscle-tendon length computed by Opensim at each time instance.

The aponeurosis strain of the GM muscle was defined as:

$$\varepsilon_A = \frac{\Delta l_A}{l_A^0} \tag{3}$$

Where l_A^0 is the initial aponeurosis length estimated at the same instance as l_T^0.

Over the entire force production range the relative moment contribution of the GM to the ankle joint net moment and the moment arm of GM were assumed constant [29]. Consequently, the normalized force was computed as the measured joint moment normalized by its maximum value during the task. Finally, a second-order polynomial model was used to fit the tendon and aponeurosis force-strain relationship for the GM muscle.

Estimation of the Tendon-aponeurosis Force-strain Relationship for Each Muscle

The tendon and the aponeurosis were considered as two elements in series (Fig. 1). These two elements in series could be represented by one element, henceforth called Tendon-Aponeurosis (T-A). In rest position, one ultrasound probe was used to measure the tendon length (l_T^0), the fascicle length and the pennation angle for the GL, GM and SOL. The aponeurosis length in the rest position (l_A^0) was estimated by using the geometric model described previously (Fig. 1). A muscle-specific ratio for the GL, GM and SOL was defined to represent the tendon length according to the T-A length such as:

$$ratio = \frac{l_T^0}{l_T^0 + l_A^0} \tag{4}$$

From this ratio, the strain for the tendon-aponeurosis complex is:

$$\varepsilon_{T-A} = \varepsilon_T \times ratio + \varepsilon_A \times (1 - ratio) \tag{5}$$

ε_T represents the tendon strain of the GM muscle and ε_A the aponeurosis strain of the GM muscle.

At each force level, the T-A strain was estimated by using equation 5, the muscle-specific ratio and the corresponding tendon and aponeurosis strain for each subject. Fig. 3 illustrates the method used to estimate the T-A force-strain relationship based on the aponeurosis and tendon force-strain relationships and the muscle specific ratio.

Calibration and Prediction Process of the EMG-driven Model

Once the T-A force strain relationship was estimated for each muscle and each subject, the next step was the muscle force estimation by using the EMG-driven model. The model used in the present study has already been extensively described [30], [31] and only a brief description is given here. The EMG-driven model used EMG, kinematic, anatomical, and net joint moment data to estimate muscle forces. The model consisted of five parts: (1) an anatomical model to estimate muscle-tendon lengths and moment

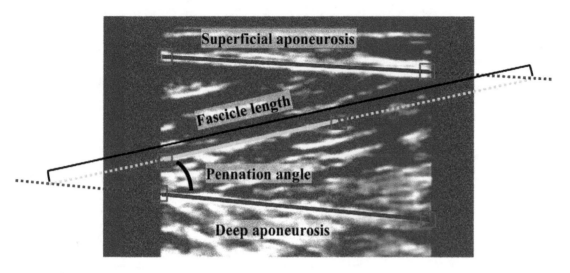

Figure 2. Illustration of method used to estimate the fascicle length and pennation angle. The proximal and distal ends of the superficial aponeurosis, deep aponeurosis, and muscle fascicle were tracked automatically at each frame. The missing part was estimated by linear interpolation.

arms, (2) an EMG-to-activation model to represent muscle activation dynamics, (3) a Hill-type model to characterize muscle-tendon contraction dynamics and estimate the forces in the muscle-tendon unit, (4) a calibration process to tune model parameters based on ankle net joint moment computed through inverse dynamics, and (5) a prediction process to compute joint moments by using adjusted model parameters (Fig. 4).

OpenSim (Simtk, Stanford, USA) was used to create an anatomical model and to scale this model based on the subject's static marker measurements (more information in Delp et al. [29]). This model included four muscle-tendon units (GL, GM, SOL and TA). Based on kinematic measurements, the muscle-tendon

lengths and flexion-extension moment arms at the ankle joint were estimated at each time instance for each subject and trial.

The raw EMGs were band-pass filtered (10–500 Hz), full-wave rectified, filtered using a zero-lag Butterworth low-pass filter (4th order, 6Hz cut-off frequency) and normalized by the maximal EMG value for each muscle obtained during isometric and dynamic tasks. Normalized EMG was transformed to muscle activation by combining a linear second-order differential equation to represent the electromechanical delay and a specific function to represent the non-linear relationship between EMG and muscle activation [29], [32].

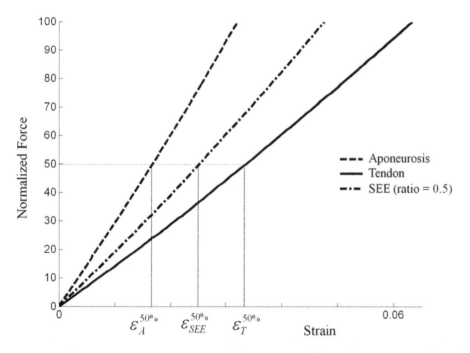

Figure 3. Estimation of Tendon-Aponeurosis force-strain relationship from tendon and aponeurosis individual force-strain relationship. At the same force level, the tendon and aponeurosis strain were estimated and combined with an experimentally-derived ratio to compute the Tendon-Aponeurosis strain (see eq. 5 in text).

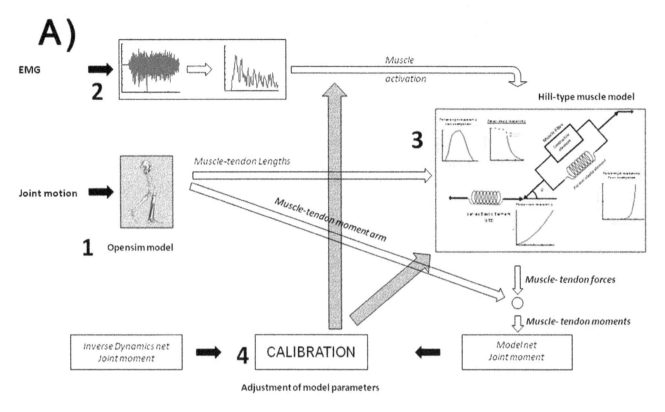

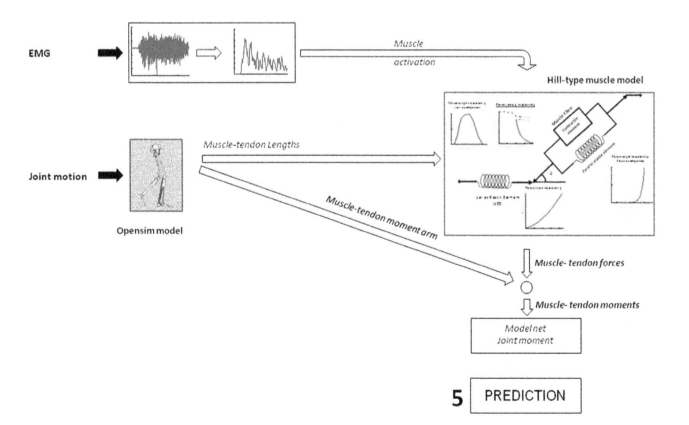

Figure 4. Description of EMG-driven model (A) Calibration and (B) Prediction process of the EMG-driven model. (1) represents the Anatomical Model used to estimate muscle-tendon lengths and moment arms, (2) an EMG-to-Activation Model to represent muscle activation dynamics, (3) a Hill-type Model to characterize muscle-tendon contraction dynamics and estimate the forces in the muscle-tendon complex, (4) a calibration process to tune model parameters based on ankle net joint moment computed by Inverse Dynamic, and (5) a prediction process to predict joint moment by using adjusted model parameters.

The muscle activations and muscle-tendon lengths for each subject were used as inputs into a Hill-type muscle model to estimate muscle forces. In the Hill-type model, the muscle fibre was represented by a contractile element, characterized by a force-length-velocity relationship, in parallel with an elastic element, characterized by a passive force-length relationship. The SEE in series with the muscle fibre was characterised by a force-strain relationship (either generic or subject-specific). During the process of muscle force estimation, the muscle fibre length and velocity were estimated at each time instance such that the muscle fibre force is equal to the SEE force. Finally, muscle forces were multiplied by the muscle-tendon moment arms and summed to determine joint net moment.

Due to the large inter-subject variability, several model parameters need to be adjusted to accurately estimate the ankle joint net moment. During the calibration process, model parameters were adjusted using constrained numerical optimization which minimized the difference between the ankle joint net moment computed by the model (M_i^{MOD}) and the ankle joint net moment estimated through Inverse Dynamics (M_i^{ID}) across the entire trial using the following objective function:

$$\min\left\{\frac{1}{n}\sum_{i=1}^{n}(M_i^{ID}-M_i^{MOD})^2\right\} \tag{6}$$

Two SEE definitions of the Hill-type model were used during the calibration process:

(1) The in-vivo subject-specific tendon-aponeurosis force-strain relationship obtained previously by using ultrasonography (henceforth referred to as SS T-A condition), and (2) the generic definition (henceforth referred to as Generic condition) given by:

$$\begin{cases} \bar{F}_{SEE}=0 & \varepsilon_{SEC} \leq 0 \\ \bar{F}_{SEE}=1480.3\,\varepsilon_{SEE}^2 & 0<\varepsilon_{SEE}<0.0127 \\ \bar{F}_{SEE}=37.5\,\varepsilon_{SEE}-0.2375 & \varepsilon_{SEE}\geq 0.0127 \end{cases} \tag{7}$$

with $\bar{F}_{SEE}$ and ε_{SEE} being the normalized SEE force and the SEE strain respectively [5].

Once the calibration process was completed on one trial of running and hopping, the adjusted model parameters were used to predict the ankle joint net moment using EMG and kinematics data from novel running and hopping trials. The predicted model moments were compared for SS T-A and Generic conditions. The data obtained from model predictions were further named *prediction*.

Data Analysis

Only the prediction process data were analysed to evaluate the robustness of the EMG-driven model (opposite to the calibration process that is more a curve fitting process). The net joint moment predicted by the model was compared with the net joint moment computed by Inverse Dynamics. R^2 represent the coefficient of determination used to indicate the closeness of fit between estimated and measured ankle net joint moment. Correlation

between model and inverse dynamics moments has been used to investigate the ability of the NMS model to predict the net joint moment [30], [31]. The R^2 is computed for each trial on the complete time history such as:

$$R^2=1-\frac{\sum_{i=1}^{n}(M_i^{ID}-\overline{M^{ID}})^2}{\sum_{i=1}^{n}(M_i^{ID}-M_i^{MOD})^2} \tag{8}$$

M_i^{ID} represents the ankle joint net moment computed through inverse dynamics and used as reference, $\overline{M_i^{ID}}$ is the average of ankle joint net moment computed by inverse dynamics, and M_i^{MOD} represents the ankle joint net moment computed by the EMG-driven model.

The residual mean square error (RMS_{error}) reflects the magnitude of the error across the complete time history and is computed as:

$$RMS_{error}=\sqrt{\frac{\sum_{i=1}^{n}(M_i^{ID}-M_i^{MOD})^2}{n}} \tag{9}$$

For each prediction trial, the following model outputs were analysed: maximal net joint moment estimated by the NMS model, maximal muscle forces, variation (maximum value–minimum value) in muscle fibre length, fibre velocity and SEE length.

Student's paired t tests were conducted on the predicted model outputs described previously for GL, GM, SOL and TA muscles. A significance level of 0.05 was set *a priori* for all comparisons and Newman-Keuls Post-Hoc testing was used when necessary.

Results

Tendon-Aponeurosis Properties

The mechanical characterization of tendon and aponeurosis was performed on the GM muscle. The aponeurosis strain was lower than the tendon strain at the same force level, showing the aponeurosis was stiffer than the tendon. Additional measurements were necessary to estimate the ratio between the tendon length and tendon-aponeurosis length. This ratio was lower for the *soleus* muscle (0.23) whereas for the GM and GL muscles the ratio was close to 0.5 highlighting a tendon length equal to the aponeurosis length (Table 1). Whereas the aponeurosis was stiffer than the tendon, the small ratio of *soleus* leads to higher stiffness of the T-A unit compared to the three others muscles (Fig. 5). Finally, the SS T-A force-strain relationships showed higher compliance compared to the generic definition currently used in NMS model (Fig. 5).

EMG-driven Model Inputs and Outputs

Figure 6 illustrates the data used as input to the EMG-driven model and the model outputs in terms of muscle forces and net

Table 1. Summary of muscle-tendon geometric parameters estimated by US in rest position or from Maganaris et al. [6] and used to estimate the muscle specific tendon-aponeurosis force-strain relationships.

	GL	GM	SOL	TA
Initial Fascicle length (mm)	70.2±2.9	59.5±3.6	43.8±4.9	–
Initial pennation angle (°)	13.2±3.2	19.4±1.7	19.4±1.2	–
Initial tendon length (mm)	222.1±32.9	209.9±34.0	61.4±14.6	–
Initial aponeurosis length (mm)	194.0±11.3	219.3±9.1	217.8±19.3	–
Ratio	0.53±0.05	0.49±0.05	0.22±0.04	0.5†

†represent the value used from Maganaris et al. [6].

ankle joint moment. The R^2 for prediction process was significantly higher for SS T-A condition (0.70±0.14) than the Generic condition (0.66±0.16). The averaged RMS_{error} was 44.8±13.4 N.m and 44.8±14.6 N.m respectively for SS T-A condition and the Generic condition. The prediction of the minimal value of the net ankle joint moment was significantly lower for SS T-A condition (-166.2±53.4 N.m) than for the Generic condition (-145.7±42.2 N.m).

The use of subject-specific tendon-aponeurosis definition led to higher muscle force estimations for the plantar-flexor group than the generic condition (4988.9±1602.5 N vs. 4246.0±992.3 N) and the *soleus* muscle (3444.8±1136.7 N vs. 2870.5±803.6 N) (Fig. 7). No significant difference was found for the other three muscles.

The EMG-driven model computed the muscle fibre length and velocity to estimate the muscle force. Compared to the generic condition, the use of SS T-A definition leads to an increase of the SEE length variation and a decrease of the fibre length and velocity variations for the *soleus* muscle (Table 2).

Discussion

In the present study, the influence of subject-specific tendon-aponeurosis properties in NMS models was investigated for variables such as the muscle forces and muscle fibre behaviour. The subject-specific tendon-aponeurosis was first estimated for the medial head of the gastrocnemius combining motion capture and two ultrasound probes, and then scaled for each muscle by using a ratio between the tendon length and the aponeurosis length in rest position. The subject-specific definition of tendon-aponeurosis unit was more compliant than the generic definition from Zajac [5] currently used in most NMS models. This subject-specific definition was then used as input into EMG-driven model to estimate muscle forces during hopping and running. The use of

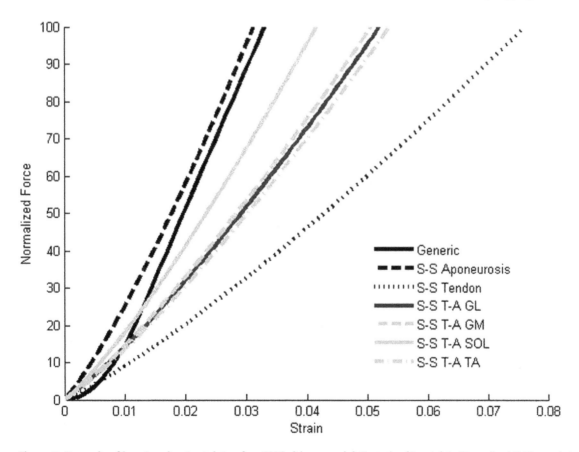

Figure 5. Example of input and output data of an EMG-driven model. Example of input data (Normalized EMG, muscle-tendon lengths and moment-arms) and output data (muscle forces and net ankle joint moment) for one subject during the contact phase of a hopping trial. The output data were obtained for both SEE definitions: the SS T-A and the generic.

Input of EMG-driven model

Output of EMG-driven model

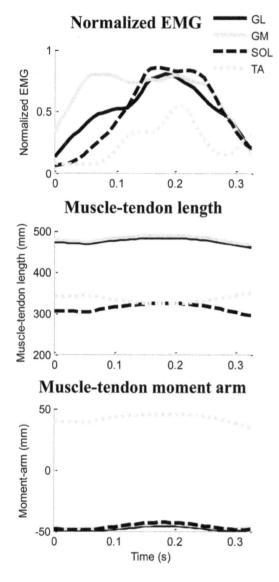

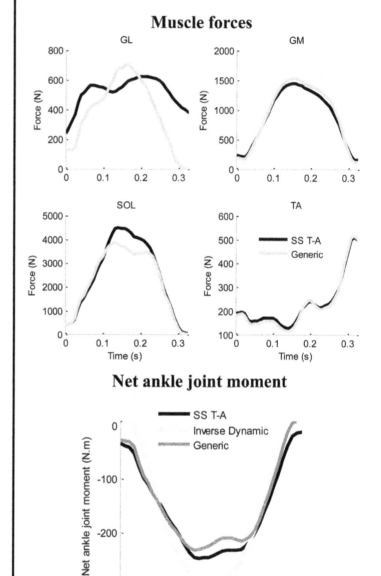

Figure 6. Force-strain relationships estimated by ultrasonography and used in Hill-type muscle model. Group averaged subject-specific tendon and aponeurosis force-strain relationships of the GM and subject-specific Tendon-Aponeurosis force-strain relationships for each muscle. The generic tendon force-strain relationship described by Zajac [5] and used for the generic calibration and prediction processes is also presented for comparison.

subject-specific tendon-aponeurosis in an EMG-Driven model leads to higher muscle force estimations.

Mechanical Characterization of T-A

The mechanical characterization of the tendon and the aponeurosis emphasize that these two components have different mechanical properties, with the aponeurosis being stiffer than tendon. This difference in properties means both the tendon

and the aponeurosis need to be defined separately. Given the different tendon and the aponeurosis stiffness, additional measurements of the GM, GL and SOL were performed to estimate the ratio between the tendon and aponeurosis lengths at rest. Based on this ratio, the tendon-aponeurosis force-strain relationship was scaled for each muscle and each subject. We hypothesized that the mechanical properties of the tendon and the aponeurosis are the same for all the studied muscles. This

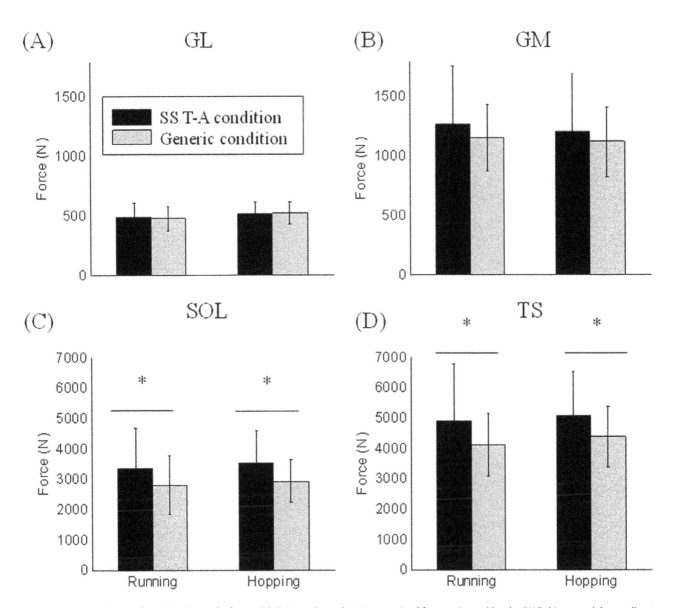

Figure 7. Comparison of maximal muscle force: SS T-A vs. Generic. Mean maximal force estimated by the EMG-driven model according to the condition, SS T-A and Generic for the GL (A), GM (B), SOL (C) and the *Triceps Surae* group (i.e., sum of GL, GM, and Sol muscles) (D). * indicates a significant difference between the conditions (SS T-A vs. Generic).

assumption seems reasonable as the tendon of the GM muscle has a common distal part with the GL and SOL muscles, suggesting a close behaviour. However, further studies on

mechanical characterization of tendon and aponeurosis for all three plantar-flexor muscles will be necessary to validate this hypothesis. A constant ratio was used for the Tibialis Anterior

Table 2. Summary of the behaviour of the muscle fibre and the tendon-aponeurosis unit in terms of variation of length and velocity.

	GL		GM		SOL	
	SS T-A	Generic	SS T-A	Generic	SS T-A	Generic
Variation of fibre velocity (mm.s⁻¹)	563±13	655±184	476±139*	599±147*	524±136*	652±137*
Variation of fibre length (mm)	24±3	27±3	19±3	22±1	22±4*	25±3*
Variation of SEE length (mm)	6±2*	4±1*	10±4*	8±2*	10±3*	7±2*

*Significative difference between SS T-A and Generic.

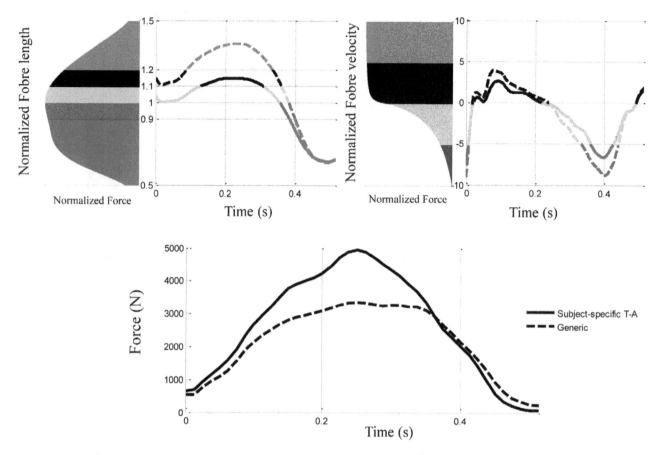

Figure 8. Normalized fibre length and velocity with corresponding muscle forces for the *soleus*. Trajectory of normalized fibre length and velocity for one subject corresponding to the *soleus*. The colours of the curve represent the different part of the force-length and force-velocity relationships cover by the normalized fibre length and velocity according to the SEE definition. The figure at the bottom represents the muscle forces according to the SEE definition.

muscle based on previous measurements [14]. The contribution of the TA to the ankle joint is small compared to the three other muscles and the lack of effect of SS T-A on TA muscle variables suggest that it's most important to be focused on the three other muscles than the TA. The ratio was close to 0.5 for the GM and GL whereas the mean value was 0.23 for the SOL. This lower ratio for the soleus leads to tendon-aponeurosis characterization stiffer than the three others muscles but still less stiff than the generic condition currently used into EMG-driven model [7]. Taken together, these results suggest a clear difference in terms of mechanical properties of the SEE for the two conditions tested in the present study (i.e., generic vs. SS T-A).

Muscle Force Estimations

Our results showed the importance of the SEE definition in muscle force estimations as the muscles forces and ankle net joint moment estimations were strongly affected during hopping and running tasks. The use of SS T-A definition in Hill-type muscle model leads to higher muscle forces for the *soleus* and the plantar-flexor group (i.e., sum of the soleus and the gastrocnemii muscles). The higher force for the plantar-flexor group explains the higher absolute value of ankle net joint moment computed by the EMG-driven model with the SS T-A definition. In addition, the use of SS T-A improves the prediction ability of the model by a 4% increase in the R^2 value.

The effect of SEE definition in Hill-type muscle model has been previously investigated through simulations [19], [30], [33]. These simulations were focused on the determination of an arbitrary value of SEE compliance maximizing either the performance or the muscle force. They have shown that the use of less stiff SEE definition in Hill-type muscle model increases either the estimation of muscle force or the squat jump performance. Whereas simulations represent an average subject with an arbitrary choice of the SEE compliance, our study combined subject-specific patterns of muscle activations from EMG, kinematic motion and external ground reaction forces and subject-specific SEE definition. The results of our study are in agreement with these previous simulations showing that an increase of SEE compliance leads to estimate higher muscle forces during highly dynamic tasks. The generic Zajac definition appears to be too stiff to well represent the SEE into Hill-type muscle model. To our knowledge, the present study is the first to report specific T-A properties that are able to maximize the muscle force production during human movement.

Decoupling Behaviour between Muscle Fibre and Muscle-tendon Unit

The force produced by the muscle fibre depends on the force-length and force-velocity relationships. In Hill-type models, the fibre behaviour is computed at each time such that the force produced by the muscle fibre is equal to the force produced by the SEE. The use of SS T-A definition leads to decrease the variation

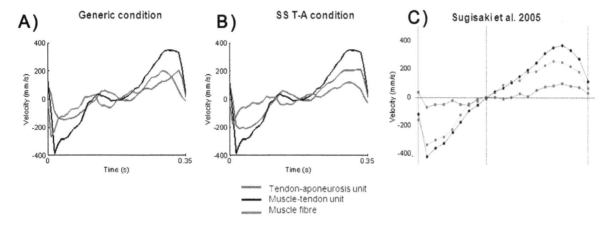

Figure 9. Decoupling behaviour between muscle fibre and muscle-tendon unit. Comparison of the velocity of the muscle fibre, the tendon-aponeurosis unit and the muscle-tendon unit from one subject on running tasks for the (A) generic and (B) SS T-A conditions and from (C) a previous experimentation with the muscle fibre velocity measured using ultrasonography. Note that the SS T-A condition leads to physiologically sound behaviour of the muscle fibre while the generic condition simply shared the muscle-tendon stretch over both the fibre and the SEE complex. Reprinted with permission.

of fibre length and velocity. According to the force-velocity relationship, this decrease of shortening velocity due to less stiff definition of the SEE increases the corresponding muscle force for the same muscle activation (Fig. 8). The decrease in fibre length moves the muscle fibre closer to its optimal force length relationship and hence closer to maximal force. This different behaviour of muscle fibre obtained by using SS T-A definition explains the higher muscle force for the soleus.

The *in vivo* measurement of muscle forces is difficult due to the invasiveness of direct measurement methods (i.e surgical implants, etc...). In the present study, the validation of the estimation of muscle forces was not directly possible. Ultrasonography has been previously used to investigate the behaviour of the muscle fibre relative to the muscle-tendon unit. During walking task in humans, Ishikawa and al. [2] have shown the presence of a decoupling between muscle fascicle and muscle-tendon unit behaviours. During highly a dynamic task such as a drop jump, this decoupling is less important but remains present [2], [4]. The use of SS T-A definition leads to a lower muscle fibre velocity and a higher SEE velocity (i.e., a strong decoupling behaviour) compared to the use of generic definition. This higher decoupling behaviour between the muscle fibre and SEE is in agreement with previous experimental recordings. Sugisaki et al. [34] have combined motion capture and ultrasonography to investigate the behaviour of muscle fibre relative to the muscle-tendon unit for the GM muscle during dynamic contractions. Figure 9 illustrates the similarity of the behaviour of the SEE and the muscle fibre when using the SS T-A definition in a NMS model relative to the experimental measurements of Sugisaki et al. [34]. The comparison with experimental measurements highlights that the use of generic Zajac definition failed to represent a physiological behaviour of muscle fibre. The conformity of our results with previous experiments provides us with confidence in our modelling methods. We hypothesize that the higher predicted muscle forces from NMS models using a subject-specific SEE definition was a more physiologically accurate approach than the use of a generic definition.

Perspectives

In this study, we were focused on the subject-specific tendon-aponeurosis force-strain relationship. Li et al. [35] have shown that the use of subject-specific optimal fibre length and pennation angle data improves the prediction of elbow movement for healthy individuals and stroke victims. The ultrasonography has also been used to estimate the subject-specific moment arm [36]. Further studies are necessary to investigate the influence of additional subject-specific muscle-tendon parameters into NMS models such as moment arm, and combined *in vivo* aponeurosis-tendon force-strain relationship, initial and optimal fibre length, and pennation angle.

Conclusion

This study highlights the importance of using subject-specific measurements in terms of SEE definition in Hill-type muscle models during dynamic tasks. Subject-specific SEE induced a 17% increase in maximal predicted muscle force. Furthermore, it resulted in improved physiologically behaviour of the muscle fibre. Moreover, the present work combined direct experimental measurements to characterize the *in vivo* properties of the tendon-aponeurosis unit with the implementation of the results in a neuromusculoskeletal model to estimate muscle forces and fibre behaviours. Based on our results, the NMS model was able to numerically replicate experimental results showing a decoupling behaviour between the fibre and the muscle-tendon unit. The mechanical properties of tendon and aponeurosis may be altered by musculoskeletal disorders such as stroke [37], [38] or by ageing [39]. The present study demonstrates that it is crucial to take into account alterations of tendon-aponeurosis mechanical properties in order to accurately treat characterize muscle function.

Author Contributions

Conceived and designed the experiments: PG GR EB. Performed the experiments: PG. Analyzed the data: PG GR. Contributed reagents/materials/analysis tools: PG. Wrote the paper: PG GR EB.

References

1. Griffiths RI (1991) Shortening of muscle fibres during stretch of the active cat medial gastrocnemius muscle: the role of tendon compliance. Journal of Physiology 436: 219–236.
2. Ishikawa M, Komi PV, Grey MJ, Lepola V, Bruggemann GP (2005) Muscle-tendon interaction and elastic energy usage in human walking. Journal of Applied Physiology 99: 603–608.
3. Ishikawa M, Niemel E, Komi PV (2005) Interaction between fascicle and tendinous tissues in short- contact stretch-shortening cycle exercise with varying eccentric intensities. Journal of Applied Physiology 99: 217–223.
4. Sousa F, Ishikawa M, Vilas-Boas JP, Komi PV (2007) Intensity- and muscle-specific fascicle behavior during human drop jumps. Journal of Applied Physiology 102: 382–389.
5. Zajac FE (1989) Muscle and tendon: properties, models, scaling, and application to biomechanics and motor control. Critical Reviews in Biomedical Engineering 17: 359–411.
6. Maganaris CN (2002) Tensile properties of in vivo human tendinous tissue. Journal of Biomechanics 35: 1019–1027.
7. Burgess KE, Pearson SJ, Breen L, Onambele GNL (2009) Tendon structural and mechanical properties do not differ between genders in a healthy community-dwelling elderly population. Journal of Orthopaedic Research 27: 820–825.
8. Duclay J, Martin A, Duclay A, Cometti G, Pousson M (2009) Behavior of fascicles and the myotendinous junction of human medial gastrocnemius following eccentric strength training. Muscle Nerve 39: 819–827.
9. Kubo K, Kanehisa H, Azuma K, Ishizu M, Kuno SY, et al. (2003) Muscle architectural characteristics in young and elderly men and women. International Journal of Sports Medicine 24: 125–130.
10. Pearson SJ, Burgess K, Onambele GNL (2007) Creep and the in vivo assessment of human patellar tendon mechanical properties. Clinical Biomechanics 22: 712–717.
11. Gerus P, Rao G, Berton E (2011) A method to characterize in vivo tendon force-strain relationship by combining ultrasonography, motion capture and loading rates. Journal of Biomechanics 44: 2333–2336.
12. Muramatsu T, Muraoka T, Takeshita D, Kawakami Y, Hirano Y, et al. (2001) Mechanical properties of tendon and aponeurosis of human gastrocnemius muscle in vivo. Journal of Applied Physiology 90: 1671–1678.
13. Stafilidis S, Karamanidis K, Morey-Klapsing G, Demonte G, Bruggemann GP, et al. (2005) Strain and elongation of the vastus lateralis aponeurosis and tendon in vivo during maximal isometric contraction. European Journal of Applied Physiology 94: 317–322.
14. Maganaris CN, Paul JP (2000) In vivo human tendinous tissue stretch upon maximum muscle force generation. Journal of Biomechanics 33: 1453–1459.
15. Maganaris CN, Paul JP (2000) Load-elongation characteristics of in vivo human tendon and aponeurosis. Journal of Experimental Biology 203: 751–756.
16. Magnusson SP, Hansen P, Aagaard P, Brond J, Dyhre-Poulsen P, et al. (2003) Differential strain patterns of the human gastrocnemius aponeurosis and free tendon, in vivo. Acta Physiologica Scandinavica 177: 185–195.
17. Tilp M, Steib S, Herzog W (2012) Length changes of human tibialis anterior central aponeurosis during passive movements and isometric, concentric, and eccentric contractions. Eur J Appl Physiol 112: 1485–1494.
18. Lieber RL, Brown CG, Trestik CL (1992) Model of muscle-tendon interaction during frog semitendinosis fixed-end contractions. Journal of Biomechanics 25: 421–428.
19. Bobbert MF (2001) Dependence of human squat jump performance on the series elastic compliance of the triceps surae: a simulation study. Journal of Experimental Biology 204: 533–542.
20. Oda T, Kanehisa H, Chino K, Kurihara T, Nagayoshi T, et al. (2007) In vivo behavior of muscle fascicles and tendinous tissues of human gastrocnemius and soleus muscles during twitch contraction. Journal of Electromyography and Kinesiololgy 17: 587–595.
21. Lichtwark GA, Wilson AM (2005) In vivo mechanical properties of the human achilles tendon during one-legged hopping. Journal of Experimental Biology 208: 4715–4725.
22. Korstanje JWH, Selles RW, Stam HJ, Hovius SER, Bosch JG (2010) Development and validation of ultrasound speckle tracking to quantify tendon displacement. Journal of Biomechanics 43: 1373–1379.
23. Fukashiro S (2006) Comparison of the muscle-tendon complex behavior in the gastrocnemius during 4 types of human vertical jumping in-vivo. International Journal of Sport and Health Science 4: 298–302.
24. Finni T, Komi PV (2002) Two method for estimating tendinous tissue elongation during human movement. Journal of Applied Biomechanics 18: 180–188.
25. Muramatsu T, Muraoka T, Kawakami Y, Shibayama A, Fukunaga T (2002) In vivo determination of fascicle curvature in contracting human skeletal muscles. Journal of Applied Physiology 92: 129–134.
26. Shin DD, Hodgson JA, Edgerton VR, Sinha S (2009) In vivo intramuscular fascicle-aponeuroses dynamics of the human medial gastrocnemius during plantarflexion and dorsiflexion of the foot. Journal of Applied Physiology 107: 1276–1284.
27. Lichtwark GA, Bougoulias K, Wilson AM (2007) Muscle fascicle and series elastic element length changes along the length of the human gastrocnemius during walking and running. Journal of Biomechanics 40: 157–164.
28. Delp SL, Anderson FC, Arnold AS, Loan P, Habib A, et al. (2007) Opensim: open-source soft- ware to create and analyze dynamic simulations of movement. IEEE Transactions on Bio-Medical Engineering 54: 1940–1950.
29. Kubo K, Kanehisa H, Kawakami Y, Fukunaga T (2001) Effects of repeated muscle contractions on the tendon structures in humans. European Journal of Applied Physiology 84: 162–166.
30. Buchanan TS, Lloyd DG, Manal K, Besier TF (2004) Neuromusculoskeletal modeling: estimation of muscle forces and joint moments and movements from measurements of neural command. Journal of Applied Biomechanics 20: 367–395.
31. Lloyd DG, Besier TF (2003) An emg-driven musculoskeletal model to estimate muscle forces and knee joint moments in vivo. Journal of Biomechanics 36: 765–776.
32. Manal K, Buchanan TS (2003) A one-parameter neural activation to muscle activation model: estimating isometric joint moments from electromyograms. Journal of Biomechanics 36: 1197–1202.
33. Domire ZJ, Challis JH (2007) The influence of an elastic tendon on the force producing capabilities of a muscle during dynamic movements. Computer Methods in Biomechanics and Biomedical Engineering 10: 337–341.
34. Sugisaki N, Kanehisa H, Kawakami Y, Fukunaga T (2005) Behavior of fascicle and tendinous tissue of medial gastrocnemius muscle during rebound exercise of ankle joint. Internation Journal of Sport and Health Science 3: 100–109.
35. Li L, Tong KY, Hu XL, Hung LK, Koo TKK (2009) Incorporating ultrasound-measured muscu- lotendon parameters to subject-specific emg-driven model to simulate voluntary elbow flexion for persons after stroke. Clinical Biomechanics 24: 101–109.
36. Manal K, Cowder JD, Buchanan TS (2010) A hybrid method for computing achilles tendon moment arm using ultrasound and motion analysis. Journal of Applied Biomechanics 26: 224–228.
37. Gao F, Ren Y, Roth EJ, Harvey R, Zhang LQ (2011) Effects of repeated ankle stretching on calf muscle-tendon and ankle biomechanical properties in stroke survivors. Clinical Biomechanics 26: 516–522.
38. Zhao H, Ren Y, Wu YN, Liu SQ, Zhang LQ (2009) Ultrasonic evaluations of achilles tendon mechanical properties poststroke. Journal of Applied Physiology 106: 843–849.
39. Karamanidis K, Arampatzis A (2005) Mechanical and morphological properties of different muscle- tendon units in the lower extremity and running mechanics: effect of aging and physical activity. Journal of Experimental Biology 208: 3907–3923.

9

The Proton Pump Inhibitor Lansoprazole Improves the Skeletal Phenotype in Dystrophin Deficient *mdx* Mice

Arpana Sali[1], Gina M. Many[1], Heather Gordish-Dressman[1], Jack H. van der Meulen[1], Aditi Phadke[1], Christopher F. Spurney[1,2], Avital Cnaan[1], Eric P. Hoffman[1], Kanneboyina Nagaraju[1]*

1 Center for Genetic Medicine Research, Children's National Medical Center, Department of Integrative Systems Biology, George Washington University School of Medicine and Health Sciences, Washington, DC, United States of America, 2 Division of Cardiology, Children's National Medical Center, Washington, DC, United States of America

Abstract

Background: In Duchenne muscular dystrophy (DMD), loss of the membrane stabilizing protein dystrophin results in myofiber damage. Microinjury to dystrophic myofibers also causes secondary imbalances in sarcolemmic ion permeability and resting membrane potential, which modifies excitation-contraction coupling and increases proinflammatory/apoptotic signaling cascades. Although glucocorticoids remain the standard of care for the treatment of DMD, there is a need to investigate the efficacy of other pharmacological agents targeting the involvement of imbalances in ion flux on dystrophic pathology.

Methodology/Principal Findings: We designed a preclinical trial to investigate the effects of lansoprazole (LANZO) administration, a proton pump inhibitor, on the dystrophic muscle phenotype in dystrophin deficient (*mdx*) mice. Eight to ten week-old female mice were assigned to one of four treatment groups (n = 12 per group): (1) vehicle control; (2) 5 mg/kg/day LANZO; (3) 5 mg/kg/day prednisolone; and (4) combined treatment of 5 mg/kg/day prednisolone (PRED) and 5 mg/kg/day LANZO. Treatment was administered orally 5 d/wk for 3 months. At the end of the study, behavioral (Digiscan) and functional outcomes (grip strength and Rotarod) were assessed prior to sacrifice. After sacrifice, body, tissue and organ masses, muscle histology, *in vitro* muscle force, and creatine kinase levels were measured. Mice in the combined treatment groups displayed significant reductions in the number of degenerating muscle fibers and number of inflammatory foci per muscle field relative to vehicle control. Additionally, mice in the combined treatment group displayed less of a decline in normalized forelimb and hindlimb grip strength and declines in *in vitro* EDL force after repeated eccentric contractions.

Conclusions/Significance: Together our findings suggest that combined treatment of LANZO and prednisolone attenuates some components of dystrophic pathology in *mdx* mice. Our findings warrant future investigation of the clinical efficacy of LANZO and prednisolone combined treatment regimens in dystrophic pathology.

Editor: Ronald Cohn, Johns Hopkins University School of Medicine, United States of America

Funding: Funding for this work was provided by Charley's Fund (http://www.charleysfund.com), the Department of Defense USAMRAA (W81XWH-05-1-0616), the Foundation to Eradicate Duchenne, Inc. (http://www.duchennemd.org), the Muscular Dystrophy Association, and the National Institutes of Health (R01-AR050478, K26OD011171, and 1U54HD053177). This work was also partially supported by the National Center for Medical Rehabilitation Research/National Institute for Neurological Disorders and Stroke (2R24HD050846-06). The funders had no role in study design, data collection and analysis, decision to publish, or preparation of the manuscript.

Competing Interests: The authors have declared that no competing interests exist.

* E-mail: knagaraju@cnmcresearch.org

Introduction

Dystrophin is located in the cytoplasmic portion of the sarcolemma and aids in muscle membrane stability and structural integrity. Dystrophin and other proteins of the dystrophin-associated complex serve as scaffolding proteins that regulate the association of proteins, such as ion channels, with the sarcolemma. Loss of dystrophin is thought to destabilize the myofiber membrane, in part, by altering the flux of ions and other proteins through the sarcolemma [1]. This is supported by observations of altered intracellular concentrations of Ca^{2+} [2], Mg^{2+} [2], K^+ [3], and Na^+ [4] within dystrophic myofibers. Such alterations in intracellular ion concentrations likely contribute to reductions in resting membrane potential, membrane resistivity, and excitability [5,6] observed in in dystrophic myofibers, which negatively affects muscle function. Further, increases in intracellular Ca^{2+} levels within dystrophic fibers induce myofiber necrosis via increasing protease activity [7].

The progression of dystrophic pathology occurs as multiple mechanical and inflammatory insults contribute to chronic degeneration-regeneration remodeling cycles. Therapies aimed at reducing muscle inflammation, i.e. glucocorticoids, remain the standard-of-care for dystrophic pathology. Despite the acknowledged efficacy and widespread use of glucocorticoids, they do not fully ameliorate dystrophic pathology. Diets high in NaCl have been shown to attenuate myofiber necrosis and serum creatine kinase levels in *mdx* mice [8], suggesting that manipulation of systemic ion concentration gradients may help alleviate dystrophic pathology. This data also suggests a need to investigate the therapeutic efficacy of compounds capable of altering sarcolemmic ion flux.

Lansoprazole, 2-[(4-trifluoroethoxy-3-methyl-2-pyridyl)methyl-sulfinyl]-1H-benzimidazole, is a 369.36 kDa substituted benzimidazole that acts as a gastric proton pump inhibitor (PPI). Lansoprazole (LANZO) reduces stomach acidity by binding to hydrogen-potassium adenosine triphosphatase (H^+/K^+-ATPase) pumps located on the apical surface of gastric parietal cells. LANZO H^+/K^+-ATPase binding inhibits parietal cell secretion of hydrogen ions into the gastric cavity. LANZO is widely used in the treatment of gastroesophageal reflux disease (GERD) and peptic ulcers. In addition to reducing gastric acidity, LANZO has been observed to attenuate inflammation in the gastric mucosa [9,10] and inhibit nitric oxide (NO) [11] production by macrophages, suggesting that an additional mechanism of LANZO action in the gut may include its anti-inflammatory properties. A similar PPI, omeprazole, has been shown to decrease the activity of immune cells in the peripheral blood after oral administration in healthy human subjects [11], suggesting LANZO may act systemically to attenuate inflammation. Inflammation is a major component of the dystrophic phenotypic in *mdx* mice and proinflammatory macrophage accumulation has been shown to lyse dystrophic fibers in an NO-dependent manner [12]. We thus sought to investigate the effects of this proton pump inhibitor on the skeletal muscle phenotype in *mdx* mice. We hypothesized that LANZO administration would attenuate the dystrophic skeletal muscle phenotype via altering ion influx and attenuating proinflammatory and apoptotic signaling cascades underlying the dystrophic pathology.

In this study, eight to ten week-old *mdx* mice were orally dosed with a saline vehicle control, LANZO, prednisolone, or a combined treatment regimen to determine the therapeutic efficacy of each treatment. After three months of treatment, dual LANZO and prednisolone administration was found to reduce serum creatine kinase levels, the number of degenerating muscle fibers, and the number of gastrocnemius inflammatory foci. Combined treatment of LANZO and prednisolone also improved *in vitro* and *in vivo* muscle force relative to vehicle control. Findings from our study, thus, warrant future investigation of the therapeutic efficacy of combined glucocorticoid and LANZO treatment regimens in the treatment of dystrophic pathology.

Materials and Methods

Animal Care

This protocol was approved by the Children's National Medical Center Institutional Animal Care and Use Committee (IACUC) guidelines (Protocol # 1206) and thereby all animals were treated according to local IACUC standards. C57BL/10ScSn-Dmdmdx/ J (*mdx*) 8–10 week-old female mice were purchased from Jackson Laboratories (Bar Harbor, ME). All mice were acclimated for 7 days prior to study initiation and individually housed in a vented cage system with 12 h alternating light-dark cycles. Mice received standard mouse chow and purified water *ad libitum*.

Study Design

Four experimental treatment groups with 12 animals per group were included in this study: (a) vehicle control group receiving saline solution (0.9% NaCl, the vehicle used for LANZO administration); (b) experimental group treated with 5 mg/kg/ day LANZO; (c) experimental group treated with 5 mg/kg/day prednisolone; and (d) combined treatment group receiving 5 mg/ kg/day prednisolone and 5 mg/kg/day LANZO. Saline and LANZO were administered via oral gavage, and prednisolone was

Table 1. Comparison of muscle and organ weights between treatment groups at time of sacrifice.

Tissue Weight	Vehicle N	Vehicle Mean ± SEM	LANZO N	LANZO Mean ± SEM	PRED N	PRED Mean ± SEM	Combined N	Combined Mean ± SEM	Overall p-value	Significantly different means
Total Body Mass* (g)	10#	24.9±0.63	12	24.0±0.33	12	24.1±0.33	12	23.9±0.54	NS	None
Gastrocnemius (mg)*	10	134.9±2.9	12	135.6±1.8	12	131.7±3.8	12	126.2±3.1	NS	None
Soleus (mg)*	10	8.2±0.4	12	8.2±0.2	12	8.3±0.3	12	8.3±0.3	NS	None
EDL (mg)*	10	10.3±0.4	12	11.4±0.4	12	11.7±0.4	12	11.1±0.2	NS	None
Heart (mg)	10	82.6±1.4	12	81.0±2.1	12	82.3±1.5	12	84.0±2.7	NS	None
Spleen (mg)	10	94.3±4.2	12	95.0±6.0	12	72.9±4.2[b, ab]	12	68.3±5.7[c, ac]	<0.001	[b]Veh vs. PRED (p = 0.038); [c]Veh vs. Combined (p = 0.007); [ab]LANZO vs. PRED (p = 0.021); [ac]LANZO vs. Combined (p = 0.003)

Footnotes:
*Body mass was significantly different between groups at baseline, therefore, baseline body mass was included as a covariate in ANOVA modeling.
#Two of the mice in the vehicle control group died before the time of sacrifice and thus 10 mice were analyzed at study completion in the untreated group.
*The muscle weights presented represent average weight between right and left muscle groups.

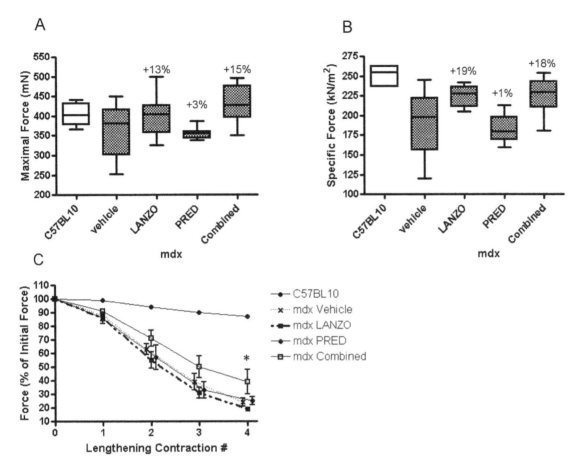

Figure 1. Effect of treatment on in vitro muscle force. The maximal (A) and specific (B) EDL muscle force was compared between vehicle control (n = 8), LANZO (n = 7), prednisolone (n = 8), and combined treatment groups (n = 9). The percent differences in maximal or specific force relative to vehicle control are presented above the error bars. No statistically significant differences in maximal muscle force were detected within treatment groups. There were statistically significant within group differences in specific muscle force (p = 0.0242), although no statistically significant between group differences were observed. (C) The EDL muscles of C57Bl/10 and *mdx* mice in each of the four treatment groups were subjected to four lengthening contractions and the decline in maximal force was tested using a mixed-effects linear regression model. Maximal force was also shown to decrease after each subsequent contraction due to the damage incurred by the lengthening contractions. *The overall decline in maximal force was significantly lower in response to repeated lengthening contractions in the combined treatment group relative to vehicle control.

administered via oral drops. Each of the treatment regimens was administered 5 days per week (Monday-Friday) for 3 months. All functional, behavioral and histological assessments were acquired and analyzed in a blinded fashion.

Treadmill Exercise

Treadmill exercise was performed on all mice before and during the 3-month treatment regimen to unmask the mild dystrophic phenotype of *mdx* mice based on previous studies demonstrating an exacerbation of the dystrophic phenotype in *mdx* mice with treadmill exercise [13]. All mice were exercised on a horizontal treadmill (Columbus Instruments, Columbus, OH) 2 days per week at a treadmill speed of 12 m/min for 30 min per day in accordance to the Treat NMD standard operating procedure for preclinical studies using *mdx* mice (http://www.treat-nmd.eu/downloads/file/sops/dmd/MDX/DMD_M.2.1.001.pdf). All exercise was performed between 0800 h and 1200 h and completed 1–2 days prior to functional testing.

Rotarod Testing

Rotarod testing was performed according to methods we have described previously [14,15,16]. Briefly, mice were trained on a

Rotarod apparatus (UgoBasile, VA, Italy) for 2 days prior to data collection on day 3. Each trial was performed twice per day, consecutively for 3 days, with a 2 h interval between sessions before and after the three-month pre-clinical trial. The latency to fall score was measured six times per trial for each mouse. The average latency to fall score was then calculated using data from each of the six trials and was expressed in seconds for each mouse tested.

Grip Strength Testing

Forelimb and hindlimb grip strength was assessed at the beginning and end of the trial in order to evaluate changes in motor strength in response to the different treatment regimens. Forelimb and hindlimb grip strength measurements were performed using a Grip Strength Meter (Columbus Instruments, Columbus, OH). Grip strength was quantified by averaging five successful hindlimb and forelimb strength measurements each recorded within a 2 min time interval in order to calculate absolute grip strength. All strength measures were then normalized to individual animal body mass to calculate normalized grip strength, expressed in kgf/kg, as described previously [16].

Table 2. Effect of treatment on functional outcomes following 3 months of treatment.

Measurement	N	Vehicle Mean ± SEM	N	LANZO Mean ± SEM	N	PRED Mean ± SEM	N	Combined Mean ± SEM	Overall p-value	Significantly different means
Body weight (g)*	10	24.9±0.63	12	24.0±0.33	12	24.1±0.33	12	23.9±0.54	NS	None
Forelimb GSM (kgf)*	10	0.102±0.003	12	0.101±0.002	12	0.102±0.003	12	0.113±0.003[ac]	0.0368	[ac]LANZO vs. Combined (p = 0.049)
Hindlimb GSM (kgf)	10	0.185±0.004	12	0.198±0.004	12	0.192±0.003	12	0.204±0.003[c]	0.0099	[c]Veh vs. Combined (p = 0.009)
Normalized Forelimb GSM (kgf/kg)*	10	4.282±0.144	12	4.279±0.120	12	4.225±0.130	12	4.553±0.120	NS	None
Normalized Hindlimb GSM (kgf/kg)*	10	7.983±0.240	12	8.420±0.208	12	7.855±0.209	12	8.065±0.217	NS	None

Footnotes:
*Baseline measurements were significantly different between groups and thus baseline measurements were used as a covariate in ANOVA models.

Behavioral Activity Measurement

Open field behavioral activity was measured using an open field Digiscan apparatus (Omnitech Electronics, Columbus, OH) in order to assess locomotor activity as described previously [16]. All mice were acclimated 60 min prior to data collection. Outcome variables included total vertical and horizontal activity, total distance traveled, movement time, and rest time. Data were collected every 10 min over a 1 h period before and after the pre-clinical trial.

Histological Evaluations

At the end of the study, all mice were euthanized via carbon dioxide exposure, and organ and tissue samples were collected for histological evaluation. After weighing, a portion of each of the dissected tissues (i.e., gastrocnemius, EDL, soleus, heart and spleen) was kept in formalin for H&E staining. The remaining portion of each tissue was embedded in OCT compound and frozen in isopentane chilled in liquid nitrogen. Sections were imaged using a Nikon E800 microscope and taken at a magnification of 20x. Five non-overlapping field images representative of the overall tissue histology were captured using digital imaging computer software (Olympus C.A.S.T. Stereology System, Center Valley, PA). All of the digital images were uploaded into Image J Software (NIH, Bethesda, MD) for analysis using a cell counter software plug-in. The number of inflammatory foci and fibrosis were assessed in the diaphragm between treatment groups. Diaphragm fibrosis was assessed by use of Picro sirius red staining with a Weigert's haematoxylin nuclear counter stain on diaphragm cross-sections. In gastrocnemius cross-sections the total number of degenerating, regenerating and inflammatory foci per field were quantified in order to assess differences between treatment groups. The average number of fibers sampled in the 5 non-overlapping cross-sections was 170, with a range of 88–300 fibers per field. Fibers displaying a loss of striations/homogenous appearance of fiber contents were counted as degenerating fibers.

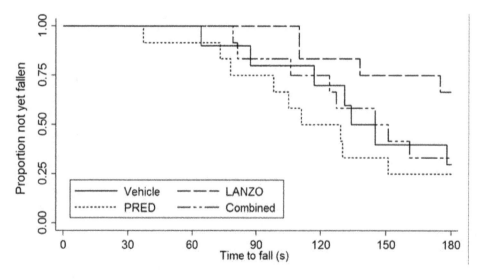

Figure 2. Effect of treatment on Rotarod latency to fall. Latency to fall time was measured between treatment groups (n = 12 per group, with the exception of the vehicle control [n = 10]) via Rotarod testing during the last week of the trial. The data analyzed is an average of six latency to fall scores where Rotarod testing was performed two times per day for 3 consecutive days after a 24 h acclimation period. Time to fall was compared between treatment groups using a log-rank test and Kaplan-Meier estimate. Although the LANZO and combined treatment groups displayed a greater median time to fall, no statistically significant differences were detected between treatment groups.

Table 3. Effect of treatment on open field behavioral (locomotor) activity.

Post-Treatment Measurement	Vehicle		LANZO		PRED		Combined		Overall p-value
	N	Median (range)	N	Median (range)	N	Median (range)	N	Median (range)	
HACTV	10	1213 (785–2212)	12	1266 (772–2021)	12	1266 (995–1963)	12	1096 (402–1963)	NS
TOTDIST	10	251 (155–841)	12	273 (114–628)	12	253 (182–516)	12	213 (64–516)	NS
MOVTIME	10	27 (16–101)	12	29 (11–74)	12	28 (20–64)	12	25 (9–64)	NS
RESTIME	10	573 (499–584)	12	571 (526–589)	12	573 (536–580)	12	576 (536–591)	NS
VACTV	10	14 (10–88)	12	14 (7–37)	12	21 (12–47)	12	21 (3–47)	NS

Legend:
HACTV = total horizontal activity; TOTDIST = total movement distance; MOVTIME = total movement time; RESTIME = total rest time; VACTV = total vertical activity.

Regenerating fibers were counted as fibers with basophilic cytoplasm, large peripheral, or central nuclei with prominent nucleoli. All cell counts per image field (degenerating/regenerating fibers and inflammatory foci) were assessed in a blinded manner as described previously [16].

Creatine Kinase Determination

Blood for creatine kinase (CK) assay was collected by cardiac puncture into preservative-free Eppendorf tubes immediately after animal sacrifice. Blood serum was isolated by centrifugation for CK activity determination by standard enzymatic assay preformed according to the manufacturer's instructions (CK10, Fisher Scientific). Enzymatic activity was calculated by measuring light absorption on a spectrometer set at 340 nm every minute for a total of 2 min at 37°C. All serum samples were run in duplicate for CK quantification.

In Vitro Force Measurement

In vitro force measurements were performed according to methods we have described previously [17]. Briefly, the EDL of the right hindlimb was surgically removed and placed vertically in 25°C bath containing buffered mammalian Ringer solution and aerated with 95% O_2–5% CO_2. Muscles were secured to the lever arm of a servomotor/force transducer by the distal tendon (model 305B, Aurora Scientific) and the proximal tendon was connected to a stationary post in the bath. The muscles were stimulated at optimal length for 300 ms. Increasing electrode frequencies were used until a plateau was achieved and recorded as the maximal force. Specific force was obtained by dividing the maximal force by the EDL cross sectional area. Additionally, the muscles were subjected to a protocol of 4 lengthening contractions separated by 1 min intervals of rest. The muscles were lengthened over 10% of their length.

Statistical Analysis

All analyses were performed using Stata V11 (College Station, TX). Results are represented as mean±SEM or median (range), where appropriate. Normality was assessed for each measurement using the Shapiro-Wilk normality test. For measurements meeting the assumption normality, analysis of variance (ANOVA) was used to compare means among groups (vehicle control, LANZO treatment, prednisolone treatment and combined treatment). *Post-hoc* pairwise group comparisons were performed where ANOVA models showed a significant F-test and the resulting group p-values were adjusted for multiple comparisons using the Sidak method. For measurements not meeting the assumption of normality (e.g. baseline open field measures), a non-parametric Kruskal-Wallis test was used to compare medians among groups. Data displaying significant p-values from the Kruskal-Wallis was further analyzed for between group differences via Wilcoxon rank-sum pair-wise comparisons. Resulting p-values were again adjusted for multiple comparisons using the Sidak method. Rotarod data was analyzed as a time to fall analysis using a log rank test of the equality of survivor functions between treatment groups. CK values were log-transformed to conform to normality. Histology measurements were compared between treatment groups using Poisson regression models for count data where appropriate. Longitudinal analysis of the repeated lengthening contractions used a mixed-effects linear regression model where mouse ID# was a random coefficient and where each treatment was compared to control only. Nominal statistical significance was set at $\alpha = 0.05$.

Results

Effect on Muscle and Organ Weight

Mice in each of the treatment groups gained body mass over the course of this three-month pre-clinical trial (Table S1). Although mice were randomly assigned to treatment groups, there were statistically significant between-group differences in mean body mass prior to treatment (not shown). Due to these differences, baseline body mass was used as a covariate when comparing between group differences in mean body mass at the end of the three-month preclinical trial. Upon analysis, no significant differences in mean body mass between groups were observed at trial's end (Tables 1 & S1). When comparing changes in mean body mass over the length of the trial, mice in the LANZO, prednisolone and combined treatment groups gained significantly less weight over the course of the study relative to the vehicle control (percent body mass gain relative to vehicle control: LANZO -23%, PRED −27%, Combined −36%) (Table S1). These findings support the efficacy of the treatment regimens as they are in agreement with our previous observations that untreated *mdx* mice gain more weight overtime than wild type littermate controls [14]. Muscle and organ weights were recorded at time of sacrifice. No significant differences in average gastrocnemius, soleus, EDL, or heart mass were observed between treatment groups (Table 1). A significantly lower mean spleen mass was observed in mice in the prednisolone and combined treatment groups relative to the vehicle control (spleen mass at time of sacrifice relative to vehicle control: PRED −22%, Combined −28%). Mice in the vehicle control and LANZO groups displayed similar spleen weights at time of sacrifice (94.3±4.2 and

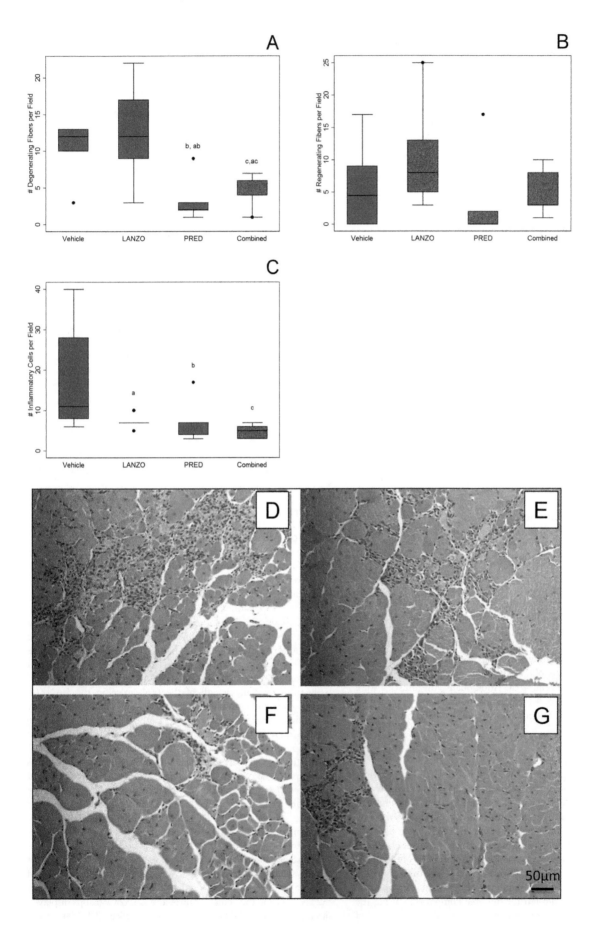

Figure 3. Effect of treatment on histological parameters between treatment groups at 20 weeks. H&E staining was performed on gastrocnemius muscle cross sections. Muscle histology (number of degenerating, regenerating and inflammatory foci per field) was averaged over five representative fields of non-overlapping fiber cross-sections (A–C). (A) Average number of degenerating fibers per field. (B) Average number of regenerating fibers per field. (C) Average number of inflammatory cell foci per field per group. (D–G) Representative gastrocnemius muscle cross sectional fields taken from vehicle control (D), LANZO-treated (E), prednisolone-treated (F), and combined treatment (G) groups.

95.0±6.0 mg, respectively) (Table 1). Additionally, the combined treatment group did not show a significant difference in mean spleen mass relative to the prednisolone treatment group (Table 1).

Effect of Treatment on Muscle Function

In vitro maximal and specific muscle force was compared between treatment groups. Maximal force was not significantly different among treatment groups (p = 0.179), although there was a non-significant 13% and 15% increase in maximal force in LANZO and combined treatment groups, respectively, relative to the vehicle control group at the trial's end (Fig. 1 A). Maximal force was not different between normal C57Bl/10 mice and vehicle treated *mdx* mice, which is consistent with previous reports [18]. However, there was a distinct reduction in EDL specific force in *mdx* mice in comparison to C57Bl/10 mice (Fig. 1 B), which is consistent with previous reports of reduced specific force in *mdx* mice [19]. *In vitro* specific force was significantly different among treatment groups (p<0.05). Although no statistically significant between group differences were observed, mice in the LANZO and combined treatment groups displayed a 19% and 18% increase in specific force, respectively, relative to the vehicle control at the trial's end (Fig. 1 B). Isolated EDL muscle was additionally subjected to four lengthening contractions in order to assess declines in maximal muscle force in response to repeated eccentric stretching. Declines in maximal EDL force in response to lengthening contractions were significantly less in the combined treatment group relative to vehicle control (Fig. 1 C).

Forelimb and hindlimb grip strength testing was performed before and after the 3-month study and on untreated (non-exercised) C57Bl/10 mice, which served as a normal reference group. In *mdx* treatment groups, absolute forelimb grip strength was significantly different between groups prior to treatment (not shown). Therefore, baseline absolute forelimb grip strength was used as a covariate in ANCOVA models when determining between group differences in post-study grip strength measures. At the end of the pre-clinical trial, mice in the combined treatment group displayed a 10% higher absolute hindlimb grip strength relative to the vehicle control (p<0.01) (Table 2). Additionally, mice in the combined treatment group displayed a 12% higher absolute forelimb grip strength relative to mice in the LANZO treatment group (p<0.05). No other statistically significant between group differences in grip strength at the time of sacrifice were observed. There were no statistically significant differences in mean change in absolute forelimb or hindlimb grip strength (post minus pre values) between treatment groups (Table S1). Normalized grip strength did not display statistically significant differences between groups at trial's end (Table 2). However, over the 3-month course of the study, mice in the prednisolone and combined treatment groups displayed an attenuated decline in normalized forelimb grip strength relative to the vehicle control (change in normalized forelimb grip strength relative to vehicle control: PRED +60% and combined +57%; p<0.05). Additionally, mice in the combined treatment group displayed a 44% attenuation in the decline of normalized hindlimb grip strength relative to the vehicle control at the trial's end (p<0.05; Table S1).

Effect of Treatment on Behavioral Outcomes

No statistically significant differences in post-treatment or changes in open field behavioral activity measures, including: total distance traveled, vertical activity, horizontal activity, movement time and rest time were detected between treatment groups (Table 3). Of note, there were no significant differences in baseline open field behavioral activity measurements (data not shown). There were no significant differences in median latency to fall time by Rotarod between groups at trial's end by log-rank test (p = 0.115) (Fig. 2). However, mice in the LANZO treatment group did display a higher median latency to fall score relative to the vehicle control. Mice in the combined treatment group displayed similar latency to fall scores as mice in the vehicle control group, while mice in the prednisolone treatment group displayed the lowest latency to fall score.

Effect of Treatment on Muscle Histology and Creatine Kinase

Muscle histology was performed on gastrocnemius cross sections at time of sacrifice to quantify the number of degenerating/ regenerating fibers and the number of inflammatory foci. Histology was compared between groups via Poisson regression on the median for count data, where appropriate. A decrease in the median number of degenerating fibers was observed in the prednisolone and combined treatment groups relative to mice receiving vehicle control (percent decrease in median number of degenerating fibers relative to vehicle: PRED −83%, p<0.01; combined: −50%, p<0.05) and LANZO treatment groups (Table 4; Fig. 3 A). No significant differences in the number of regenerating fibers were observed between any of the treatment groups (Table 4; Fig. 3 B). The median number of inflammatory foci per gastrocnemius cross sectional field was reduced in all three of the treatment groups relative to vehicle control (decrease in inflammatory foci per field relative to vehicle control: LANZO −36%, p<0.01; PRED −36%, p<0.05; combined −55% p<0.001) (Table 4; Fig. 3 C). Mice in the combined treatment group displayed the lowest amount of median inflammatory foci per gastrocnemius cross sectional field. Representative H&E stained gastrocnemius cross-sections are displayed in Fig. 3 D–G.

There were no significant between group differences in the mean number of inflammatory foci or fibrosis per diaphragm cross sectional field. However, the mean number of inflammatory foci was decreased ~22% in the diaphragm of mice receiving combined treatment relative to vehicle control (Table 4). Additionally, a non-significant ~14% decrease in the mean number of fibrotic regions was observed in the diaphragm of mice in the combined treatment group relative to vehicle control (Table 4).

Sera was obtained via cardiac venipuncture at time of sacrifice and analyzed in duplicate via enzymatic assay. Mice in the combined treatment group displayed a ~64% reduction in mean serum CK relative to vehicle control (p<0.05) (Fig. 4). Mice in the prednisolone treatment group displayed a ~54% reduction in mean serum CK relative to untreated control, but this did not reach statistical significance. No significant differences in mean serum CK were observed between any of the other treatment groups. However, upon removal of two outliers in the Vehicle and

Table 4. Effect of treatment on histological outcomes following 3 months of treatment.

Measurement	Vehicle		LANZO		PRED		Combined		Significantly different means/medians
	N	Median (Range)	N	Median (Range)	N	Median (Range)	N	Median (Range)	
Degenerating fibers per field (gastrocnemius)**	6	12 (3–13)	5	12 (3–33)	5	2 (1–9)[b, ab]	5	6 (1–7)[c, ac]	[b]Veh vs. PRED (p=0.002); [c]Veh vs. Combined (p=0.018); [ab]LANZO vs. PRED (p=0.001); [ac]LANZO vs. Combined (p=0.005)
Regenerating fibers per field (gastrocnemius)**	6	5 (0–17)	5	8 (3–25)	5	0 (0–17)	5	3 (1–10)	NONE
Inflammatory foci per field (gastrocnemius)**	6	11 (6–40)	5	7 (5–10)[a]	5	7 (3–17)[b]	5	5 (3–7)[c]	[a]Veh vs. LANZO (p=0.008); [b]Veh vs. PRED (p=0.012); [c]Veh vs. Combined (p<0.001)
Inflammatory foci per field (diaphragm)	6	59±16	6	56±16	6	57±17	6	46±15	NONE
Fibrosis (diaphragm)	5	22.0±4.7	5	24.2±9.6	5	18.5±3.9	5	18.9±3.7	NONE

Footnotes:
**Histology compared between groups using Poisson regression.

LANZO groups, no statistical differences remained among treatment groups.

Discussion

Skeletal muscle excitability is regulated by ionic gradients. Following membrane depolarization, activation of the Na^+/K^+-ATPase proton pump restores resting Na^+ and K^+ gradients and helps maintain muscle excitability for repeated contractions [20]. Due to alterations in membrane stability and ion conductivity in dystrophic muscle, we sought to investigate the effects of the proton pump inhibitor LANZO on the dystrophic phenotype in *mdx* mice. The main finding of our study was that combined LANZO and prednisolone treatment improved some components of the dystrophic phenotype in dystrophin deficient *mdx* mice. Attenuation of the dystrophic phenotype in the combined treatment group relative to the vehicle control was indicated by observations of: 1) a decreased number of degenerating fibers and inflammatory foci per gastrocnemius cross sectional field; 2) attenuated declines in normalized forelimb and hindlimb grip strength; 3) attenuated declines in maximal *in vitro* EDL force in response to repeated lengthening contractions. LANZO administration decreased declines in body mass and reduced the number of muscle inflammatory foci. LANZO administration also appeared to improve specific and maximal gastrocnemius muscle force, although this did not reach statistical significance. The effects of LANZO and prednisolone were not additive, mice in the combined treatment group did display greater improvements in muscle force in response to repeated eccentric contractions and a reduced number of muscle inflammatory foci relative to the prednisolone treatment group.

The beneficial effects of dual LANZO and prednisolone administration are likely multifold. LANZO belongs to a class of proton pump inhibitors (PPIs) that become active in weakly acidic environments. LANZO has been suggested to bind to other classes of proton pumps, including the Na^+/K^+-ATPase [21]. However, the ability of the dose of LANZO used in this study to induce *in vivo* inhibition of proton pumps extragastrically has not been thoroughly investigated. We hypothesize that the mechanisms by which combined LANZO and prednisolone treatment improve the dystrophic phenotype in *mdx* mice may include: 1) reduced inflammatory cell recruitment to the skeletal muscle; 2) altered ion conductivity of skeletal muscle Na^+/K^+-ATPase and chloride ion channels; 3) decreased apoptotic signaling cascades promoting myonecrosis.

Off-label use of LANZO has been more thoroughly investigated in the treatment of cancer, wherein LANZO has been suggested to have anti-inflammatory and anti-metastatic effects. De Milito *et al.* observed that PPI administration promotes B cell apoptosis in acute B cell lymphatic leukemia via altering tumor lysosomes and extracellular pH [22]. The anti-metastatic effects of LANZO administration are also supported by a Phase I/II trial by Spungnini *et al.* who observed improved tumor outcomes in animals receiving combined treatment of LANZO and chemo-therapeutics [23]. The ability of LANZO to inhibit tumor metastasis is suggested to occur via LANZO-mediated inhibition of V-ATPases, which are upregulated in metastatic cancers and contribute to maintenance of the metastatic tumor microenvironment and the Warburg effect via proton extrusion [23]. Both V- and H^+/K^+-ATPases are inhibited by disulfide binding to cysteine residues on their α subunits [24]. This supports the role of LANZO action on various classes of ATPases. Like the H^+/K^+-ATPase, the Na^+/K^+-ATPase is a class IIC P-type ATPase which is expressed in skeletal muscle. LANZO has also been observed to

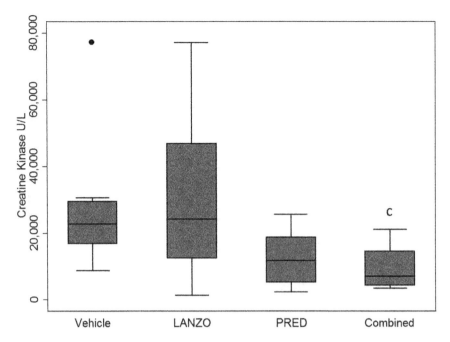

Figure 4. Effect of treatment on creatine kinase. Serum CK levels at time of sacrifice between vehicle control (n = 9), LANZO (n = 11), prednisolone (n = 12), and combined treatment (n = 11) groups. There were three mice for which a cardiac venipuncture was not obtained due to technical difficulties. All sera was obtained via cardiac venipuncture and analyzed in duplicate via enzymatic assay. Statistical analysis was performed on log-transformed data. Upon removal of two outliers in the vehicle and LANZO groups, no statistical differences remained among treatment groups (not shown).

inhibit the Na^+/K^+-ATPase, albeit at a higher IC_{50} than it inhibits the H^+/K^+-ATPase [21]. The H^+/K^+-ATPase and Na^+/K^+-ATPase pumps are highly homologous and display species conservation in their catalytic α subunit cysteine residues (LANZO binding sites) [25]. In the skeletal muscle, the Na^+/K^+-ATPase pump resides at the sarcolemma and t-tubule system, where it functions to restore membrane potential following contraction via ATP-mediated Na^+ extrusion and K^+ import. It is conceivable that LANZO may improve components of the dystrophic phenotype by binding to the skeletal muscle Na^+/K^+-ATPase and altering ion influx. Dystrophic fibers display an accumulation of intracellular calcium, which promotes myonecrosis [7] and reduces skeletal muscle force [26] via altering excitation-relaxation coupling [27]. Dietary NaCl supplementation has been shown to attenuate myofiber necrosis and reduce serum CK concentrations in *mdx* mice [8]. As predicted by the Nernst equation, an increase in intracellular Na^+ that may occur via LANZO-mediated Na^+/K^+ ATPase pump inhibition may reduce intracellular Ca^{2+} influx. A reduction in intracellular Ca^{2+} would thus reduce myofiber lysis and improve the dystrophic phenotype in *mdx* mice. Such alterations in Ca^{2+} ionic flux due to LANZO administration may also affect macrophage polarization and NO production as macrophage production of NO is enhanced in the presence of Ca^{2+} ionophores [28]. Contrary to this hypothesis of Na^+-mediated Ca^{2+} extrusion, an increase in intracellular Na^+ levels may increase intracellular Ca^{2+} by decreasing the electrogenic potential of the Na^+/Ca^{2+} exchanger. This is supported by findings from Allen *et al.* who observed that elevated intercellular Na^+ promotes Ca^{2+} influx in myocytes [29]. Thus, the beneficial effects of combined LANZO and prednisolone administration may occur by mechanisms other than regulation of Na^+ and Ca^{2+} influx and warrant further investigation. In dystrophic fibers, decreases in membrane resistivity increase membrane conductivity of a variety of ions including Cl^- [3]. Increases in Cl^-

conductance alter skeletal muscle membrane excitability [30]. Increased Cl^- ion flux in fibroblasts surrounding myofibers of *mdx* mice has also been shown to worsen the dystrophic phenotype [31]. LANZO has been observed to inhibit gastric chloride ion channels [32]. Our findings of an attenuated decline in *in vitro* muscle force in response to repeated eccentric contractions in mice given combined LANZO and prednisolone treatment could thus be due to altered Cl^-, Na^+ or Ca^{2+} conductance and subsequent enhanced muscle excitability in response to LANZO administration. Declines in *in vitro* muscle force in response to eccentric contractions have been attributed to failure in E–C coupling and thus our findings support a potential role for LANZO in improving dystrophic muscle excitability [33]. Further research investigating the kinetics of oral LANZO administration on skeletal muscle ATPases will help elucidate the potential mechanisms of LANZO action.

Another putative beneficial effect of LANZO on the dystrophic phenotype may be due to its anti-inflammatory properties. Macrophage pre-treatment with LANZO decreases nitric oxide (NO) synthesis and cell viability in response to stimulation by LPS [34]. Further, pretreatment of monocytes with LANZO has been shown to decrease LPS-induced $TNF\alpha$ and IL-1β expression via decreasing IκB-α and ERK phosphorylation [35]. A similar PPI, omeprazole, has been shown to decrease neutrophil chemotaxis and ROS production [36]. Further, omeprazole has been shown to decrease peripheral blood neutrophil phagocytic activity and oxidation 4 hours after oral administration in healthy human subjects [11]. Since the mechanisms of actions between different classes of PPI are similar, we hypothesize that oral LANZO administration may attenuate the dystrophic phenotype in *mdx* mice by reducing neutrophil recruitment and respiratory burst and by skewing of muscle macrophages away from a proinflammatory M1 macrophage phenotype. This is supported as populations of iNOS expressing muscle macrophages have been suggested to contribute to muscle cell lysis in *mdx* mice and shifts in muscle macrophage activation from a proinflammatory to anti-inflammatory/regenerative phenotype improve dystrophic pathology [12]. Further, depletion of neutrophils has been shown to attenuate components of the dystrophic phenotype in *mdx* mice [37].

LANZO irreversibly binds to cysteine moieties and its serum half-life is ~1.5 hours. Due to the rapid catabolism of LANZO by the gastric environment and metabolism by the liver, the effects of LANZO administration are likely less pronounced in the skeletal muscle relative to the gastric epithelia. Therefore, we hypothesize that dual LANZO and prednisolone administration was efficacious due to partial inhibition of Na^+/K^+-ATPase pumps and chloride channels. The beneficial effects of dual LANZO and prednisolone administration were not additive. Glucocorticoids, like prednisolone, upregulate Na^+/K^+-ATPases [38]. We thus believe that the combined treatment was more efficacious than prednisolone administration alone because of the ability of LANZO to reduce elevated skeletal muscle Na^+/K^+-ATPase activity, due to prednisolone treatment, and further decreasing neutrophil and macrophage cytoxcity. Additional investigation of the dose-dependent effects of combined LANZO and prednisolone treatment are thus warranted as higher doses of LANZO may be more efficacious in the treatment of dystrophic pathology.

References

1. Carlson CG (1998) The dystrophinopathies: an alternative to the structural hypothesis. Neurobiology of disease 5: 3–15.
2. Bertorini TE, Bhattacharya SK, Palmieri GM, Chesney CM, Pifer D, et al. (1982) Muscle calcium and magnesium content in Duchenne muscular dystrophy. Neurology 32: 1088–1092.
3. Kerr LM, Sperelakis N (1983) Effects of pH on membrane resistance in normal and dystrophic mouse skeletal muscle fibers. Experimental neurology 82: 203–214.
4. Dunn JF, Bannister N, Kemp GJ, Publicover SJ (1993) Sodium is elevated in mdx muscles: ionic interactions in dystrophic cells. Journal of the neurological sciences 114: 76–80.
5. Sellin LC, Sperelakis N (1978) Decreased potassium permeability in dystrophic mouse skeletal muscle. Experimental neurology 62: 605–617.
6. De Luca A, Pierno S, Camerino DC (1997) Electrical properties of diaphragm and EDL muscles during the life of dystrophic mice. The American journal of physiology 272: C333–340.
7. Tidball JG, Spencer MJ (2000) Calpains and muscular dystrophies. The international journal of biochemistry & cell biology 32: 1–5.
8. Yoshida M, Yonetani A, Shirasaki T, Wada K (2006) Dietary NaCl supplementation prevents muscle necrosis in a mouse model of Duchenne muscular dystrophy. American journal of physiology Regulatory, integrative and comparative physiology 290: R449–455.
9. Isomoto H, Nishi Y, Kanazawa Y, Shikuwa S, Mizuta Y, et al. (2007) Immune and Inflammatory Responses in GERD and Lansoprazole. Journal of clinical biochemistry and nutrition 41: 84–91.
10. Hinoki A, Yoshimura K, Fujita K, Akita M, Ikeda R, et al. (2006) Suppression of proinflammatory cytokine production in macrophages by lansoprazole. Pediatric surgery international 22: 915–923.
11. Zedtwitz-Liebenstein K, Wenisch C, Patruta S, Parschalk B, Daxbock F, et al. (2002) Omeprazole treatment diminishes intra- and extracellular neutrophil reactive oxygen production and bactericidal activity. Critical care medicine 30: 1118–1122.
12. Villalta SA, Nguyen HX, Deng B, Gotoh T, Tidball JG (2009) Shifts in macrophage phenotypes and macrophage competition for arginine metabolism affect the severity of muscle pathology in muscular dystrophy. Human molecular genetics 18: 482–496.
13. De Luca A (2008) Use of treadmill and wheel exercise for impact on mdx mice phenotype. Treat-NMD Neuromuscular Network Ver. 2.
14. Spurney CF, Gordish-Dressman H, Guerron AD, Sali A, Pandey GS, et al. (2009) Preclinical drug trials in the mdx mouse: assessment of reliable and sensitive outcome measures. Muscle & nerve 39: 591–602.
15. Spurney CF, Knoblach S, Pistilli EE, Nagaraju K, Martin GR, et al. (2008) Dystrophin-deficient cardiomyopathy in mouse: expression of Nox4 and Lox are associated with fibrosis and altered functional parameters in the heart. Neuromuscular disorders : NMD 18: 371–381.
16. Guerron AD, Rawat R, Sali A, Spurney CF, Pistilli E, et al. (2010) Functional and molecular effects of arginine butyrate and prednisone on muscle and heart in the mdx mouse model of Duchenne Muscular Dystrophy. PloS one 5: e11220.

Conclusions

Our findings suggest that combined LANZO and prednisolone treatment provides slightly improved therapeutic efficacy in treating the dystrophic skeletal muscle phenotype in *mdx* mice relative to prednisolone treatment alone. Complications of DMD may include other symptoms that may be improved with LANZO administration, such as delayed gastric emptying, gastric inflammation, smooth muscle fibrosis and dilation [39,40]. Due to the therapeutic benefits of LANZO on the dystrophic phenotype, future investigation of the clinical efficacy of dual LANZO and prednisolone administration in human trials may be warranted.

Supporting Information

Table S1 Changes in body mass and functional outcomes before and after treatment. The mean change (final-baseline) in each parameter tested is presented for all treatment groups.

Author Contributions

Conceived and designed the experiments: KN AS HG CS EH AC JvdM. Performed the experiments: AS CS JvdM AP. Analyzed the data: KN JvdM HG GM CS AC. Wrote the paper: KN GM JvdM HG.

17. Rayavarapu S, Van der Meulen JH, Gordish-Dressman H, Hoffman EP, Nagaraju K, et al. (2010) Characterization of dysferlin deficient SJL/J mice to assess preclinical drug efficacy: fasudil exacerbates muscle disease phenotype. PloS one 5: e12981.
18. Gehrig SM, Ryall JG, Schertzer JD, Lynch GS (2008) Insulin-like growth factor-I analogue protects muscles of dystrophic mdx mice from contraction-mediated damage. Experimental physiology 93: 1190–1198.
19. Consolino CM, Brooks SV (2004) Susceptibility to sarcomere injury induced by single stretches of maximally activated muscles of mdx mice. Journal of applied physiology 96: 633–638.
20. Clausen T (2003) Na+-K+ pump regulation and skeletal muscle contractility. Physiological reviews 83: 1269–1324.
21. Ito K, Kinoshita K, Tomizawa A, Inaba F, Morikawa-Inomata Y, et al. (2007) Pharmacological profile of novel acid pump antagonist 7-(4-fluorobenzyloxy)-2,3-dimethyl-1-{[(1S,2S)-2-methyl cyclopropyl]methyl}-1H-pyrrolo[2,3-d]pyridazine (CS-526). The Journal of pharmacology and experimental therapeutics 323: 308–317.
22. De Milito A, Iessi E, Logozzi M, Lozupone F, Spada M, et al. (2007) Proton pump inhibitors induce apoptosis of human B-cell tumors through a caspase-independent mechanism involving reactive oxygen species. Cancer research 67: 5408–5417.
23. Spugnini EP, Baldi A, Buglioni S, Carocci F, de Bazzichini GM, et al. (2011) Lansoprazole as a rescue agent in chemoresistant tumors: a phase I/II study in companion animals with spontaneously occurring tumors. Journal of translational medicine 9: 221.
24. Feng Y, Forgac M (1994) Inhibition of vacuolar H(+)-ATPase by disulfide bond formation between cysteine 254 and cysteine 532 in subunit A. The Journal of biological chemistry 269: 13224–13230.
25. Maeda M (1994) Gastric proton pump (H+/K(+)-ATPase): structure and gene regulation through GATA DNA-binding protein(s). Journal of biochemistry 115: 6–14.
26. Chin ER, Allen DG (1996) The role of elevations in intracellular [Ca2+] in the development of low frequency fatigue in mouse single muscle fibres. The Journal of physiology 491 (Pt 3): 813–824.
27. Lamb GD, Junankar PR, Stephenson DG (1995) Raised intracellular [Ca2+] abolishes excitation-contraction coupling in skeletal muscle fibres of rat and toad. The Journal of physiology 489 (Pt 2): 349–362.
28. Denlinger LC, Fisette PL, Garis KA, Kwon G, Vazquez-Torres A, et al. (1996) Regulation of inducible nitric oxide synthase expression by macrophage purinoreceptors and calcium. The Journal of biological chemistry 271: 337–342.
29. Allen DG, Eisner DA, Lab MJ, Orchard CH (1983) The effects of low sodium solutions on intracellular calcium concentration and tension in ferret ventricular muscle. The Journal of physiology 345: 391–407.
30. Allard B (2006) Sarcolemmal ion channels in dystrophin-deficient skeletal muscle fibres. Journal of muscle research and cell motility 27: 367–373.
31. Pato CN, Davis MH, Doughty MJ, Bryant SH, Gruenstein E (1983) Increased membrane permeability to chloride in Duchenne muscular dystrophy fibroblasts and its relationship to muscle function. Proceedings of the National Academy of Sciences of the United States of America 80: 4732–4736.

32. Schmarda A, Dinkhauser P, Gschwentner M, Ritter M, Furst J, et al. (2000) The gastric H,K-ATPase blocker lansoprazole is an inhibitor of chloride channels. British journal of pharmacology 129: 598–604.

33. Ingalls CP, Warren GL, Williams JH, Ward CW, Armstrong RB (1998) E-C coupling failure in mouse EDL muscle after in vivo eccentric contractions. Journal of applied physiology 85: 58–67.

34. Nakagawa S, Arai Y, Kishida T, Hiraoka N, Tsuchida S, et al. (2012) Lansoprazole Inhibits Nitric Oxide and Prostaglandin E(2) Production in Murine Macrophage RAW 264.7 Cells. Inflammation 35: 1062–1068.

35. Tanigawa T, Watanabe T, Higuchi K, Machida H, Okazaki H, et al. (2009) Lansoprazole, a Proton Pump Inhibitor, Suppresses Production of Tumor Necrosis Factor-alpha and Interleukin-1beta Induced by Lipopolysaccharide and Helicobacter Pylori Bacterial Components in Human Monocytic Cells via Inhibition of Activation of Nuclear Factor-kappaB and Extracellular Signal-Regulated Kinase. Journal of clinical biochemistry and nutrition 45: 86–92.

36. Wandall JH (1992) Effects of omeprazole on neutrophil chemotaxis, super oxide production, degranulation, and translocation of cytochrome b-245. Gut 33: 617–621.

37. Hodgetts S, Radley H, Davies M, Grounds MD (2006) Reduced necrosis of dystrophic muscle by depletion of host neutrophils, or blocking TNFalpha function with Etanercept in mdx mice. Neuromuscular disorders : NMD 16: 591–602.

38. Devarajan P, Benz EJ Jr (2000) Translational regulation of Na-K-ATPase subunit mRNAs by glucocorticoids. American journal of physiology Renal physiology 279: F1132–1138.

39. Leon SH, Schuffler MD, Kettler M, Rohrmann CA (1986) Chronic intestinal pseudoobstruction as a complication of Duchenne's muscular dystrophy. Gastroenterology 90: 455–459.

40. Bensen ES, Jaffe KM, Tarr PI (1996) Acute gastric dilatation in Duchenne muscular dystrophy: a case report and review of the literature. Archives of physical medicine and rehabilitation 77: 512–514.

10

The Importance of Synergy between Deep Inspirations and Fluidization in Reversing Airway Closure

Graham M. Donovan[1]*, James Sneyd[1], Merryn H. Tawhai[2]

1 Department of Mathematics, University of Auckland, Auckland, New Zealand, **2** Auckland Bioengineering Institute, University of Auckland, Auckland, New Zealand

Abstract

Deep inspirations (DIs) and airway smooth muscle fluidization are two widely studied phenomena in asthma research, particularly for their ability (or inability) to counteract severe airway constriction. For example, DIs have been shown effectively to reverse airway constriction in normal subjects, but this is impaired in asthmatics. Fluidization is a connected phenomenon, wherein the ability of airway smooth muscle (ASM, which surrounds and constricts the airways) to exert force is decreased by applied strain. A maneuver which sufficiently strains the ASM, then, such as a DI, is thought to reduce the force generating capacity of the muscle via fluidization and hence reverse or prevent airway constriction. Understanding these two phenomena is considered key to understanding the pathophysiology of asthma and airway hyper-responsiveness, and while both have been extensively studied, the mechanism by which DIs fail in asthmatics remains elusive. Here we show for the first time the synergistic interaction between DIs and fluidization which allows the combination to provide near complete reversal of airway closure where neither is effective alone. This relies not just on the traditional model of airway bistability between open and closed states, but also the critical addition of previously-unknown oscillatory and chaotic dynamics. It also allows us to explore the types of subtle change which can cause this interaction to fail, and thus could provide the missing link to explain DI failure in asthmatics.

Editor: Bard Ermentrout, University of Pittsburgh, United States of America

Funding: The authors acknowledge the support of the National Institutes of Health (NIH) under grant HL103405. The funders had no role in study design, data collection and analysis, decision to publish, or preparation of the manuscript.

Competing Interests: The authors have declared that no competing interests exist.

* E-mail: g.donovan@auckland.ac.nz

Introduction

Deep inspirations (DIs) and airway smooth muscle fluidization are two phenomena which have the potential to counteract severe airway constriction. This is of particular interest as this mediating effect is often found in normal subjects, but impaired in asthmatics (i.e. [1,2]). Thus understanding their impairment may be central to understanding the pathophysiology of asthma. We consider the interactions between DIs and fluidization, and show that synergies between the two can be critical for effective reversal of severe airway constriction. As such, failure of this interaction may explain the impairment of DI effectiveness in asthmatics. Moreover, our method of analysis lends itself naturally to exploring other modes of failure, such as a reduction in parenchymal tethering effectiveness.

The effect of DIs has been the subject of extensive research, with many studies drawing a distinction between asthmatic and normal subjects on the basis of their response to DI. For example it has been shown that DIs are protective against bronchoconstriction in normals, whereas they fail to limit bronchoconstriction in asthmatics. Normal subjects who are prevented from taking DIs develop a bronchoconstrictive response similar to that seen in asthmatics [3–5] and DIs fail to limit bronchoconstriction in asthmatics, where they are effective in normals [6,7]. A distinction is drawn between a bronchoprotective effect, wherein DIs are taken prior to constriction (and limit subsequent constriction), and bronchodilation, where DIs are taken during constriction (and dilate constricted airways). In addition to the failure of

bronchoprotection, asthmatics also display limited bronchodilation due to DI as compared to normals [1,2].

Fluidization is the response of biological tissues in response to oscillatory or transient strain, typically characterized by a reduction in stiffness, exerted force, and an increase in hysteresivity (i.e. [8,9]), and as such has been suggested as a potentially powerful mechanism for countering bronchoconstriction. In this work we will consider fluidization of ASM in response to the transient strain of a deep inspiration, which renders the muscle less able to generate constricting force. As such, fluidization in response to a DI is one potential route to bronchodilation, and interactions between the two are a potentially crucial area for understanding the effectiveness (or failure) of the combination in counteracting airway constriction.

We explore the interactions between DIs and fluidization by considering a minimal new mathematical model of a single airway, based on a combination of canonical models in the field. The constituent parts are the Lambert model [10] for the passive stiffness of the airway wall itself; the Lai-Fook model [11], describing the so-called *tethering* forces external to the airway wall from the lung parenchyma; the Laplace law, describing changes in the constricting pressure as the airway narrows; and a ring of activated airway smooth muscle surrounding and constricting the airway. These models are well-established and many studies exist combining some elements, for example Macklem's combination of the Laplace law and linear parenchyma [12], Affonce & Lutchen's study combining airway wall mechanics with linear parenchyma

[13], a series of papers considering the combination of the Lambert model and airflow [14–16] and the mechanics study of Moreno *et al.* [17]. Similar ideas have also been incorporated into experimental control [18,19]. Bistability also appears in the terminal airway model of Anafi and Wilson [20], and in the extension to an airway tree by Venegas *et al.* [21], though it is important to note that it is driven by flow, which does not appear in this model. (See 'Discussion' for more on this point.)

Such models are often combined and in the process solved iteratively (i.e. [21,22]), for example first calculating airway radius as a function of transmural pressure using the Lambert model, followed by the calculation of transmural pressure as a function of radius due to the combination of the Laplace law and Lai-Fook parenchymal tethering model. Instead of this two-step approach, we opt to describe the combination of the models as an iterated map, removing the intermediate step of calculating the transmural pressure and instead taking an initial airway radius as input and providing a new, updated radius as output. Thus the airway map, formulated fully in 'Methods', may be understood in the following basic form

$$r_{n+1} = \Phi(r_n; f, P_{tp}) \qquad (1)$$

where r is the airway radius, and Φ maps one value of r to another; the subscripts denote the iteration of the map. The map depends parametrically on the airway smooth muscle force f and tethering coefficient (or transpulmonary pressure) P_{tp}; the former describes the force attempting to constrict the airway, and the latter is the coefficient of the restoring, tethering forces attempting to hold it open. (We adopt the term 'tethering coefficient' to describe generically the pressure-dependent coefficient of the increase in tethering force due to airway constriction. Please see 'Methods' and Eq. 4 for a more detailed discussion of this coefficient.)

One essential idea in the study of airway dynamics is the concept of hysteresis and a bistability between open and closed states, which has been previously explored by a number of authors (i.e. [10,13,20,21]). This is a central idea in this field in that it provides a mechanism which might account for clustered ventilation defects, wherein some portions of a constricted lung are severely constricted, while other regions are normally- or even hyper-ventilated. The airway map exhibits not only the previously studied bistability but also oscillatory dynamics, and in some regimes undergoes a period-doubling cascade leading to chaos [23]. While chaotic behavior has been found in particle mixing in the lung (i.e. [24]) and a coupled tree of airways [21,25] where the dynamics are driven by flow, we show here for the first time that it also occurs in a minimal model of an individual airway in isolation, without flow. Moreover, these map dynamics are central to the synergistic interactions between DIs and fluidization which make the combination so potent.

Results

With the airway model formulated as an iterated map describing airway radius, we have the tools necessary to study its behavior as important parameters are varied; in this case we are principally interested in the strength of ASM constriction, as controlled by the parameter f, and the strength of parenchymal tethering, as controlled by the parameter P_{tp} (see 'Methods'). We begin by holding the tethering coefficient (P_{tp}) fixed and varying the applied ASM force (f). Initially, for $P_{tp}/P_{tp0} = 0.5$, we find the typical well-known bistability and hysteresis loop (Fig. 1, a), allowing for both closed and open states to coexist for some range of f (i.e. [13], here for f/f_0 ranging from approximately 0.1 to

0.7). Beginning at zero force, the airway is open, and stays open with force increasing up to approximately $f/f_0 \approx 0.7$ where a sharp transition to closure occurs. Retracing from the closed state by decreasing applied force results in the closed state persisting all the way back to $f/f_0 \approx 0.1$. In this range the open and closed states both exist. However, upon increasing the tethering strength to $P_{tp}/P_{tp0} = 0.75$, we find not only this bistability, but also an oscillatory regime beginning around $f/f_0 = 0.6$ leading into a period-doubling cascade to chaos [23] (Fig. 1, b). A zoom to show detail of this route to chaos is given in panel d. The variations observed in the oscillatory and chaotic regime are also significant, ranging from an entirely open airway to one quite severely constricted.

One way to attempt to address the origin of these behaviors is to look at the balance of the static loads between 1) the airway wall itself and 2) the combination of the ASM force and parenchymal tethering. These static load curves are given in Fig. 1, panel c, for each of the two cases above, specifically at $f/f_0 = 0.675$ where the behavior is either bistable or chaotic (depending on the choice of P_{tp}). The solid black curve gives the Lambert airway wall model [10], and the dashed curves the ASM/parenchyma static load (blue for the bistable case, red in the chaotic case). In principle, from this analysis, one might expect each situation to have three solutions, one at each point of intersection near zero transmural pressure, and another at the intersection representing closure near zero radius and large negative transmural pressure (not shown). However, this is not the case and demonstrates the need to consider the problem as a map, as otherwise the stability is ignored and important dynamics can be overlooked. In fact in the case of the blue curve there are two stable and one unstable equilibria, as shown in panel a, and for the red curve there are no stable equilibria at all (panels b and d).

While these examples demonstrate the existence of rich dynamics, the dependence upon tethering coefficient P_{tp} calls for a two-parameter bifurcation study to understand the influence of both the constricting and restoring forces. Varying both f and P_{tp} now simultaneously, we can no longer plot the value of each point obtained from the map but instead classify the results into categories as follows: one stable fixed point, airway open; one fixed point, airway closed; bistability; oscillations, period 2; oscillations, period 4; oscillations, period 8; chaos. Each of these cases occur in one or more regions of the (f, P_{tp})-plane. By analysing the map we can find the boundaries between each of these regions, given in Fig. 2 (a). Color coding corresponding to the categories above is given in the figure legend.

We can clearly see that for values of P_{tp}/P_{tp0} less than approximately 0.58, the traditional view exists: a single, open, fixed point for small values of f, followed by a region of bistability, and finally for sufficiently large f only a single closed state (as in Fig. 1 (a)). Right of this line, however, the new behavior emerges. Initially period-two oscillations emerge, then progressing through a period-doubling cascade to chaos. At the end of chaos, the closed state again prevails; (we have colored this grey, rather than black, to reflect that while empirically only the closed state exists, formally there are three fixed points here, each sufficiently small as to be considered closed states.) While the existence of this route to chaos in this model is new and interesting in its own right, most importantly it explains the synergistic interaction between DIs and fluidization which result in effective bronchodilation.

Consider the path in parameter space marked out by the points A, B, C and D (Fig. 2, (b)), and suppose that we begin with a population of severely constricted airways at A – only the single closed state exists here. This point we think of as analogous to a severely constricted lung. The path of a DI combined with

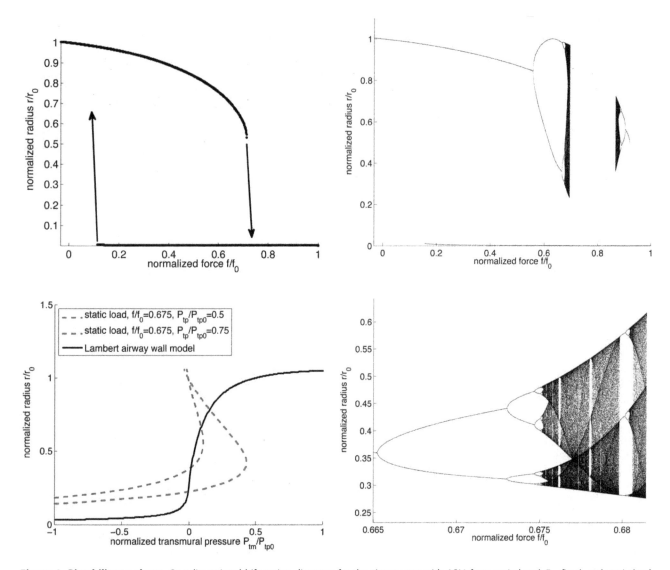

Figure 1. Bistability to chaos. One-dimensional bifurcation diagrams for the airway map with ASM force varied and P_{tp} fixed, and static load curves. Top left panel: the traditional view of bistability and hysteresis found when $P_{tp}/P_{tp0} = 0.5$. Beginning at zero force, the airway is open with increasing force up to approximately $f/f_0 \approx 0.7$ where a sharp transition to closure occurs. Retracing from the closed state by decreasing applied force results in the closed state persisting all the way back to $f/f_0 \approx 0.1$. In this range the open and closed states both exist. Top right: period-doubling route to chaos found when $P_{tp}/P_{tp0} = 0.75$. Bottom left: static load curves and Lambert airway wall model. The solid black curve gives the Lambert airway wall mode [10] for an order 5 airway. The dashed lines give the static load determined by Eq. 3 for each of the cases in the upper panels – the blue curve corresponds to the simple bistability of the $P_{tp}/P_{tp0} = 0.5$ case in the top left, while the red curve represents the case with the oscillations and chaos of the $P_{tp}/P_{tp0} = 0.75$ case in the top right (see text). Bottom right: detailed view of top right panel.

fluidization, then, might be approximated as A-B-C-D, with an increase in P_{tp} as the DI is drawn (to B), a decrease in ASM force due to fluidization induced by the DI strain (to C), and a decrease again in pressure as the breath is exhaled (to D). As D is in the bistable region, in principle here our population may now be entirely closed, entirely open, or anywhere in between. What is important is the dependence of this closed fraction *on the path taken*. The pseudo-dynamics of a population of airways along this path (see 'Methods') are computed and given in Fig. 2 (c), showing the initially closed population beginning to open as the maneuver progresses. Initially a small number of closed airways jump into the open state upon moving into the bistable region, with a gradual increase as the path moves through the period-doubling cascade and into chaos. As the path moves back out of chaos (toward C) and traverses the cascade in reverse, the rate of opening increases

dramatically, as can be seen from the red closed fraction line, and continues as the breath is exhaled (to D). At the end of the maneuver, more than 90% of the airways have been reopened. The combination of a DI and fluidization together is thus highly effective at reversing airway closure.

Contrast this with the direct path A–D, with the same reduction in force but without the DI itself; this is equivalent to fluidization alone. The pseudo-dynamics of this path are given in Fig. 2 (d). Here some small fraction of points do move into the open state along the path, but without the progression through the period-doubling cascade and the band of chaos, more than 95% of the airways remain in the closed state. Thus despite beginning and ending at the same points, one can have either a near-complete reopening from closure, or near-complete failure.

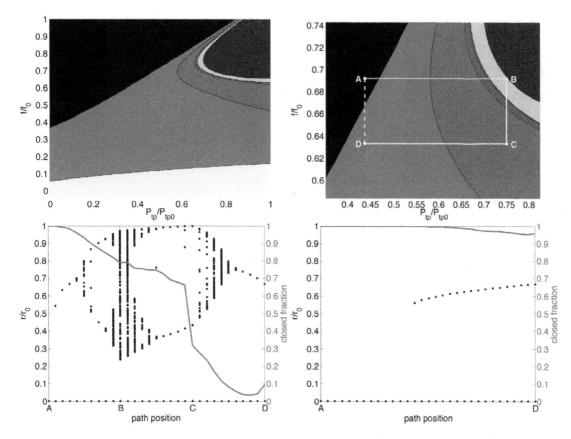

Figure 2. 2D bifurcation sets and pseudo-dynamics. Top left: 2D bifurcation set for the airway map, color-coded by behavior. Yellow: one fixed point, airway open; red: bistability; black: one fixed point, airway closed; blue: oscillations, with darker shades for longer period oscillations; green: chaos; grey: three fixed points, all near closure. Top right: detail showing the path of DI pseudo-dynamics. Bottom left: Pseudo-dynamics for full DI path (A-B-C-D). Left axis, black dots: airway radii for 1000 samples, each dot corresponding to an airway at each path position. Right axis, red line: fraction of closed airways in the sample. Throughout the maneuver airways gradually open, with a near-complete opening of closed airways at the conclusion. Bottom right: Pseudo-dynamics for direct force reduction without DI (A–D). Along this path, without the DI, near-total closure persists.

Of course, a DI alone without fluidization is equivalent to the path A-B-A. Independent of any opening which occurs along this path, upon return to point A all airways must be in the closed state – this is the only fixed point there, and so the closed fraction must be 1. Thus the airway map demonstrates the much greater power of a DI and fluidization together, as compared to either alone. It is worth noting that the precise location of point B in the chaotic band is not critical; the general requirements for reopening are that the path traverses the oscillatory or chaotic bands, and that the terminal point be in the bistable region. The specific path given here is in this sense generic.

If the effectiveness of a DI is dependent upon synergies with fluidization, then what can this tell us about the possible mechanisms for DI failure in asthmatics? While the map does not in itself suggest a specific distinction between normals and asthmatics, it does raise the prospect that the difference may be quite subtle. Consider, for example, the hypothesis that parenchymal tethering is less effective in asthmatics, relative to normals. One manifestation of this hypothesis could be that the nonlinear coefficient of tethering (see Eq. (4), 'Methods') is reduced. As an illustration, we reduce this coefficient from its standard value (1.5, as in [11]) to 0.5 and recompute both the bifurcation sets and DI pseudo-dynamics resulting from this modified model, with the results given in Fig. 3. Now this path begins and ends in the region with only the closed state available; thus the end result of the DI maneuver must be that all airways are

closed. It is also instructive to observe that even in the portion of the path which traverses the bistable region, more than 85% of the airways remain closed. Thus the decreased tethering force has eliminated the reversal of airway closure from a DI, and limited even the transient effects. While this arbitrary modification is not directly indicative of the difference between normals and asthmatics, it is an illustration both of the type of subtle phenomena which may account for the difference, and the power of this type of analysis to shed light on the many proposed hypotheses – particularly in light of recent controversy surrounding the role of DIs and fluidization in limiting airway constriction in intact airways; see 'Discussion'.

Discussion

Looking at the problem of airway constriction as an iterated map is a new way of analyzing airway behavior. It has yielded critical insight into the relationship between DIs and ASM fluidization, which helps to explain the importance of synergy between the two in reversing airway closure. In addition, it is a powerful new tool for the study of the myriad hypothesized differences between asthmatic and normal subjects. We have illustrated, with a simple example of reduced parenchymal tethering nonlinearity, the possibility of a relatively subtle change significantly altering the DI and fluidization dynamics (such that reversal of several airway constriction no longer results from the

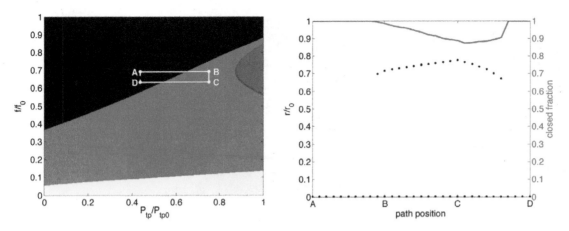

Figure 3. Bifurcation set and DI pseudo-dynamics, with modified parenchymal tethering nonlinearity (see text). By reducing the degree of nonlinear tethering, the DI and ASM fluidization combination fail completely in reversing airway closure. Even transient dilation is limited, with more than 85% of airways remaining in the closed state throughout.

DI-fluidization synergy). While it is merely an example, rather than a concrete hypothesis, it does demonstrate the ability of the airway map to quickly and easily test the effect of many such theories.

We have also shown that airway states, including both the previously-known (open, closed, and bistable) and the new states (oscillatory and chaotic), can be found in a model which does not include a force-length relationship, ASM dynamics, or ventilation. The static bistability in a single airway is in keeping with the findings of Affonce and Lutchen [13], who demonstrated the potential of the bistability to contribute to airway hyper-reactivity. The Anafi and Wilson model [20] also exhibits a well-known bistability, which has in common some elements with the model presented here, but also key differences. It remains possible that the Anafi-Wilson terminal airway model would exhibit a similar bistability to that shown here, based on the elastic mechanics alone in the absence of flow; however this has not been shown and remains the subject of speculation. Similarly their terminal airway model was extended by Venegas *et al.* [21] into a symmetrically branching airway tree. This extended model was shown to exhibit chaotic switching driven by parallel flow and the interacting structure of multiple airways. Here we have shown for the first time that such chaotic behavior can occur in a minimal single airway model, even in the absence of ventilation, and moreover that these chaotic and oscillatory dynamics yield a potential explanation of synergy between deep inspirations and fluidization.

The findings here should also be considered in light of recent controversy surrounding the role of DIs and fluidization in bronchodilation, due to discrepancy between tissue strip and excised airway studies [4,26–28]. We have shown here that synergy between fluidization (or, in fact, a reduction in ASM force by any cause) and DI in airway reopening. However, the idea that fluidization may not bear primary responsibility is certainly worth considering. The methods of analysis presented here are useful tools for evaluating other hypothesis as well.

One significant limitation of the airway map model is that no proper attempt is made to account for the dynamics of ASM itself – ASM force is modelled in the simplest possible fashion, as a prescribed, exerted force. As such, ASM fluidization can only be represented by a simple reduction in exerted force, rather than a process occurring over time. This is a significant assumption, as many potentially important phenomena are ascribed to ASM dynamics (i.e. [29]), and we have previously shown the ability of

ASM dynamics to modulate transitions between open and closed airway states [22]. While many models of ASM dynamics are available in the literature (i.e. [30–33]), modifying the model and analysis presented here to include such effects is as yet an unsolved problem. This remains an important area for future work.

We have assumed throughout that the force-length relationship is constant. Though our formulation easily allows for an approximation to the experimental data (i.e. [34–37]), we have not done so at this stage for two reasons. The first is that properly accounting for the force-length relationship requires a full dynamic model, the difficulties with which are discussed in the preceding paragraph. Secondly, under a simple, static force-length relationship (i.e. [22]), the critical behaviour is driven by the force exerted at very short lengths far from the adapted length, which must typically be extrapolated from the experimental data. In the absence of a dynamic model and detailed data at the short end of the force-length curve, the best assumption is a constant relationship. It is interesting to note that bistable behavior does occur in this model in the absence of ASM force-length dependence, much as it has previously been shown that flow and compensatory pathways are not required [13]. Thus there are several mooted mechanisms driving bistability, each of which could plausibly explain observed heterogeneity and patchy ventilation defects when coupled with a suitable organizing principle. However, we have shown more than just a new route to bistability, but also new oscillatory and chaotic dynamics which were previously unknown and lead to a possible explanation of synergy between fluidization and deep inspiration.

Methods

The 1D continuous map is constructed by combination of the Lambert model [10], which relates airway transmural pressure P and radius r as

$$r(P) = \begin{cases} \sqrt{R_i^2(1-P/P_1)^{-n_1}}, & P \leq 0 \\ \sqrt{r_{imax}^2 - (r_{imax}^2 - R_i^2)(1-P/P_2)^{-n_2}}, & P > 0 \end{cases} \quad (2)$$

where the parameters $R_i, r_{imax}, P_1, P_2, n_1$ and n_2 depend upon airway order [22] and are given explicitly at the end of this section. Throughout we have used an order 5 airway; results are similar for other small caliber airways. The transmural pressure P is given by

$$P(r) = P_{base} - f\frac{F_a(r)}{r} + \tau(r) \qquad (3)$$

where P_{base} is the base transmural pressure, the second term reflects active muscle force f (along with the force-length relationship $F_a(r)$) and the Laplace law $1/r$ dependence, and the third term is the parenchymal tethering. Following the Lai-Fook model [11] we have

$$\tau(r) = 1.4P_{tp}\left(\left(\frac{R_{ref}-r}{R_{ref}}\right) + 1.5\left(\frac{R_{ref}-r}{R_{ref}}\right)^2\right) \qquad (4)$$

where the reference radius R_{ref} is taken according to Eq. 2 at a transmural pressure of 10 cmH$_2$O. The leading coefficient of Eq. 4 bears further discussion. We adopt the notation of Lai-Fook [11], using P_{tp} and referring to it as the *tethering coefficient*. In [11] this is the transpulmonary pressure, by way of its connection with the parenchymal shear modulus μ, where $\mu = 0.7P_{tp}$. In the formulation of Anafi and Wilson [20] the symbol P_A is used instead, in the context of flow-driven behaviour. We adopt the notation of the former as the most natural for a model in the absence of flow.

Thus by substituting Eq. 4 into 3, and then into 2 we obtain the composite function $r(P(r))$ and call this

$$r_2 = r(P(r_1)) := \Phi(r_1; f, P_{tp}), \qquad (5)$$

and thus the combined model may be thought of as a 1D iterated map. We include explicitly the parametric dependence on f and P_{tp} as these are the bifurcation parameters used here. The full explicit form in terms of r_1 is then given by

$$r_2 = \Phi(r_1; f, P_{tp}) =$$
$$\begin{cases} \sqrt{R_i^2(1 - (P_{base} - f\frac{F_a(r_1)}{r_1} + 1.4P_{tp}((\frac{R_{ref}-r_1}{R_{ref}}) + 1.5(\frac{R_{ref}-r_1}{R_{ref}})^2))/P_1)^{-n_1}}, \\ \qquad \text{for} \left(P_{base} - f\frac{F_a(r_1)}{r_1} + 1.4P_{tp}((\frac{R_{ref}-r_1}{R_{ref}}) + 1.5(\frac{R_{ref}-r_1}{R_{ref}})^2)\right) \le 0 \\ \sqrt{r_{imax}^2 - (r_{imax}^2 - R_i^2)(1 - (P_{base} - f\frac{F_a(r_1)}{r_1} + 1.4P_{tp}((\frac{R_{ref}-r_1}{R_{ref}}) + 1.5(\frac{R_{ref}-r_1}{R_{ref}})^2))/P_2)^{-n_2}}, \\ \qquad \text{for} \left(P_{base} - f\frac{F_a(r_1)}{r_1} + 1.4P_{tp}((\frac{R_{ref}-r_1}{R_{ref}}) + 1.5(\frac{R_{ref}-r_1}{R_{ref}})^2)\right) > 0. \end{cases} \qquad (6)$$

Note that continuity of the piecewise function is ensured by the definition of P_2 [10,22]. It is also important to observe that the smooth muscle force f is treated in the simplest possible way, as a prescribed, exerted constant force. In fact, this is an entirely static model and time does not appear at all. While more sophisticated models of ASM are available (i.e. [30–32]), including such dynamics significantly complicates the analysis. See 'Discussion' for more detail. The baseline transmural pressure P_{base} is taken to

be 10 cmH$_2$O throughout. We assume no force-length relationship, that is $F_a \equiv R_{ref}$. The implications of, and reasons for this assumption are addressed in 'Discussion'.

The one-dimensional bifurcation diagrams in Fig. 1 are made by brute force iteration of the map, starting from 5 evenly spaced seeds between 0 and 2 mm. If the iterations converge to a fixed point with a tolerance of 10^{-5} mm, that point is plotted alone; if there is no convergence after 2000 iterations, the last 200 points are all plotted together.

The static load curves of Fig. 1 (c) were created using Eqs. 2, 3 and 4 as follows. The solid curve representing the Lambert airway wall model comes from Eq. 2 alone. The static load curves are obtained by substituting Eq. 4 into 3.

The boundaries of the 2D bifurcation sets in Fig. 2 are computed by the more sophisticated methods used to analyze such maps. For example, boundaries between one fixed point and bistability (yellow-red, and red-black) occur where

$$\Phi(r^*; f, P_{tp}) = r^*, \qquad (7)$$

$$\Phi'(r^*; f, P_{tp}) = 1, \qquad (8)$$

the prime denotes differentiation with respect to r and r^* is the fixed point [38]. These, and similar equations for the other boundaries [38,39] must be solved numerically by a technique known as numerical continuation, which allows solutions to be followed as parameters change [40]. For purposes of classifying fixed points in bifurcation sets (i.e. is the fixed point open or closed?) we use a threshold of 41% of reference radius (0.15 mm for an order 5 airway with $R_{ref} = 0.363$ mm).

The pseudo-dynamics in Fig. 2 are computed by sampling 1000 separate and independent airways, each of which begins at point A and make 10 steps along each segment of the path. At each step, each airway is perturbed by an additive Gaussian random variable and then iterated in the map 30 times. This value is then taken to be the new radius for the airway at that step. The additive random variables have zero mean and standard deviation 0.06 mm, which is 16.6% of R_{ref} for an order 5 airway.

The parameter values used throughout are $R_i = 0.096$ mm, $r_{imax} = 0.384$ mm, $P_1 = 0.2768$ cmH$_2$O, $P_2 = -33.21$ cmH$_2$O, $n_1 = 1$, $n_2 = 8$, $R_{ref} = 0.363$ mm, $f_0 = 15$ cmH$_2$O, and $P_{tp0} = 20$ cmH$_2$O. These are taken from [22] for an order 5 airway.

Acknowledgments

The authors acknowledge the helpful advice of Claire Postlethwaite with regard to map analysis.

Author Contributions

Analyzed the data: GMD JS MHT. Contributed reagents/materials/analysis tools: GMD JS MHT. Wrote the paper: GMD.

References

1. Fish J, Ankin M, Kelly J, Peterman V (1981) Regulation of bronchomotor tone by lung ination in asthmatic and nonasthmatic subjects. Journal of Applied Physiology 50: 1079–1086.
2. Salome C, Thorpe C, Diba C, Brown N, Berend N, et al. (2003) Airway re-narrowing following deep inspiration in asthmatic and nonasthmatic subjects. European Respiratory Journal 22: 62.
3. Skloot G, Permutt S, Togias A (1995) Airway hyperresponsiveness in asthma: a problem of limited smooth muscle relaxation with inspiration. Journal of Clinical Investigation 96: 2393.
4. Chapman D, King G, Berend N, Diba C, Salome C (2010) Avoiding deep inspirations increases the maximal response to methacholine without altering sensitivity in non-asthmatics. Respiratory Physiology & Neurobiology 173: 157–163.
5. Chapman D, Berend N, King G, Salome C (2011) Effect of deep inspiration avoidance on ventilation heterogeneity and airway responsiveness in healthy adults. Journal of Applied Physiology 110: 1400.

6. Kapsali T, Permutt S, Laube B, Scichilone N, Togias A (2000) Potent bronchoprotective effect of deep inspiration and its absence in asthma. Journal of Applied Physiology 89: 711.

7. Scichilone N, Permutt S, Togias A (2001) The lack of the bronchoprotective and not the bronchodilatory ability of deep inspiration is associated with airway hyperresponsiveness. American Journal of Respiratory and Critical Care Medicine 163: 413.

8. Fabry B, Maksym GN, Butler JP, Glogauer M, Navajas D, et al. (2001) Scaling the microrheology of living cells. Physical Review Letters 87: 148102.

9. Trepat X, Deng L, An S, Navajas D, Tschumperlin D, et al. (2007) Universal physical responses to stretch in the living cell. Nature 447: 592–595.

10. Lambert R, Wilson T, Hyatt R, Rodarte J (1982) A computational model for expiratory flow. J Appl Physiol 52: 44–56.

11. Lai-Fook S (1979) A continuum mechanics analysis of pulmonary vascular interdependence in isolated dog lobes. J Appl Physiol 46: 419–429.

12. Macklem P (1996) A theoretical analysis of the effect of airway smooth muscle load on airway narrowing. American Journal of Respiratory and Critical Care Medicine 153: 83–89.

13. Affonce D, Lutchen K (2006) New perspectives on the mechanical basis for airway reactivity and airway hypersensitivity in asthma. J Appl Physiol 101: 1710–1719.

14. Wiggs B, Moreno R, Hogg J, Hilliam C, Pare P (1990) A model of the mechanics of airway narrowing. Journal of Applied Physiology 69: 849–860.

15. Lambert R, Wiggs B, Kuwano K, Hogg J, Pare P (1993) Functional significance of increased airway smooth muscle in asthma and copd. Journal of Applied Physiology 74: 2771–2781.

16. Lambert R, Paré P (1997) Lung parenchymal shear modulus, airway wall remodeling, and bronchial hyperresponsiveness. Journal of Applied Physiology 83: 140–147.

17. Moreno R, Hogg J, Paré P (1986) Mechanics of airway narrowing. The American Review of Respiratory Disease 133: 1171.

18. Latourelle J, Fabry B, Fredberg J (2002) Dynamic equilibration of airway smooth muscle contraction during physiological loading. Journal of Applied Physiology 92: 771–782.

19. Oliver M, Fabry B, Marinkovic A, Mijailovich S, Butler J, et al. (2007) Airway hyperresponsiveness, remodeling, and smooth muscle mass: right answer, wrong reason? American Journal of Respiratory Cell and Molecular Biology 37: 264.

20. Anafi RC, Wilson TA (2001) Airway stability and heterogeneity in the constricted lung. J Appl Physiol 91: 1185–1192.

21. Venegas JG, Winkler T, Musch G, Melo MFV, Layfield D, et al. (2005) Self-organized patchiness in asthma as a prelude to catastrophic shifts. Nature 434: 777–782.

22. Politi A, Donovan G, Tawhai M, Sanderson M, Lauzon A, et al. (2010) A multiscale, spatially distributed model of asthmatic airway hyper-responsiveness. Journal of Theoretical Biology 266: 614–624.

23. Feigenbaum M (1983) Universal behavior in nonlinear systems. Physica D: Nonlinear Phenomena 7: 16–39.

24. Tsuda A, Laine-Pearson F, Hydon P (2011) Why chaotic mixing of particles is inevitable in the deep lung. Journal of Theoretical Biology 286: 57–66.

25. Winkler T, Venegas J (2011) Self-organized patterns of airway narrowing. Journal of Applied Physiology 110: 1482.

26. LaPrad AS, Szabo TL, Suki B, Lutchen KR (2010) Tidal stretches do not modulate responsiveness of intact airways in vitro. J Appl Physiol 109: 295–304.

27. Noble PB, Hernandez JM, Mitchell HW, Janssen LJ (2010) Deep inspiration and airway physiology: human, canine, porcine, or bovine? J Appl Physiol 109: 938–939.

28. LaPrad AS, Szabo TL, Suki B, Lutchen KR (2010) Reply to Noble, Hernandez, Mitchell, and Janssen. J Appl Physiol 109: 940–941.

29. An S, Bai T, Bates J, Black J, Brown R, et al. (2007) Airway smooth muscle dynamics: a common pathway of airway obstruction in asthma. European Respiratory Journal 29: 834–860.

30. Mijailovich S, Butler J, Fredberg J (2000) Perturbed equilibria of myosin binding in airway smooth muscle: bond-length distributions, mechanics, and atp metabolism. Biophysical Journal 79: 2667–2681.

31. Wang I, Politi A, Tania N, Bai Y, Sanderson M, et al. (2008) A mathematical model of airway and pulmonary arteriole smooth muscle. Biophysical Journal 94: 2053–2064.

32. Bates J, Bullimore S, Politi A, Sneyd J, Anafi R, et al. (2009) Transient oscillatory force-length behavior of activated airway smooth muscle. American Journal of Physiology-Lung Cellular and Molecular Physiology 297: L362–L372.

33. Donovan G, Bullimore S, Elvin A, Tawhai M, Bates J, et al. (2010) A continuous-binding cross-linker model for passive airway smooth muscle. Biophysical Journal 99: 3164–3171.

34. Gunst S, Stropp J (1988) Pressure-volume and length-stress relationships in canine bronchi in vitro. Journal of Applied Physiology 64: 2522.

35. Wang L, Pare P, Seow C (2001) Effect of chronic passive length change on airway smooth muscle length-tension relationship. Journal of Applied Physiology 90: 734–740.

36. Bai T, Bates J, Brusasco V, Camoretti-Mercado B, Chitano P, et al. (2004) On the terminology for describing the length-force relationship and its changes in airway smooth muscle. Journal of applied physiology (Bethesda, Md: 1985) 97: 2029.

37. Chin L, Bossé Y, Pascoe C, Hackett T, Seow C, et al. (2012) Mechanical properties of asthmatic airway smooth muscle. European Respiratory Journal 40: 45–54.

38. Strogatz S (1994) Nonlinear dynamics and chaos: with applications to physics, biology, chemistry, and engineering. Studies in nonlinearity. Westview Press.

39. Murray J (2002) Mathematical biology. Number v. 2 in Interdisciplinary applied mathematics. Springer.

40. Allgower E, Georg K (2003) Introduction to numerical continuation methods, volume 45. Society for Industrial Mathematics.

11

Estimation of Individual Muscle Force Using Elastography

Killian Bouillard, Antoine Nordez*, François Hug

University of Nantes, Laboratory «Motricité, Interactions, Performance» (EA 4334), Nantes, France

Abstract

Background: Estimation of an individual muscle force still remains one of the main challenges in biomechanics. In this way, the present study aimed: (1) to determine whether an elastography technique called Supersonic Shear Imaging (SSI) could be used to estimate muscle force, (2) to compare this estimation to that one provided by surface electromyography (EMG), and (3) to determine the effect of the pennation of muscle fibers on the accuracy of the estimation.

Methods and Results: Eleven subjects participated in two experimental sessions; one was devoted to the shear elastic modulus measurements and the other was devoted to the EMG recordings. Each session consisted in: (1) two smooth linear torque ramps from 0 to 60% and from 0 to 30% of maximal voluntary contraction, for the *first dorsal interosseous* and the *abductor digiti minimi*, respectively (referred to as "ramp contraction"); (2) two contractions done with the instruction to freely change the torque (referred to as "random changes contraction"). Multi-channel surface EMG recordings were obtained from a linear array of eight electrodes and the shear elastic modulus was measured using SSI. For ramp contractions, significant linear relationships were reported between EMG activity level and torque ($R^2 = 0.949 \pm 0.036$), and between shear elastic modulus and torque ($R^2 = 0.982 \pm 0.013$). SSI provided significant lower $RMS_{deviation}$ between measured torque and estimated torque than EMG activity level for both types of contraction (1.4 ± 0.7 *vs.* 2.8 ± 1.4% of maximal voluntary contraction for "ramp contractions", $p < 0.01$; 4.5 ± 2.3 *vs.* 7.9 ± 5.9% of MVC for "random changes contractions", $p < 0.05$). No significant difference was reported between muscles.

Conclusion: The shear elastic modulus measured using SSI can provide a more accurate estimation of individual muscle force than surface EMG. In addition, pennation of muscle fibers does not influence the accuracy of the estimation.

Editor: Jose A. L. Calbet, University of Las Palmas de Gran Canaria, Spain

Funding: This work was supported by the Association Française contre les Myopathies (AFM - contract 14597), the Région des Pays de la Loire (2010_11120), and the Fonds Européen de Développement Régional. The funders had no role in study design, data collection and analysis, decision to publish, or preparation of the manuscript.

Competing Interests: The authors have declared that no competing interests exist.

* E-mail: antoine.nordez@univ-nantes.fr

Introduction

Estimation of individual muscle force could provide considerable insight into neuromuscular physiology, motor control, biomechanics, and robotics. It can also contribute to improved diagnosis and management of both neurological and orthopaedic diseases [1]. However, due to muscle redundancy, this estimation represents one of the main challenges in biomechanics. Classically, muscle activity level is evaluated by surface electromyography (EMG), but several limitations inherent to this technique can preclude an accurate estimation of muscle force [2,3]. In addition, although several modelling approaches have been proposed in the literature to estimate muscle force with or without EMG data [1,4,5], these models cannot be fully validated because of the lack of accurate *in vivo* experimental procedures [1].

Because of the non-linearity of the mechanical properties of biological tissues, muscle stress is linked to its elastic modulus [6]. In this way, a linear relationship between muscle stiffness and muscle force has been established in isolated frog muscle [7]. Ford et al. [8] considered that, for isometric contractions, the number of active cross bridges could be the source of both tension and active stiffness of the muscle. Consequently, muscle stiffness could

provide an estimation of muscle force during contraction. However, classical methods used to study the elastic behavior of muscle *in vivo* (e.g., quick release, sinusoidal perturbation) assess the global mechanical properties at a joint level [9,10] without any differentiation of the different structures (i.e., muscle, tendon, or joint) and of the various muscles involved in the task. This problem could be solved by using a new elastographic technique, called supersonic shear imaging (SSI) [11,12]. This technique consists of calculating shear elastic modulus by measuring the local shear wave velocity propagation from a remote mechanical vibration. It has been shown to provide reliable measurements of shear elastic modulus at rest (Lacourpaille L. et al., submitted) and during contraction [13].

Therefore, the aim of this study was to determine whether SSI could be used to estimate individual muscle force and to compare this estimation to that obtained with surface EMG. For that purpose, it was necessary to investigate a task involving a muscle without synergist, i.e., a task in which the measured torque is produced by only one muscle. Thus, we studied isometric index abduction (mainly involving the *first dorsal interosseous* [14]), and isometric little finger abduction (mainly involving the *abductor digiti minimi* [15]). Since shear elastic modulus can be sensitive to the orientation of muscle fibers [16], the other aim of this study was to determine the effect of the pennation of muscle fibers on the relationship between shear elastic modulus and torque. Because the *first dorsal interosseous* is bi-pennated and the *abductor digiti minimi* is fusiform, these two muscles could provide interesting information on the influence of muscle architecture on the relationship between shear elastic modulus and torque.

Materials and Methods

Participants

Eleven healthy males volunteered to participate in this study (25 ± 2.7 years; 179.3 ± 7.9 cm; 75.4 ± 9.1 kg). Participants were informed of the purpose of the study and methods used before providing written consent. The experimental design of the study was approved by the Ethical Committee of Nantes Ouest IV (reference: n°CPP-MIP-001) and was conducted in accordance with the Declaration of Helsinki (last modified in 2004).

Measurements

Ergometer. A homemade ergometer was used to measure the torque produced by index finger abduction and little finger abduction (Fig. 1). Briefly, the subjects were seated with their right elbows flexed to 120° (180° corresponds to the full extension of the elbow), and the pronated forearm was supported by a platform; all fingers were extended with the palm facing down. The hand and fingers #3 to #5 or #2 to #4 (for index abduction and little finger abduction, respectively) were immobilized with Velcro straps to prevent any movement during the contractions (Fig. 1). The lateral side of the index finger or little finger was in contact with a rigid interface, with the proximal interphalangeal joint aligned with the force sensor (SML-50, Interface, Arizona, USA). As depicted in Fig. 1, the thumb was not restrained during index abduction in order to avoid compensation with the *adductor pollicis brevis* involved in the closing of the index-thumb hodler. Participants were instructed to not move the thumb during the index abduction.

Electromyography. Multi-channel surface EMG recordings were obtained from the *first dorsal interosseous* and the *abductor digiti minimi* using an adhesive linear array of eight electrodes with 5-mm inter-electrode distances (Spesmedica, Battipaglia, Italy). The electrode array was located over the muscle belly (for both muscles) and followed the direction of muscle fibers (for the fusiform muscle, the *abductor digiti minimi*). A reference electrode was placed at the level of the wrist. Prior to electrode placement, the skin was cleaned with alcohol in order to minimize impedance. To ensure proper skin-electrode contact, 20 µL of conductive gel were inserted into the cavities of the electrode. Signals were amplified (x 500, EMG-USB, LISIN-OttinoBiolettronica, Turin, Italy), band-pass filtered (6–400 Hz), digitized at a sampling rate of 4096 Hz, and stored by a computer.

Elastography. For measurements of shear elastic modulus, an Aixplorer ultrasonic scanner (Version 4.2, Supersonic Imagine, Aix en Provence, France) was used in the SSI mode (musculo-skeletal preset). As described by Bercoff et al. [11], the system consisted of a transient and remote mechanical vibration generated by radiation force induced by a focused ultrasonic beam (i.e., "pushing beam"). Each pushing beam generated a remote vibration that resulted in the propagation of a transient shear wave. Then, an ultrafast echographic imaging sequence was performed to acquire successive raw radio-frequency data at a very high frame rate (up to 20 kHz). A one-dimensional cross correlation of successive radio-frequency signals was used to determine the shear wave velocity (V_s) along the principle axis of the probe using a time-of-flight estimation. Then, considering a linear elastic behavior, a shear elastic modulus (μ) was calculated using V_s as follows:

$$\mu = \rho V_s^2 \tag{1}$$

where ρ is the density of muscle (1,000 kg/m³).

Note that the linear [11,17–20] and purely elastic [18,20] behaviors are classically considered in most of the studies of muscle elastography.

A. Abductor digitimi minimi   B. First dorsal interosseous

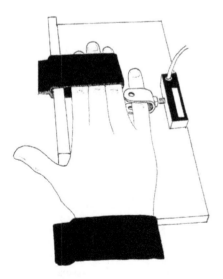
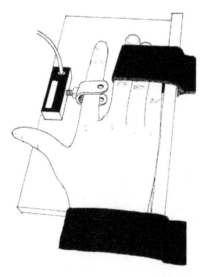

Figure 1. Experimental setup. The right pronated forearm was supported on a platform and all fingers were extended with the palm facing down. The hand and fingers 2 to 4 for little finger abduction (A) or 3 to 5 for index abduction (B) were immobilized with Velcro straps to prevent any movement and compensation during contractions. The little finger (A) or lateral side of the index finger (A) was in contact with a rigid interface, with the proximal interphalangeal joint aligned with the force sensor.

A. Abductor digitimi minimi

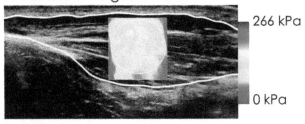

266 kPa

0 kPa

B. First dorsal interosseous

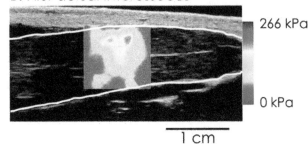

266 kPa

0 kPa

1 cm

Figure 2. Typical example of shear elastic modulus measurement of the *abductor digiti minimi* (A) and the *first dorsal interosseous* (B). These data were obtained in a representative subject during the "ramp contraction". The colored region represents the shear elasticity map with the scale to the right of the figure. The shear elastic modulus (in kPa) was averaged over the greatest muscular area avoiding aponeurosis.

Measurements were made from the *first dorsal interosseous* and *abductor digiti minimi* muscles. For each of these muscles, the probe was aligned carefully with the direction of shortening of the muscle. Maps of the shear elastic modulus were obtained at 1 Hz (i.e., maximal sampling frequency of the device) with a spatial resolution of 1x1 mm (Fig. 2). The shear elasticity map was chosen as large as possible (about from 1×1.5 cm to 1.5×1.5 cm, depending on the muscle depth/thickness) to obtain a representative averaged shear elastic modulus value.

Protocol

The experimental protocol was divided into three sessions. The first session was devoted to the familiarization. The second and third sessions were separated by 48 hours; one was devoted to the SSI measurements, and the other was devoted to the EMG recordings (randomly assigned). Each of these two sessions proceeded in two stages (randomly assigned); one stage was devoted to index abduction (i.e., measurement of the *first dorsal interosseous*), the other stage was devoted to little finger abduction (i.e., measurement of the *abductor digiti minimi*). First, for each muscle, maximal isometric voluntary contractions (MVC) were measured during three maximal contractions lasting 3 s that were separated by 2 min of recovery. The largest of the three forces was considered as the maximum voluntary force and was used to normalize subsequent submaximal contractions. Then, participants were asked to perform one smooth linear torque ramp (refered to as "ramp contraction" in this report) of 30 s from 0 to 60% of the previously determined MVC for index abduction and from 0 to 30% of MVC for little finger abduction. These ranges were the maximal range of torque that can be developed without saturation of the SSI measurement (discussed below) assessed during a preliminary experiment. To control the ramping of the

torque, the participants had to follow a visual feedback displayed on a monitor placed in front of them. After a 5-min recovery period, the subjects performed a new 30-s contraction with the instruction to randomly and slowly change the torque throughout the trial (referred to as "random changes contraction" in this report). They were instructed to develop torque within the range used during the ramp contraction (i.e., between 0 and 60% of MVC for the *first dorsal interosseous* and between 0 and 30% for the *abductor digiti minimi*), and to explore all of this range of torque. During each contraction, depending on the session, shear elastic modulus or surface EMG were recorded and synchronized with torque measurements.

To determine whether hysteresis can interfere in the ability to accurately estimate muscle force, two participants performed an additional experiment consisting of up-going/down-going ramps cycles (i.e., 20-s linear increase of the torque until 30% (*abductor digiti minimi*) or 60% (*first dorsal interosseous*) of MVC, followed by linear 20-s decrease).

Data analysis

Data processing was performed using MATLAB® scripts (The Mathworks, Natick, USA). Prior to data analysis, the raw EMG signals were checked, and putative channels corresponding to the muscle/tendon junction were removed from further analysis (0 to 2 channels, depending on the subject/muscle). Then, for each remaining channel, EMG was Root Mean Squared (RMS) using a time-averaging period of 1 s and averaged across all the channels to obtain a representative EMG activity of the whole muscle. As recommended by Keenan et al. [21], EMG RMS was normalized to the maximal value achieved over 150 ms during MVC contractions to limit signal cancellation.

SSI recordings were exported from software (Version 4.2, Supersonic Imagine, Aix en Provence, France) in "mp4" format, sequenced in "jpeg." An average value of shear elastic modulus over the largest muscular region available on the shear elastic modulus map, excluding aponeurosis from the analyzed region, was calculated for each map, i.e., each second (Fig. 2). Due to limitations of the current version of the ultrasonic scanner, shear elastic modulus measurements saturated at 266 kPa, limiting the range of analysis for most of the participants. If one value in the analyzed region reached 266 kPa, the mean value of this region (for both "ramp" and "random changes" contractions) and all the following values (for only "ramp contractions") were discarded from further analysis.

According to the literature, the relationships between EMG RMS and torque obtained for "ramp contractions" were fitted using a linear model (eq. 2) [22–24]. Based on pilot experiments that showed an excellent correlation between the shear elastic modulus and torque, linear fits (eq. 2) were also performed for the relationship between shear elastic modulus and torque. This model was chosen because it is the simplest one that could be used in the future to assess muscle force in a redundant system. a and b coefficients were classically calculated by minimization of the squared difference between the predicted ($T_{predicted}$) and the measured ($T_{measured}$) torque values during "ramp contractions".

$$T_{predicted,i} = aX_i + b \qquad (2)$$

where X is the EMG RMS (in % of MVC) or the shear elastic modulus (in kPa) and i the index of the shear elastic modulus or RMS EMG sampled at 1 Hz.

The coefficient of determination (R^2) and the $RMS_{deviation}$ (eq. 3) were calculated to assess goodness of fit and the error of estimation for both EMG and SSI measurements.

$$RMS_{deviation} = \frac{\sqrt{\sum_{i=1}^{n} \left(T_{measured,i} - T_{predicted,i}\right)^2}}{n} \quad (3)$$

Previously determined "a" and "b" coefficients (eq. 2) were used to estimate the torque during the "random change contractions" for both EMG and SSI measurements. $RMS_{deviation}$ was also calculated (eq. 3) to quantify the error of estimation during these contractions.

To quantify hysteresis in the two tested participants, relationships between shear elastic modulus and torque were plotted for up-going and down-going conditions. Normalized area of the hysteresis defined as the normalized difference between the areas under the up-going ramp relationship and under the down-going ramp relationship was calculated.

Statistical analysis

Data distributions consistently passed the Kolmogorov-Smirnov normality test (Statistica®V6, Statsoft, Maison-Alfort, France), and thus the values are reported as mean±standard deviation throughout the text and the figures.

Two-way repeated-measure ANOVAs (random factor - participant, between subject factor – method and muscle) were used to test the effect of the method (i.e., EMG and SSI) and of the muscle (i.e., *first dorsal interosseous* and *abductor digiti minimi*) on both the coefficient of determination and $RMS_{deviation}$ for "ramp" and "random changes contraction". The level of significance was set as $p < 0.05$.

Results

Range of analysis

Of the 22 "ramp contractions" (2 muscles×1 ramp×11 subjects), the saturation level of the shear elastic modulus at 266 kPa was reached 15 times before the end of the ramp. Consequently, "ramp contractions" were analyzed up to 39.1±12.6% of MVC (range: 23.8-55.4% of MVC) for *first dorsal interosseous* and up to 25.3±4.2 % of MVC (range: 16.3-32.2% of MVC) for *abductor digiti minimi*.

EMG RMS/torque and shear elastic modulus/torque relationships

For both *first dorsal interosseous* and *abductor digiti minimi*, Fig. 3 depicts a typical example of the relationship between EMG RMS and torque and between shear elastic modulus and torque.

Mean R^2 of the linear regressions fitted to EMG RMS/torque data was 0.961±0.032 (range: 0.881–0.992) for the *first dorsal interosseous* and 0.936±0.036 (range: 0.847–977) for the *abductor digiti minimi*. The mean $RMS_{deviation}$ linked to this fitting was 3.0±1.5% of MVC (range: 1.1–5.1% of MVC) for the *first dorsal interosseous* and 2.7±1.5% of MVC (range: 1.0–5.9% of MVC) for the *abductor digiti minimi*.

The linear regressions fitted to shear elastic modulus/torque data led to R^2 values greater than 0.95 for both muscles of all subjects. More precisely, mean R^2 was 0.986±0.007 (range: 0.976–0.997) for the *first dorsal interosseous* and 0.977±0.016 (range: 0.951–995) for the *abductor digiti minimi*. $RMS_{deviation}$ was 1.7±0.8% of MVC (range: 0.4–2.9% of MVC) for the *first dorsal interosseous* and 1.05±0.44% of MVC (range: 0.6–1.9 % of MVC) for the *abductor digiti minimi*.

Accuracy of torque estimation

For both *first dorsal interosseous* and *abductor digiti minimi*, Fig. 4 depicts a typical example of the torque measurements and the torque estimations during "random changes contractions".

Estimation of torque during "random change contractions" used linear regression equations as calibrations and thus combined two sources of deviation: one from linear fitting and the other one from torque estimation. Using EMG RMS, mean $RMS_{deviation}$ of the torque estimation was 7.3±3.5% of MVC (range: 4.0–13.3% of MVC) for the *first dorsal interosseous* and 9.2±7.7% of MVC (range: 1.9–28.2% of MVC) for the *abductor digiti minimi*. Using the shear elastic modulus, mean $RMS_{deviation}$ of the torque estimation was 5.8±2.3% of MVC (range: 1.3–9.2% of MVC) for the *first dorsal interosseous* and 3.2±1.3% of MVC (range: 1.7–6.0% of MVC) for the *abductor digiti minimi*.

Comparison between SSI and EMG

ANOVA revealed a main effect of "method" on both the coefficient of determination and on the $RMS_{deviation}$ of the linear fitting obtained during the "ramp contractions." More precisely, we

A. Abductor digitimi minimi

Subject #7

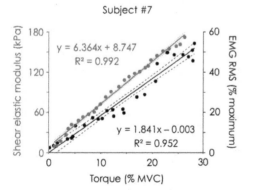

B. First dorsal interosseous

Subject #1

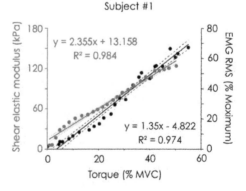

Figure 3. Typical EMG RMS/torque and shear elastic modulus/torque relationships calculated during "ramp contraction". Linear regressions (and their 95% of confidence interval in dashed lines) between normalized EMG RMS and torque (black dots/lines) and between shear elastic modulus and torque (red or grey dots/lines) are depicted for both the the *abductor digiti minimi* (A) and the *First dorsal interosseous* (A). MVC, Maximal Voluntary Contraction; EMG RMS, Root mean square value of the electromyographic signal.

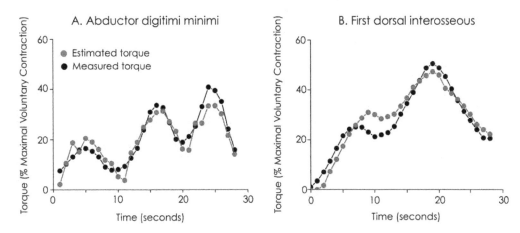

Figure 4. Typical example of torque estimation using supersonic shear imaging. Shear elastic modulus and torque (black dots/lines) measurements were obtained during "random changes contraction". Torque estimation (red or grey dots/lines) was performed using the equation of the linear regression obtained for "ramp contraction" (Eq 2 in the manuscript). Torque measurements and torque estimations are depicted for both the *abductor digiti minimi* (A) and the *first dorsal interosseous* (B).

found a significantly greater R^2 ($p < 0.001$) and a significantly lower $RMS_{deviation}$ ($p < 0.001$) for shear elastic modulus/torque relationships compared to RMS EMG/torque relationships (Fig. 5). ANOVA also revealed a main effect of "method" on the $RMS_{deviation}$ for "random changes contractions". $RMS_{deviation}$ was significantly lower ($p < 0.05$) for shear elastic modulus than for EMG RMS (Fig. 5).

Effect of the pennation of muscle fibers

ANOVA revealed no main effect of "muscle" on the coefficients of determination of the linear regressions obtained for the "ramp contractions" ($p = 0.10$) or on $RMS_{deviations}$ for

both "ramp contractions" ($p = 0.17$) and "random change contractions" ($p = 0.61$).

Hysteresis

Figure 6 depicts an individual example of the negligible hysteresis calculated for shear elastic modulus measurements. For subject #1, hysteresis was 4.15% for *abductor digiti minimi* and −6.87% for *first dorsal interosseous*; for subject #2, it was 4.3% for *abductor digiti minimi* and 2.8% for *first dorsal interosseous*.

Discussion

The present study reported linear relationships between EMG activity level and torque and between shear elastic modulus and torque for both the *first dorsal interosseous* (from 0 to about 40% of MVC) and the *abductor digiti minimi* muscles (from 0 to 25% of MVC). The results also showed that estimation of individual muscle force is more accurate using shear elastic modulus measured with SSI than surface EMG.

The *first dorsal interosseous* is responsible of about 93% of the force produced during index finger abduction [14]. Subjects with a transfer of the *abductor digiti minimi* are not able to perform a little finger abduction [15]. Consequently, one could reasonably consider that the measured torque was produced by only one muscle in both tasks. In other words, the measured external torque can be considered as the individual muscle torque. This condition resolves the indeterminacy problem of load sharing (due to muscle redundancy), which usually complicates the relationship between individual muscle torque and the external global torque. For instance, Nordez and Hug [13] reported the shear elastic modulus/torque relationship during an isometric elbow flexion involving various synergist muscles. Because changes in load sharing can occur during this task (Bouillard K., et al., submitted), they were unable to establish the relationship between modulus and individual muscle torque. To the best of our knowledge, the present study is the first to report robust linear regression between the shear elastic modulus and individual muscle torque. Using magnetic resonance imaging, other authors measured the muscle shear elastic modulus during contraction [25,26]. However, due to the long acquisition time (up to 1 min) of this technique, these studies

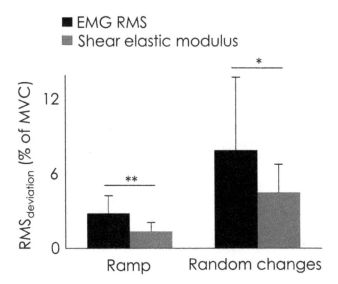

Figure 5. Accuracy of individual muscle force estimation. $RMS_{deviation}$ between estimated torque and measured torque was calculated for "ramp contractions" and "random changes contractions" from both EMG RMS and shear elastic modulus. *: $p < 0.05$ **: $p < 0.01$ MVC, Maximal Voluntary Contraction.

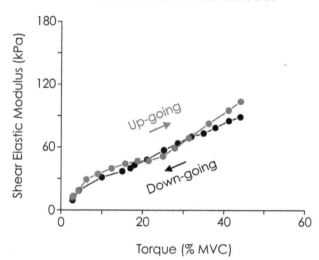

Figure 6. Illustration of the absence of hysteresis. Two subjects performed up-going/down-going ramps cycles (i.e., 20-s linear increase of the torque until 30% (*abductor digiti minimi*) or 60% (*first dorsal interosseous*) of maximal voluntary contraction (MVC) directly followed by linear 20-s decrease). The relationship between shear elastic modulus and torque is depicted for the *abductor digiti minimi* (A) and the *first dorsal interosseous* (A) and. The results show that there was no hysteresis effect on the relationship between shear elastic modulus and torque.

tested only a few torque levels and thus were not able to provide robust shear elastic modulus/torque relationships. Taking into account the high coefficients of determination (i.e., $R^2 > 0.95$ in all of the cases) and the low deviation (i.e., $RMS_{deviation} < 2.9\%$ of MVC in all of the cases) reported herein, the relationship between shear elastic modulus and individual muscle torque seems to be fitted correctly by linear regression. Furthermore, we can reasonably extend our results to individual muscle force, confirming expectations that a stiffness measurement can provide an estimation of muscle force [7,8]. Thus, individual muscle force can be simply estimated using SSI and a linear calibration.

In accordance with previous studies, relationships between EMG activity level and muscle torque were fitted well by a linear model for both the *first dorsal interosseous* [22,23] and the *abductor digiti minimi* [24], at least over the torque ranges examined in present study. However, statistical analysis showed a significantly lower $RMS_{deviation}$ obtained from shear elastic modulus compared to EMG activity level for both "ramp contractions" and "random changes contractions." This demonstrates that SSI provides a more precise estimation of muscle force than EMG.

Note that estimation of muscle force during "random changes contractions" using SSI could be affected by hysteresis on the ascending (i.e., torque increase) and descending (i.e., torque decrease) shear elastic modulus/torque relationship (i.e., higher shear elastic modulus values during the ascending phase compared to the descending phase). To determine whether this phenomenon could have influenced the measurement of shear elastic modulus, an additional experiment was performed on two subjects. Fig. 6 clearly shows that there was no hysteresis effect on the shear elastic modulus/torque relationship. This was confirmed by the calculation of the normalized area of the hysteresis. Since hysteresis was demonstrated for EMG activity level/torque relationship [27], this result can also explain the more accurate estimation of individual muscle force using SSI compared to EMG.

Regarding the influence of the angle between muscle fascicules and the SSI probe on the measurements of shear elastic modulus

[16], we tested the effect of muscle architecture on the precision of the estimation of muscle torque. In this way, the present study reported data for a bi-pennated muscle (i.e., the *first dorsal interosseous*, pennation angle $\approx 15°$) [28], and a fusiform muscle (i.e., the *abductor digiti minimi*). The accuracy of the estimation of individual muscle force using both SSI and EMG was not significantly different between muscles. It must be acknowledged that, due to saturation limitation, the experiments were not performed on the same range of torque for both muscles (i.e., $39.1\pm12.6\%$ of MVC for the *first dorsal interosseous* vs. $25.3\pm4.2\%$ of MVC for the *abductor digiti minimi*). However, the same range of values of the shear elastic modulus was tested. Overall, this conclusion should be confirmed in other conditions because it might be specific to the present experimental procedure (task and muscle).

Conclusions and perspectives

The present study focused on tasks involving only one synergist muscle to show that the shear elastic modulus measured using SSI can provide an accurate estimation of individual muscle force until 40% of MVC and during isometric contraction. Further investigations should associate moment arm measurements (e.g., using magnetic resonance imaging) to shear elastic modulus measurements to estimate individual muscle forces more directly during more complex movement, allowing us to precisely quantify the load sharing among all the synergists. In addition, the shear elastic modulus measurement using SSI would provide a unique way to validate the numerous models implemented to estimate muscle force [1].

Acknowledgments

The authors thank Jean Hug for drawing Fig. 1.

Author Contributions

Conceived and designed the experiments: KB AN FH. Performed the experiments: KB. Analyzed the data: KB. Contributed reagents/materials/analysis tools: KB AN FH. Wrote the paper: KB AN FH.

References

1. Erdemir A, McLean S, Herzog W, van den Bogert AJ (2007) Model-based estimation of muscle forces exerted during movements. ClinBiomech (Bristol, Avon) 22: 131–154.

2. Farina D, Merletti R, Enoka RM (2004) The extraction of neural strategies from the surface EMG. J ApplPhysiol 96: 1486–1495.

3. Hug F (2011) Can muscle coordination be precisely studied by surface electromyography? J ElectromyogrKinesiol 21: 1–12.

4. Buchanan TS, Lloyd DG, Manal K, Besier TF (2004) Neuromusculoskeletal modeling: estimation of muscle forces and joint moments and movements from measurements of neural command. J ApplBiomech 20: 367–395.

5. Zajac FE, Neptune RR, Kautz SA (2003) Biomechanics and muscle coordination of human walking: part II: lessons from dynamical simulations and clinical implications. Gait Posture 17: 1–17.

6. Fung Y-cheng (1993) Biomechanics: mechanical properties of living tissues. Springer. 590 p.

7. Mason P (1977) Dynamic stiffness and crossbridge action in muscle. BiophysStructMech 4: 15–25.

8. Ford LE, Huxley AF, Simmons RM (1981) The relation between stiffness and filament overlap in stimulated frog muscle fibres. J Physiol (Lond) 311: 219–249.

9. Cornu C, Goubel F, Fardeau M (2001) Muscle and joint elastic properties during elbow flexion in Duchenne muscular dystrophy. J Physiol (Lond) 533: 605–616.

10. Weiss PL, Hunter IW, Kearney RE (1988) Human ankle joint stiffness over the full range of muscle activation levels. J Biomech 21: 539–544.

11. Bercoff J, Tanter M, Fink M (2004) Supersonic shear imaging: a new technique for soft tissue elasticity mapping. IEEE Trans UltrasonFerroelectr Freq Control 51: 396–409.

12. Shinohara M, Sabra K, Gennisson J-L, Fink M, Tanter M (2010) Real-time visualization of muscle stiffness distribution with ultrasound shear wave imaging during muscle contraction. Muscle Nerve 42: 438–441.

13. Nordez A, Hug F (2010) Muscle shear elastic modulus measured using supersonic shear imaging is highly related to muscle activity level. J ApplPhysiol 108: 1389–1394.

14. Chao EY (1989) Biomechanics of the hand: a basic research study. World Scientific. 208 p.

15. Lebreton E (2010) Hypothenar eminence. Chir Main 29: 213–223.

16. Gennisson J-L, Deffieux T, Macé E, Montaldo G, Fink M, et al. (2010) Viscoelastic and anisotropic mechanical properties of in vivo muscle tissue assessed by supersonic shear imaging. Ultrasound Med Biol 36: 789–801.17.

17. Gennisson J-L, Catheline S, Chaffaï S, Fink M (2003) Transient elastography in anisotropic medium: application to the measurement of slow and fast shear wave speeds in muscles. J Acoust Soc Am 114: 536–541.

18. Catheline S, Gennisson JL, Delon G, Fink M, Sinkus R, et al. (2004) Measuring of viscoelastic properties of homogeneous soft solid using transient elastography: an inverse problem approach. J Acoust Soc Am 116: 3734–3741.

19. Nordez A, Gennisson JL, Casari P, Catheline S, Cornu C (2008) Character-ization of muscle belly elastic properties during passive stretching using transient elastography. J Biomech 41: 2305–2311.

20. Deffieux T, Montaldo G, Tanter M, Fink M (2009) Shear wave spectroscopy for in vivo quantification of human soft tissues visco-elasticity. IEEE Trans Med Imaging 28: 313–322.

21. Keenan KG, Farina D, Maluf KS, Merletti R, Enoka RM (2005) Influence of amplitude cancellation on the simulated surface electromyogram. J ApplPhysiol 98: 120–131.22.

22. Milner-Brown HS, Stein RB (1975) The relation between the surface electromyogram and muscular force. J Physiol (Lond) 246: 549–569.

23. Lawrence JH, De Luca CJ (1983) Myoelectric signal versus force relationship in different human muscles. J ApplPhysiol 54: 1653–1659.

24. Del Santo F, Gelli F, Ginanneschi F, Popa T, Rossi A (2007) Relation between isometric muscle force and surface EMG in intrinsic hand muscles as function of the arm geometry. Brain Res 1163: 79–85.

25. Dresner MA, Rose GH, Rossman PJ, Muthupillai R, Manduca A, et al. (2001) Magnetic resonance elastography of skeletal muscle. J MagnReson Imaging 13: 269–276.

26. Basford JR, Jenkyn TR, An K-N, Ehman RL, Heers G, et al. (2002) Evaluation of healthy and diseased muscle with magnetic resonance elastography. Arch Phys Med Rehabil 83: 1530–1536.

27. Orizio C, Baruzzi E, Gaffurini P, Diemont B, Gobbo M (2010) Electromyogram and force fluctuation during different linearly varying isometric motor tasks. J ElectromyogrKinesiol 20: 732–741.

28. Infantolino BW, Challis JH (2010) Architectural properties of the first dorsal interosseous muscle. J Anat 216: 463–469.

12

Distinct Disease Phases in Muscles of Facioscapulohumeral Dystrophy Patients Identified by MR Detected Fat Infiltration

Barbara H. Janssen[1]*, **Nicoline B. M. Voet**[2], **Christine I. Nabuurs**[1], **Hermien E. Kan**[1,3], **Jacky W. J. de Rooy**[1], **Alexander C. Geurts**[2], **George W. Padberg**[4], **Baziel G. M. van Engelen**[4], **Arend Heerschap**[1]

1 Department of Radiology, Radboud University Medical Center, Nijmegen, The Netherlands, 2 Department of Rehabilitation, Radboud University Medical Center, Nijmegen, The Netherlands, 3 Department of Radiology, Leiden University Medical Centre, Leiden, The Netherlands, 4 Department of Neurology, Radboud University Medical Center, Nijmegen, The Netherlands

Abstract

Facioscapulohumeral muscular dystrophy (FSHD) is an untreatable disease, characterized by asymmetric progressive weakness of skeletal muscle with fatty infiltration. Although the main genetic defect has been uncovered, the downstream mechanisms causing FSHD are not understood. The objective of this study was to determine natural disease state and progression in muscles of FSHD patients and to establish diagnostic biomarkers by quantitative MRI of fat infiltration and phosphorylated metabolites. MRI was performed at 3T with dedicated coils on legs of 41 patients (28 men/13 women, age 34–76 years), of which eleven were re-examined after four months of usual care. Muscular fat fraction was determined with multi spin-echo and T1 weighted MRI, edema by TIRM and phosphorylated metabolites by 3D ^{31}P MR spectroscopic imaging. Fat fractions were compared to clinical severity, muscle force, age, edema and phosphocreatine (PCr)/ATP. Longitudinal intramuscular fat fraction variation was analyzed by linear regression. Increased intramuscular fat correlated with age ($p<0.05$), FSHD severity score ($p<0.0001$), inversely with muscle strength ($p<0.0001$), and also occurred sub-clinically. Muscles were nearly dichotomously divided in those with high and with low fat fraction, with only 13% having an intermediate fat fraction. The intramuscular fat fraction along the muscle's length, increased from proximal to distal. This fat gradient was the steepest for intermediate fat infiltrated muscles (0.07 ± 0.01/cm, $p<0.001$). Leg muscles in this intermediate phase showed a decreased PCr/ATP ($p<0.05$) and the fastest increase in fatty infiltration over time (0.18 ± 0.15/year, $p<0.001$), which correlated with initial edema ($p<0.01$), if present. Thus, in the MR assessment of fat infiltration as biomarker for diseased muscles, the intramuscular fat distribution needs to be taken into account. Our results indicate that healthy individual leg muscles become diseased by entering a progressive phase with distal fat infiltration and altered energy metabolite levels. Fat replacement then relatively rapidly spreads over the whole muscle.

Editor: Jan Kassubek, University of Ulm, Germany

Funding: This work was supported by the Prinses Beatrix Spierfonds [WAR08-15] (https://www.prinsesbeatrixspierfonds.nl), ZonMW [89000003 (http://www.zonmw.nl/en/), the FSHD Global Research Foundation (http://www.fshdglobal.org/), and the FSH Society (http://www.fshsociety.org/). The funders had no role in study design, data collection and analysis, decision to publish, or preparation of the manuscript.

Competing Interests: The authors have declared that no competing interests exist.

* E-mail: Barbara.Janssen@radboudumc.nl

Introduction

Facioscapulohumeral muscular dystrophy (FSHD) is the third most common hereditary muscular disorder [1]. The disease is characterized by progressive asymmetric weakness and fatty infiltration of skeletal muscles. In recent years it was demonstrated that FSHD is associated with a contraction of D4Z4 repeats on chromosome 4q35 [2], leading to lost repression of DUX4, a protein that exerts toxic effects on muscle cells [3].

Even though the most important genetic event for the disease seems to be identified, a causative treatment is not yet available [4]. Progress is hampered because the trigger for DUX4 expression and the further unfolding of disease processes leading to fatty infiltration and muscle weakness are not known. Thus clarification of the underlying mechanisms is expected to offer clues for a more targeted approach in the search for treatment [5]. Understanding these mechanisms first requires that some key questions concerning the process of fatty infiltration are addressed. What is the natural distribution of fatty infiltration? How is this related to clinical severity, to muscle weakness and to energy metabolism? Is there prevalence for specific muscles to be affected and does fatty infiltration vary within muscles? What is the natural progression over time and what are predictive signs of progression?

To answer these questions and to evaluate treatment effectiveness, the use of a non-invasive quantitative imaging method, such as MRI, is essential. Unlike biopsies, MRI is not limited to a single location, and longitudinal data can be collected without risk for the patient. MR of fatty infiltration in muscles has been used to study muscular disorders like Duchenne muscular dystrophy [6,7]. We have introduced a quantitative MRI measure of fatty infiltration in muscles based on T2 relaxation time analysis and demonstrated its value in a preliminary study of FSHD patients [8]. Phosphorus MR spectroscopy has been used extensively to investigate the energy status of diseased muscles [9–15]. Recently it was also introduced in a pilot study with FSHD patients [16].

Until now quantitative MR imaging studies were performed in limited numbers of patients. However, because of the variability in age of onset and in degree of disease severity [17], a study of its pathophysiology requires the participation of a relatively large number of well described patients. The main aim of this study was to determine natural disease state and progression by quantitative MRI of skeletal muscles in the legs of a large, well-characterized cohort of genetically confirmed FSHD patients. In particular we wanted to address the aforementioned pathophysiological questions to ultimately uncover clues on disease mechanism and to establish MRI biomarkers with prognostic and predictive value for personalized assessments.

Materials and Methods

Patients and Study Design

We recruited 41 FSHD patients from the local neurology department (28 men/13 women, age 21–81 years, see Table 1 for patients demographics). Of 36 patients the upper leg ('thigh') was examined, they were selected from a group of patients that were entering a clinical trial to assess the effects of rehabilitation intervention [18]. In addition we included the MR exams of the lower leg of five patients from a previous study [8], which were re-analyzed in the exact same way as the MR exams of the aforementioned patients (vide infra).

Eleven patients (8 men/3 women, age 34–76 years) were randomly selected, from the group that underwent an MR examination of the thigh, for a follow-up measurement after a period of four months. During this period these patients were instructed to maintain a normal level of activity ('usual care').

All patients were clinically and genetically diagnosed with FSHD and able to walk independently (ankle-foot orthoses and canes were accepted). Patients were all unrelated except for one mother and son (patients #7 and #37). Disease severity was assessed with the Ricci score [19] and maximum voluntary isometric extension (quadriceps) and flexion (hamstrings) of the knee were measured with a quantitative fixed myometry testing system [20]. Ethical approval was obtained from the Radboud university medical center review board, and written informed consent was obtained from all subjects.

MR Methods

MR measurements were performed on a 3T MR system (TIM Trio, Siemens, Erlangen, Germany). Subjects were positioned feet first supine inside the magnet bore. Images were acquired with a home-built proton birdcage radiofrequency coil (inner diameter 25 cm).

In 36 patients, the least affected thigh, according to the subject's own experience was examined, unless there were contraindications (e.g. a previous fracture or recent injury). A fish oil capsule was positioned at one third of the distance between the spina iliaca anterior superior and the patella and served as a landmark for exact matching of the imaging slices between the baseline and follow-up measurements. For the MR examinations of leg, the upper end of the proton coil was positioned at the center of the patella.

MR imaging. Scout images were made in three orthogonal directions to position MRI slices for subsequent scans. The transmit frequency was set on the water resonance and the transmitter voltage was adjusted to the load.

Table 1. Patient demographics.

Patient nr.	Ricci-score	Sex	Age (years)	FSHD duration (years)
1	0	f	21	15
2	1.5	f	25	2
3	1.5	m	31	5
4*	2	m	34	3
5*	3	m	34	9
6	1.5	m	38	17
7	2	m	38	16
8*	3	m	39	19
9	1	f	42	5
10	3.5	m	44	32
11*	2	m	48	14
12	4	m	49	40
13	3.5	m	50	14
14	1.5	f	50	1
15	1.5	f	51	6
16*	4	m	52	19
17*	3.5	m	53	9
18	4.5	f	54	24
19*	3	f	55	1
20*	1.5	m	55	21
21	2	f	56	2
22	2	f	56	22
23	3.5	m	57	17
24	4	m	57	41
25	4	m	58	41
26*	2	f	59	22
27	3	m	59	41
28	4	m	60	9
29	3	m	61	22
30	3.5	m	61	17
31	4	f	63	31
32	4	m	64	15
33	4	m	66	30
34	3	m	66	9
35*	4.5	f	66	49
36	3	m	66	6
37	3	f	68	12
38	2	m	69	na
39	3	m	69	19
40*	3.5	m	76	4
41	3.5	m	81	3

*Underwent two MR exams four months apart.
na = not available.

All imaging was performed in the transversal plane centered on the middle femur for the thigh, or the largest circumference for the leg.

T1 weighted spin echo (SE) MR images were acquired first (field of view (FOV) 175×175 mm; base resolution 384; repetition time

(TR) 530 ms; echo time (TE) 16 ms; slices 23; slice thickness 4 mm; gap 0.4 mm).

Turbo Inversion Recovery Magnitude (TIRM) images were collected with an inversion time (IT) to null the fat signals (FOV 175×175 mm; base resolution 256; TR 4000 ms; TE 41 ms; IT 22 ms; slices 23; slice thickness 4 mm; gap 0.4 mm) to visualize edema [21–23]. To avoid inflow artifacts from venous and arterial blood, saturation bands were placed above the upper and below the lower slice [24].

Subsequently, multi SE MR images were acquired (FOV 175×175 mm; base resolution 256; TR 3000 ms; 16 equally spaced TE's 7.7–123.2 ms; slices 5–8, limited by specific absorption rate; slice thickness 6 mm; gap 9 mm).

Phosphorus MR spectroscopic imaging (^{31}P MRSI). A ^{31}P quadrature insert surface coil covered the quadriceps muscles of the thigh, and for the leg measurements a circularly polarized half volume ^{31}P coil covered the calf musculature. A 3D ^{31}P MRSI dataset was acquired after imaging (FOV 150×150×200 mm; matrix-size 14×14×8 quadriceps/10×10×8 calf, TR 1000 ms; BIR45 adiabatic pulse for excitation; 12 averages; weighted k-space acquisition; nominal voxel volume 8.6 ml quadriceps/16.6 ml calf). Datasets were interpolated to a matrix size of 16×16×8.

Data Analysis

MR imaging. Each of the investigated muscles (see Fig. 1) was analyzed separately. T1weighted images were scored for fatty infiltration using the four grade scale of Lamminen [25], by one experienced musculoskeletal radiologist (J.W.J.R). When a different score was awarded to the proximal and distal images the average score was used.

Muscle area was assessed by drawing regions of interest (ROI's) for every muscle on the center slice of the T2weighted MRI. Fat and muscle fractions were quantified from the multi SE MR images as described earlier [8]. Note that normal fat fraction for healthy muscle does not exceed 10% [26]. This method is not suitable when edema is present, as it will affect the tissues transverse relaxation properties. In those cases, T1 signal intensity (SI) and TIRM SI of the individual muscles were quantified by carefully drawing ROI's in ImageJ (http://rsb.info.nih.gov/ij/) and normalized to bone marrow SI.

To assess natural progression fat fraction differences were normalized to a period of one year for every patient (for every muscle) by dividing these fractions by the exact number of days between the baseline and follow up measurement, multiplied by 365.25.

^{31}P MRSI. From the middle slice of the 3D-MRSI dataset with the largest circumference, representative voxels were assigned to a specific muscle according to the corresponding T1weighted image overlaid with the MRSI grid. Only spectra with a sufficient signal-to-noise-ratio (SNR) (Cramer Rao Lower Bound (γATP) <30%) were included for further analysis.

Free induction decays were zero-filled to double the number of points and apodized by 8 Hz with a Lorentzian line shape and manually phased using jMRUI 4.0 [27]. Peak areas were obtained from inorganic phosphate (Pi), PCr (fitted to a Lorentzian line shape), and ATP (fitted to a Gaussian line shape), using the AMARES algorithm [28] with prior knowledge on the relative line width, frequency and amplitude.

Metabolite ratios: PCr/ATP and Pi/ATP were evaluated to avoid coil profile variations. The pH was calculated from the Pi-PCr frequency shift [29]. The value of each parameter was averaged for all analyzed voxels in one muscle and this value was used for further analysis.

Statistics

Statistical analyses were performed with Prism 5.0 (GraphPad Software, San Diego, California, USA). Non-parametric one-way-ANOVA (Kruskal-Wallis test) was used to investigate differences in the average fat fraction between muscles, with Dunn's Multiple Comparison Test as post-hoc test. One-tailed correlation analyses were performed between fat fraction and patients' age, duration of disease, radiological score, Ricci-scores, maximum voluntary force, PCr/ATP, Pi/ATP, and pH. Linear regression analysis was used to assess the distribution of fatty infiltration over the length of the muscle. Outcome parameters in this analyses are the slope of the line, indicating the direction of fatty infiltration over the length of the muscle, and the coefficient of determination (R^2), indicating to what extent fat fraction increases or decreases linearly over the length of the muscle. One-way ANOVA was used to investigate dependence of fat fraction progression on initial muscle fraction. T1 SI difference was compared between muscles normal and hyperintense TIRM images with a one-tailed t-test, and correlation was investigated with linear regression.

Results

Muscular Fat Infiltration, Edema, Clinical Grading and Muscle Strength in FSHD

Fat infiltration in skeletal muscles is visible as hyperintense areas on T1 weighted MR images (Fig. 1A–C). This may be accompanied by edema, which can be identified independently from fatty infiltration by TIRM images (Fig. 1D). In 41 FSHD patients we investigated 446 leg muscles, of which 4.3% showed edema, which was mostly present in the quadriceps muscles.

The quantitative assessment of muscular fat fraction revealed that 262 of the remaining 427 muscles were normal or mildly fat infiltrated (<0.25 fat fraction), 54 were intermediately fat infiltrated (between 0.25 and 0.75 fat fraction) and 111 muscles were severely infiltrated (>0.75 fat fraction). A fat fraction distribution plot resulted in a typical hourglass shape (Fig. 2A). Significant differences were observed in average fat fractions of thigh muscles (p<0.01), in particular the semimembranosus had a significant higher fat fraction than the vastus lateralis and vastus medialis (Fig. 2B).

Average fat fraction correlated positively with patients' age (p<0.05, $R^2 = 0.15$) (Fig. 3A) and FSHD duration (p<0.0001, $R^2 = 0.54$), (Fig. 3B). Slopes of the correlations were not significantly different between muscles (Fig. S1 and S2). The average yearly increase in fatty infiltration was 0.8±0.4% for age and 1.9±0.3% for FSHD duration. The average fat fraction showed a strong correlation with radiological scores (p<0.0001, $R^2 = 0.70$) (Fig. 3C) and with overall clinical Ricci score for FSHD severity (p<0.0001, $R^2 = 0.90$) (Fig. 3D). The fat fraction deviated from normal at Ricci score 2 (a subclinical event as this score excludes leg muscle involvement) and further increased at higher Ricci scores. Muscle fraction multiplied by the muscle area significantly correlated with muscle strength for the quadriceps and hamstring (p<0.0001, $R^2 = 0.57$) (Fig. 3E).

Intramuscular Fat Distribution

Visual inspection of MR images revealed that the fat fraction was often not evenly distributed over the length of the muscle (Fig. 4). Muscle with an intermediate fat fraction showed the steepest fatty infiltration gradient over the length of the muscle (7±1% cm^{-1}, mean±SEM). This value was significantly higher compared to muscles that were normal or mildly fat infiltrated (1.3±0.3% cm^{-1}, p<0.0001) and those that were heavily

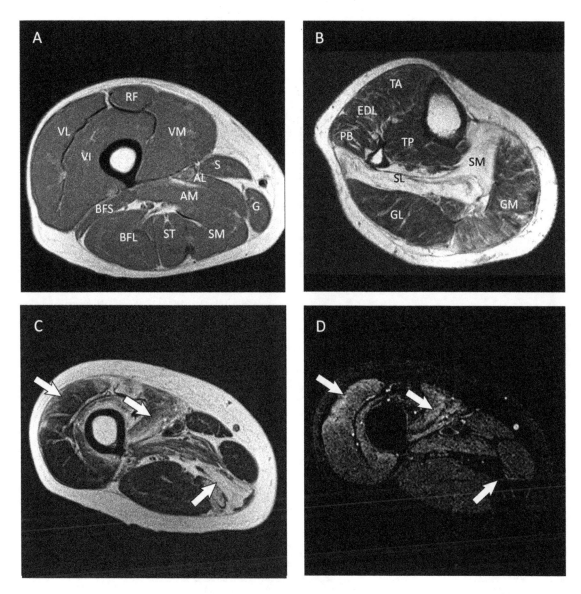

Figure 1. Typical transversal T1 weigthed and TIRM MR images of FSHD patients. (A) Transverse T1 weigthed image of the thigh of a male FSHD patient (age 38), showing fatty infiltration (hyperintense signal) in the semimembranosus and semitendinosus muscles. **(B)** Transverse T1 weighted image of the leg of a male FSHD patient (age 66 year). Fatty infiltration of the soleus muscles is clearly visible. **(C)** Transverse T1 weighted image of the thigh of a 39-year-old male FSHD patient. **(D)** Corresponding TIRM image. The semi-membranosus is clearly fat infiltrated (grey striped arrow), this results in a nulled signal on the corresponding TIRM image. In contrast, the vastus lateralis and vastus intermedius show hyperintense signal in the TIRM images (white arrows) reflecting edema or inflammation. The different muscles in the thigh (Fig. 1.A) and calf (Fig. 1.B) are indicated by the following abbreviations: rectus femoris (RF), vastus lateralis (VL), vastus intermedius (VI), vastus medialis (VM), sartorius (S), adductor longus (AL), adductor magnus (AM), gracillis (G), semi membranosus (SM), semi tendinosus (ST), biceps femoris long head (BFL) and biceps femoris short head (BFS), tibialis anterior (TA), extensor digitorum, longus (EDL), peroneus brevis (PB), tibialis posterior (TP), soleus medialis (SOM), soleus lateralis (SL), gastrocnemius medialis (GM) and gastrocnemius lateralis (GL).

infiltrated by fat $(1.1\pm0.1\% \text{ cm}^{-1}, p<0.0001)$. Overall fat fraction rose from proximal to distal.

Natural Progression of Fatty Infiltration

The natural progression of fatty infiltration was investigated for 85 muscles of eleven patients. An average increase in fat fraction of 0.054 ± 0.12 per year was observed. In intermediately affected muscles (n = 12) the progression of fatty infiltration was much faster $(0.18\pm0.15$ per year) as compared to heavily fat infiltrated muscles $(0.00\pm0.10$ per year, n = 20) and to normal to mildly infiltrated muscles $(0.043\pm0.10$ per year, n = 53). Natural progression in fat

infiltration depended on the initial muscle fraction $(p<0.01)$ and appeared to increase from distal to proximal (Fig. 4).

Six muscles, in two patients, showed hyperintensity on the baseline TIRM images, indicating edema. The T1 SI difference between baseline and follow up exam, representing fat infiltration, was significantly different in muscles with hyperintense signal on baseline TIRM images compared to TIRM normal muscles (n = 14) of the same patients $(p<0.01)$ (Fig. 5). Linear regression analysis showed a trend between the TIRM SI and the difference in T1 SI $(p<0.1, R^2 = 0.1)$.

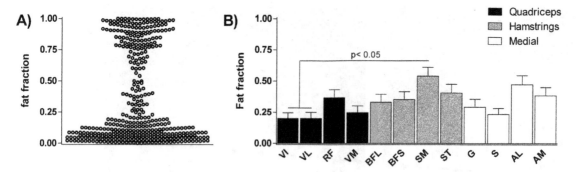

Figure 2. Distribution of naturally occuring fat fraction of the thigh muscles of a large cohort of FSHD patients. (**A**) Fat fraction distribution over all muscles. Fat fraction of 0 signifies 100% muscle, 1 indicates 100% fat. Muscles with an intermediary fat fraction (>0.25 and <0.75) are observed, in ~13% of the investigated muscles. (**B**) Involvement of individual thigh muscles in FSHD. Average fat fraction of 36 patients. Error bars (SEM) reflect the high variability in this fraction between patients. The SM appears to be the most affected muscle of the upper leg, having a significantly higher average fat fraction (0.54±0.41) compared to the VL or VI (0.20±0.29, 0.20±0.27, respectively). Note that fat fractions are not Gaussian distributed therefore reporting only mean±error values is not a good representation of the data.

High-energy Phosphate Metabolites

Analysis of phosphate metabolites by ^{31}P MRS revealed that the PCr/ATP ratio correlated with the fat fraction of the specific muscle (quadriceps $p<0.05$, $R^2 = 0.06$, calf $p<0.01$, $R^2 = 0.33$). This PCr/ATP ratio is significantly decreased in the intermediately fat infiltrated muscles compared to muscles with a normal fat fraction ($p<0.05$), but was not further decreased in muscles with a high fat fraction (Fig. 6A). The PCr/ATP ratio also correlated with muscle force ($p<0.001$, Fig. 6B).

Discussion

In this study we identified three distinct phases of fat infiltration in lower limb muscles of FSHD patients by quantitative MR. An analysis of the average fat fraction for all individual muscles uncovered an hourglass pattern of many muscles with either very

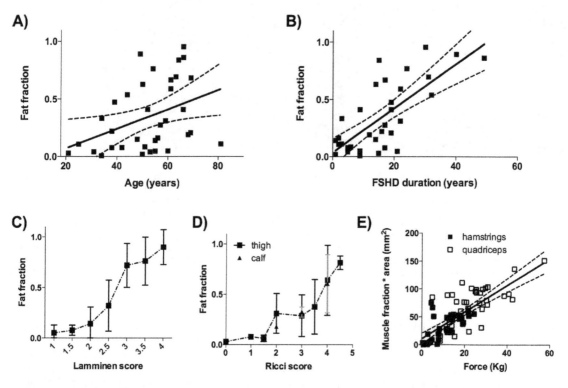

Figure 3. Correlation of fat or muscle fraction, determined by quantitative MRI, with clinical scores. (**A**) Correlation between age of the patient and average fat fraction of the thigh ($p<0.05$, $R^2 = 0.15$). (**B**) Average fat fraction of the thigh and FSHD duration are highly correlated ($p<0.0001$, $R^2 = 0.54$). (**C**) Fat fraction highly correlates with the radiological Lamminen score of the corresponding muscle ($p<0.0001$, $R^2 = 0.70$). (**D**) Quantitative fat fraction of lower limb correlates with patients Ricci score ($p<0.0001$, $R^2 = 0.90$). Fat fraction starts to increase above normal levels at Ricci score 2. The high standard deviation depicted in the error bars signifies the large variation in fat fraction determined in the limb and the appointed Ricci score. (**E**) Correlation between muscle fraction (1-fat fraction) and force of quadriceps and hamstring muscle groups ($p<0.0001$ and $R^2 = 0.76$).

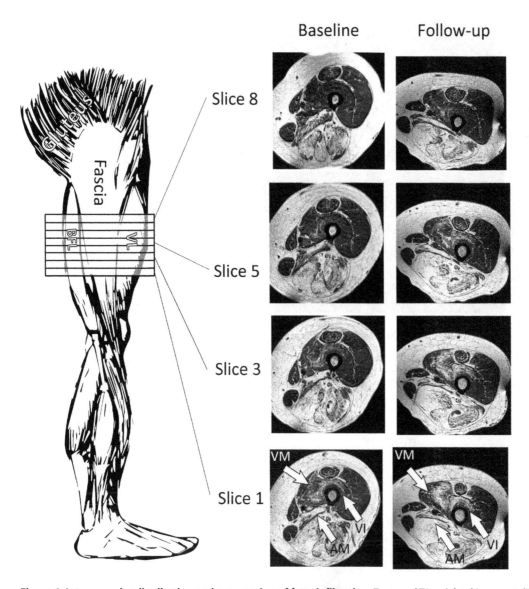

Figure 4. Intramuscular distribution and progression of fatty infiltration. Transveral T1 weighted images at different positions of the thigh of a FSHD patient. Baseline measurement (left panels) reveals an uneven distruibution over the length of the muscle with an increasing fat infiltration from proximal (top) to distal (bottom), especially prominent in the VM, VI, AM. This fatty gradient was largest in intermediate fat infiltrated muscles, as was shown by the linear regression analyses. These intermediately fat infiltrated muscles also showed the largest increase in fatty infiltration over time. From the follow-up measurement (right panels) it is clear to see that fat is increasing distally. AM = adductor magnus; BFL = biceps femoris long head; VI = vastus intermedius; VL = vastus lateris; VM = vastus medialis.

low or high fat, and few muscles with an intermediate fat fraction. This quasi-binary distribution has not been reported for other muscular dystrophies [7] and may be FSHD specific. The intermediate phase is most characteristic, showing a relative steep fat gradient over the length of the muscles, an altered energy metabolism and rapid progression of fatty infiltration.

For other dystrophies often average values of all subjects or muscles are presented, which obscures the presence of a specific distribution. The average fat fraction as calculated over all investigated muscles in this study (0.3±0.1), actually only was present in 36 out of 427 muscles. Fat fractions were highest in the semi membranosus, semi tendinosus and adductor muscles as has been previously described by Wattjes et al. [21]. The vastus muscles were largely preserved.

We found that in leg muscles the intramuscular fat fraction increased linearly from proximal to distal, as was also observed in

a pilot study of only the lower leg [8]. The steepest fat gradient occurred in the intermediate affected muscles indicating that these muscles are progressing towards a complete fat infiltrated state. This interpretation is supported by the follow-up measurements, which revealed that intermediate affected muscles were most prone to increase their fat-muscle ratio. In these muscles the average increase of this ratio was about 10% in four months. This may seem fast for a disease that is characterized by slow progression, but we observed it in only a relative small fraction of muscles. The quasi-binary fat distribution of muscles in FSHD patients mentioned above also indicates that relative rapid transitions occur. Moreover, a sudden disease progression within individual muscles is in accordance with the often reported observation in FSHD patients of periods of rapid deterioration of single muscles or muscle groups, interrupting long stable periods [30,31]. In some cases the lower performance of a single muscle

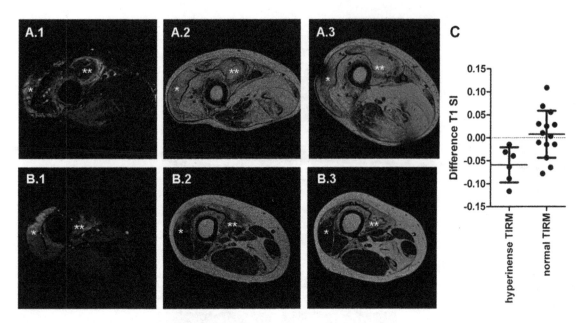

Figure 5. The presence of edema, as identified by TIRM imaging, correlates with increased fatty infiltration, as reflected in changes in T1 weighted images. (**A**) TIRM and T1 weighted images of a 76 year-old male FSHD patient. (**B**) TIRM and T1 weighted images of a 39 year-old male FSHD patient. (**A–B.1**) VL(*) and VM(**) muscles of two FSHD patients show hyperintensity on TIRM images, indicating edema. (**A–B.2**) Baseline T1 weighted images. (**A–B.3**) Follow-up T1 weighted images showing an increase of fatty infiltration after about 4 months in the VL(*) and VM(**) muscles. (**C**) SI difference between baseline and follow-up T1 weighted images is significantly different in TIRM hyperintense FSHD muscles (N = 6) compared to TIRM normal FSHD muscles (n = 14) (p<0.01).

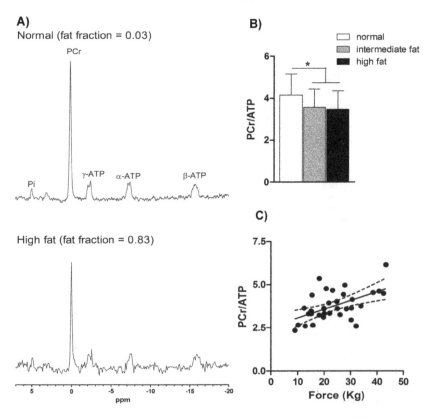

Figure 6. High-energy phosphates in the different stages of fatty infiltration and correlation with muscle force. (**A**) Representative phosphorous MR spectra of VL muscle of FSHD patients, upper with a normal fat fraction, lower with a high fat fraction. (**B**) PCr/ATP decreases with fat fraction (mean±SD). In intermediately fat infiltrated muscles the PCr/ATP is already decreased significantly from 4.15±1.00 to 3.57±0.88. Completely fat infiltrated muscles do not show a further decrease of this ratio. (**C**) Significant correlation between PCr/ATP and muscle strength (p<0.001, R^2 = 0.29). Pi = inorganic phosphate; PCr = phosphocreatine; ATP = adenosine triphosphate.

may be compensated by unaffected synergistic muscles, which would clinically mask its dysfunction [32,33]. Assuming that replacement of muscular tissue by fat occurs at a constant rate after entering this intermediate phase, fat replacement of entire muscles will, on the average, be completed within approximately three and a half years. This can be relevant for prognostication and monitoring therapy effectiveness in FSHD. There is no report on fat gradients over the length of muscles in other neuromuscular disorders, which may be FSHD specific. Recently, a muscular fatty content gradient was also found in inherited poly-neuropathy, but this was not associated with disease progression [34].

The low percentage of muscles involved in a rapid progression towards complete fatty infiltration indicates that this process is triggered by an infrequent event. The nature of this event is unknown, but the initial relatively high distal level of fatty infiltration and the differences between muscles suggests a local origin. This is in agreement with findings that only 0.1% of muscle nuclei express DUX4 in FSHD patients [35]. A recent paper by Tassin and colleagues [36] describes a model of initiation and propagation of a transcriptional cascade, which provides an elegant explanation for our observation of a gradient of fatty infiltration and fast progression in intermediate fat infiltrated muscles. In this model the activation of the DUX4 gene in (one or) few myonuclei yields DUX4 protein molecules that diffuse into the cytoplasm towards neighboring nuclei where they activate target genes, which causes expansion into a transcriptional cascade of deregulation. Because of the multinucleated nature of myofibers this model predicts a gradient of deregulation over the length of muscles. The amplification of DUX4 gene activation into a transcriptional cascade may also explain the fast progression observed in the intermediate fat infiltrated muscles. Preferential involvement of particular muscles (e.g. semi membranosus) and distal initiation may hide clues towards the initial DUX4 gene activation trigger. Our finding that MR-visible fat content increases more in the case of initial edema supports the involvement of inflammation in early disease onset, as TIRM positive muscles are associated with muscle inflammation [21–23,37–39]. However, whether inflammation is cause or consequence of DUX4 transcription in the initiation process remains unclear.

The correlation between increased fat fraction and lower strength of skeletal muscles is coherent with the loss of muscle mass and also explains the (weak) relation with the age of the patients. Clinical severity scores (Lamminen [25] and Ricci [19]) strongly correlated with fat fraction, but abnormal high fat fractions were also present in lower limb muscles without clinical symptoms, as was observed in patients with Ricci score 2 (excludes lower limb involvement). Thus, imaging fatty infiltration is a potential tool to predict clinical muscle affliction [32,33]. The extent of edema in our study (4.3%) is somewhat lower than reported in two recent FSHD studies, that however, included more muscles per patient and more severely affected patients [23,40].

The lower PCr/ATP ratios observed in intermediately fatty infiltrated muscles suggest an early change in high-energy phosphate metabolism in disease development. Lower steady state PCr/ATP ratios were also found in muscles of Becker and Duchenne patients [10,41]. This may represent a lower cellular (phospho)creatine pool due to a lower energy state. Alternatively, it may represent a change in fiber type composition, if the fraction of oxidative fibers, which have lower PCr/ATP ratio's [42,43], increase due to preferred involvement of type II fibers. This is supported by histological findings of biopsies, showing more dominant type I fibers among the remaining fibers in FSHD affected muscles [44] and is also congruent with the correlation between PCr/ATP and muscle force.

Taking muscle biopsies remains the gold standard to examine muscular dystrophies, but this is invasive, painful, restricted to a limited number of biopsy sites and only provides focal information. As observed in the present and a previous study [8] fatty infiltration is very heterogeneous, both between and within muscles, which demonstrates the need to know in advance which (part of a) muscle is affected, to acquire representative tissue. Our study indicates that MRI guidance in taking muscle biopsies is needed. Other common imaging techniques have disadvantages, such as radiation exposure in computer tomography, or poor signal to noise and limited penetration depth in ultrasound. In clinical trials muscle strength is often assessed to evaluate treatment effects, but this may show a placebo effect [45]. Muscular fat fraction determined by MRI does not involve a placebo effect.

A limitation of our study was the lack of including a component for the presence of edema in the T2 analysis. However, we identified muscles with edema by TIRM and excluded the very small fraction of edematous muscles from this T2 analysis. Progression of fatty infiltration in these muscles was then derived from T1 images. Furthermore, we chose to investigate lower extremity muscles in these patients even though FSHD is a disease known to first involve the facial and scapular muscles. However, for this study we aimed for the highest image quality, which could be achieved with a dedicated coil for the lower extremity. To compare different disease phases we had to introduce fat fraction cut-off values, for which we chose 25% and 75% of fatty infiltration. Shifting these values by ±5% did not change the main results of this study.

In conclusion, this study established fat fraction as assessed by MR imaging as an objective quantitative and sensitive biomarker for muscular affliction in FSHD, detecting even subclinical muscle involvement. This MR biomarker may serve to predict disease progression, to guide biopsies and to evaluate treatments to preserve or improve muscle performance. Importantly, in these applications the intramuscular fat distribution may have to be taken into account. Our data suggest a specific sequence of events that leads towards full muscle pathology in FSHD, in which muscles first progress from normal to being distally fat infiltrated, with an altered metabolic profile, after which fat rapidly infiltrates the whole muscles. This process of disease unfolding may direct new treatment strategies.

Supporting Information

Figure S1 Correlation between fat fractions and age for the individual thigh muscles. Solid line gives best linear correlation with 95% confidence interval indicated by the dotted lines. Slopes of the lines were statistically tested to identify possible differences between the muscles. However analyses showed no significant differences. VL = vastus lateralis, VI = vastus intermedius, RF = rectus femoris, VM = vastus medialis, BFS biceps femoris short head, BFL = biceps femoris long head, S = sartorius, G = gracillis, ST = semit endinosus, SM = semi membranosus, AM = adductor magnus, AL = adductor longus.

Figure S2 Correlation between fat fractions and disease duration for the individual thigh muscles. Solid line gives best linear correlation with 95% confidence interval indicated by the dotted lines. Slopes of the lines were statistically tested to identify possible differences between the muscles. However analyses showed no significant differences. VL = vastus lateralis, VI = vastus intermedius, RF = rectus femoris, VM = vastus medialis, BFS biceps femoris short head, BFL = biceps femoris long head, S = sartorius, G = gracillis, ST = semi tendinosus, SM = semi membranosus, AM = adductor magnus, AL = adductor longus.

Acknowledgments

We thank Rob J.W. Arts for helping with data processing and Jos IJspeert for performing the force measurements.

Author Contributions

Conceived and designed the experiments: AG BE GP AH. Performed the experiments: BJ NV CN HK. Analyzed the data: BJ NV CN HK JR. Wrote the paper: BJ NV CN HK JR AG GP BE AH.

References

1. Padberg GW (1982) Facioscapulohumeral Disease. Leiden, The Netherlands: University of Leiden Thesis.
2. Lemmers RJ, van d, Klooster R, Sacconi S, Camano P, et al. (2010) A unifying genetic model for facioscapulohumeral muscular dystrophy. Science 329: 1650–1653.
3. van der Maarel SM, Tawil R, Tapscott SJ (2011) Facioscapulohumeral muscular dystrophy and DUX4: breaking the silence. Trends Mol Med 17: 252–258.
4. Pandya S, King WM, Tawil R (2008) Facioscapulohumeral dystrophy. Phys Ther 88: 105–113.
5. Tawil R (2008) Facioscapulohumeral muscular dystrophy. Neurotherapeutics 5: 601–606.
6. Gaeta M, Messina S, Mileto A, Vita GL, Ascenti G, et al. (2012) Muscle fat-fraction and mapping in Duchenne muscular dystrophy: evaluation of disease distribution and correlation with clinical assessments. Preliminary experience. Skeletal Radiol 41: 955–961.
7. Wren TA, Bluml S, Tseng-Ong L, Gilsanz V (2008) Three-point technique of fat quantification of muscle tissue as a marker of disease progression in Duchenne muscular dystrophy: preliminary study. AJR Am J Roentgenol 190: W8–12.
8. Kan HE, Scheenen TWJ, Wohlgemuth M, Klomp DWJ, van Loosbroek-Wagenmans I, et al. (2009) Quantitative MR imaging of individual muscle involvement in facioscapulohumeral muscular dystrophy. Neuromuscul Disord 19: 357–362.
9. Heerschap A, den Hollander JA, Reynen H, Goris RJ (1993) Metabolic changes in reflex sympathetic dystrophy: a 31P NMR spectroscopy study. Muscle Nerve 16: 367–373.
10. Banerjee B, Sharma U, Balasubramanian K, Kalaivani M, Kalra V, et al. (2010) Effect of creatine monohydrate in improving cellular energetics and muscle strength in ambulatory Duchenne muscular dystrophy patients: a randomized, placebo-controlled 31P MRS study. Magn Reson Med 28: 698–707.
11. Barbiroli B, Funicello R, Iotti S, Montagna P, Ferlini A, et al. (1992) 31P-NMR spectroscopy of skeletal muscle in Becker dystrophy and DMD/BMD carriers. Altered rate of phosphate transport. J Neurol Sci 109: 188–195.
12. Barnes PR, Kemp GJ, Taylor DJ, Radda GK (1997) Skeletal muscle metabolism in myotonic dystrophy A 31P magnetic resonance spectroscopy study. Brain 120 (Pt 10): 1699–1711.
13. Grehl T, Müller K, Vorgerd M, Tegenthoff M, Malin JP, et al. (1998) Impaired aerobic glycolysis in muscle phosphofructokinase deficiency results in biphasic post-exercise phosphocreatine recovery in 31P magnetic resonance spectroscopy. Neuromuscul Disord 8: 480–488.
14. Lodi R, Muntoni F, Taylor J, Kumar S, Sewry CA, et al. (1997) Correlative MR imaging and 31P-MR spectroscopy study in sarcoglycan deficient limb girdle muscular dystrophy. Neuromuscul Disord 7: 505–511.
15. Trenell MI, Thompson CH, Sue CM (2006) Exercise and myotonic dystrophy: a 31P magnetic resonance spectroscopy and magnetic resonance imaging case study. Ann Neurol 59: 871–872.
16. Kan HE, Klomp DWJ, Wohlgemuth M, van Loosbroek-Wagemans I, van Engelen BGM, et al. (2010) Only fat infiltrated muscles in resting lower leg of FSHD patients show disturbed energy metabolism. NMR Biomed 23: 563–568.
17. Statland JM, Tawil R (2011) Facioscapulohumeral muscular dystrophy: molecular pathological advances and future directions. Curr Opin Neurol 24: 423–428.
18. Voet NBM, Bleijenberg G, Padberg GW, van Engelen BGM, Geurts ACH (2010) Effect of aerobic exercise training and cognitive behavioural therapy on reduction of chronic fatigue in patients with facioscapulohumeral dystrophy: protocol of the FACTS-2-FSHD trial. BMC Neurol 10: 56–56.
19. Ricci E, Galluzzi G, Deidda G, Cacurri S, Colantoni L, et al. (1999) Progress in the molecular diagnosis of facioscapulohumeral muscular dystrophy and correlation between the number of KpnI repeats at the 4q35 locus and clinical phenotype. Ann Neurol 45: 751–757.
20. van der Kooi EL, Vogels OJM, van Asseldonk RJGP, Lindeman E, Hendriks JCM, et al. (2004) Strength training and albuterol in facioscapulohumeral muscular dystrophy. Neurology 63: 702–708.
21. Wattjes MP, Kley RA, Fischer D (2010) Neuromuscular imaging in inherited muscle diseases. Eur Radiol 20: 2447–2460.
22. Tasca G, Pescatori M, Monforte M, Mirabella M, Iannaccone E, et al. (2012) Different molecular signatures in magnetic resonance imaging-staged facioscapulohumeral muscular dystrophy muscles. PLoS One 7: e38779.

23. Frisullo G, Frusciante R, Nociti V, Tasca G, Renna R, et al. (2011) CD8(+) T cells in facioscapulohumeral muscular dystrophy patients with inflammatory features at muscle MRI. J Clin Immunol 31: 155–166.
24. Felmlee JP, Ehman RL (1987) Spatial presaturation: a method for suppressing flow artifacts and improving depiction of vascular anatomy in MR imaging. Radiology 164: 559–564.
25. Lamminen AE (1990) Magnetic resonance imaging of primary skeletal muscle diseases: patterns of distribution and severity of involvement. Br J Radiol 63: 946–950.
26. Kuk JL, Saunders TJ, Davidson LE, Ross R (2009) Age-related changes in total and regional fat distribution. Ageing Res Rev 8: 339–348.
27. Naressi A, Couturier C, Devos JM, Janssen M, Mangeat C, et al. (2001) Java-based graphical user interface for the MRUI quantitation package. MAGMA 12: 141–152.
28. Vanhamme L, van den Boogaart A, Van Huffel S (1997) Improved method for accurate and efficient quantification of MRS data with use of prior knowledge. J Magn Reson 129: 35–43.
29. Taylor DJ, Bore PJ, Styles P, Gadian DG, Radda GK (1983) Bioenergetics of intact human muscle. A 31P nuclear magnetic resonance study. Mol Biol Med 1: 77–94.
30. Tawil R, Van Der Maarel SM (2006) Facioscapulohumeral muscular dystrophy. Muscle Nerve 34: 1–15.
31. Richards M, Coppee F, Thomas N, Belayew A, Upadhyaya M (2012) Facioscapulohumeral muscular dystrophy (FSHD): an enigma unravelled? Hum Genet 131: 325–340.
32. Sookhoo S, Mackinnon I, Bushby K, Chinnery PF, Birchall D (2007) MRI for the demonstration of subclinical muscle involvement in muscular dystrophy. Clin Radiol 62: 160–165.
33. Fischmann A, Hafner P, Fasler S, Gloor M, Bieri O, et al. (2012) Quantitative MRI can detect subclinical disease progression in muscular dystrophy. J Neurol 259: 1648–1654.
34. Gaeta M, Mileto A, Mazzeo A, Minutoli F, Di Leo R, et al. (2011) MRI findings, patterns of disease distribution, and muscle fat fraction calculation in five patients with Charcot-Marie-Tooth type 2 F disease. Skeletal Radiol 41: 515–524.
35. Snider L, Geng LN, Lemmers RJ, Kyba M, Ware CB, et al. (2010) Facioscapulohumeral dystrophy: incomplete suppression of a retrotransposed gene. PLoS Genet 6: e1001181.
36. Tassin A, Laoudj-Chenivesse D, Vanderplanck C, Barro M, Charron S, et al. (2013) DUX4 expression in FSHD muscle cells: how could such a rare protein cause a myopathy? J Cell Mol Med 17: 76–89.
37. McMahon CJ, Wu JS, Eisenberg RL (2010) Muscle edema. AJR Am J Roentgenol 194: W284–292.
38. May DA, Disler DG, Jones EA, Balkissoon AA, Manaster BJ (2000) Abnormal signal intensity in skeletal muscle at MR imaging: patterns, pearls, and pitfalls. Radiographics 20 Spec No: S295–315.
39. Friedman SD, Poliachik SL, Otto RK, Carter GT, Budech CB, et al. (2013) Longitudinal features of stir bright signal in FSHD. Muscle Nerve 31: 155–166.
40. Friedman SD, Poliachik SL, Carter GT, Budech CB, Bird TD, et al. (2012) The magnetic resonance imaging spectrum of facioscapulohumeral muscular dystrophy. Muscle Nerve 45: 500–506.
41. Kemp GJ, Taylor DJ, Dunn JF, Frostick SP, Radda GK (1993) Cellular energetics of dystrophic muscle. J Neurol Sci 116: 201–206.
42. Kushmerick MJ, Moerland TS, Wiseman RW (1992) Mammalian skeletal muscle fibers distinguished by contents of phosphocreatine, ATP, and Pi. Proc Natl Acad Sci U S A 89: 7521–7525.
43. Takahashi H, Kuno SY, Katsuta S, Shimojo H, Masuda K, et al. (1996) Relationships between fiber composition and NMR measurements in human skeletal muscle. NMR Biomed 9: 8–12.
44. Dubowitz V, Sewry CA (2007) Chapter 14: Muscular dystrophies and allied disorders V: facioscapulohumeral dystrophy, myotonic dystrophy, oculopharyngeal muscular dystrophy. Muscle biopsy : a practical approach United States: Elsevier Health Sciences.
45. Statland JM, McDermott MP, Heatwole C, Martens WB, Pandya S, et al. (2013) Reevaluating measures of disease progression in facioscapulohumeral muscular dystrophy. Neuromuscul Disord 23: 306–312.

13

Temperature Sensitivity of the Pyloric Neuromuscular System and Its Modulation by Dopamine

Jeffrey B. Thuma*, Kevin H. Hobbs, Helaine J. Burstein, Natasha S. Seiter, Scott L. Hooper

Department of Biological Sciences, Ohio University, Athens, Ohio, United States of America

Abstract

We report here the effects of temperature on the p1 neuromuscular system of the stomatogastric system of the lobster (*Panulirus interruptus*). Muscle force generation, in response to both the spontaneously rhythmic *in vitro* pyloric network neural activity and direct, controlled motor nerve stimulation, dramatically decreased as temperature increased, sufficiently that stomach movements would very unlikely be maintained at warm temperatures. However, animals fed in warm tanks showed statistically identical food digestion to those in cold tanks. Applying dopamine, a circulating hormone in crustacea, increased muscle force production at all temperatures and abolished neuromuscular system temperature dependence. Modulation may thus exist not only to increase the diversity of produced behaviors, but also to maintain individual behaviors when environmental conditions (such as temperature) vary.

Editor: Wolfgang Blenau, Goethe University Frankfurt, Germany

Funding: This work was funded by NIH grant 5RC1DA028494-02 and NSF grant IOS-0958926. The funders had no role in study design, data collection and analysis, decision to publish, or preparation of the manuscript.

Competing Interests: The authors have declared that no competing interests exist.

* E-mail: thuma@ohio.edu

Introduction

Ectotherms have lower energy requirements than endotherms because they do not actively maintain a constant body temperature. Taking advantage of this opportunity, at least for ectotherms inhabiting environments with wide temperature variations, requires that life-critical processes function across the temperature range typical of their habitat. Tidal and freshwater crustacea experience wide daily and seasonal temperature changes, and hence would be expected to have evolved temperature compensation mechanisms. Indeed, the firing phase relationships of the pyloric neural network of the crab (*Cancer borealis*) are maintained across a wide temperature range, and modeling suggests this maintenance requires neuron conductances to have similar temperature coefficients [1].

Maintaining normal behavior also requires that neuromuscular function be maintained as temperature varies, but much prior work suggests that crustacean neuromuscular function is strongly temperature-dependent. In crayfish [2,3,4] and barnacle [5], warming causes muscle resting membrane potential to hyperpolarize. EJP amplitude, facilitation, and decay time constant vary with temperature in crayfish [2,3,4] and crab [6,7]. In the crayfish *Orconectes limosus*, contraction force in response to muscle depolarization by current injection increases with warming [8], whereas in the crayfish *Astacus leptodactylus* force induced by motor neuron stimulation decreases with warming [2,3,4]. These data were mostly obtained in leg muscles. Nonetheless, this temperature sensitivity in other crustacean muscles prompted us to test whether pyloric neuromuscular function, and thus stomach activity, may also not be maintained as animal temperature changes, even if correctly-phased pyloric network rhythmic activity is.

We have performed considerable work on force generation in lobster (*Panulirus interruptus*) pyloric muscles [9,10,11,12,13,14,15,16]. However, this work did not examine the effects of temperature on neuromuscular function. We show here that pyloric neuromuscular function is highly temperature sensitive, that exogenous dopamine application can overcome this sensitivity, and that dopamine could therefore potentially help maintain muscle function *in vivo*. These data suggest that modulation may function not only to change behavior, but also to maintain it as environmental conditions change.

Materials and Methods

Spontaneous Muscle Activity

Spiny lobsters (*Panulirus interruptus*) were obtained from Marinus Scientific (Long Beach, CA) and maintained in aquaria with chilled (9–15°C), circulating, artificial seawater. Stomachs were dissected in the standard manner for muscle preparations [10,17]. The p1 muscle was freed from the surrounding tissue except for the origin on the lateral ossicle and a small piece of hard connective tissue on the medial end to use as an attachment point for the transducer. The pyloric movement pattern is as yet unknown. However, the p1 muscle is one of the largest pyloric muscles, and the largest of the three muscles innervated by the Lateral Pyloric (LP) neuron. It is thus likely to play an important role in generating pyloric movements. Great care was taken to ensure that muscle innervation remained intact. The muscle was then hooked to a Dual Mode Lever System transducer (Aurora Scientific, Inc) and set to its rest length (approximately 8 mm [16]) by using a ruler and adjusting the height of the micromanipulator to which the transducer was attached. Prior work has shown that pyloric muscles generate substantial contractions in response to motor neuron input at their rest lengths [10,11,12,13,14,15,16]. All experiments were performed in the isometric regime.

During the dissection the preparation was frequently bathed with oxygenated, chilled ($\sim$10°C) *Panulirus* saline (in mM: 479 NaCl, 12.8 KCl, 13.7 CaCl$_2$, 3.9 Na$_2$SO$_4$, 10 MgSO$_4$, 10.9 dextrose, 11.1 Tris base, 5.1 maleic acid, pH 7.4–7.6; Fisher Scientific). During the experiment the preparation was continuously perfused with oxygenated (100% oxygen), chilled (9–16°C) saline. The p1 muscle innervation by the LP neuron runs through the lateral ventricular nerve (lvn). A small "window" was cut through the stomach tissue to expose a 10–15 mm length of the lvn just rostral to the p1 muscle. A small piece of Sylgard was placed under the lvn for support and held in place with minutien pins. Extracellular nerve recordings of pyloric network activity were made using stainless steel pin electrodes on the lvn insulated with petroleum jelly and an A-M Systems amplifier.

Saline temperature was changed by varying the length of perfusion tubing immersed in an ice water bath. Perfusion tubing immersion length was varied by the experimenter as necessary to obtain gradual, continuous warming but on the cooling phase the entire length of tubing was typically re-immersed in the ice water bath in a single step. This resulted in the warming phases occurring more slowly than the cooling phases. Saline temperature was monitored using a Physitemp Instruments BAT-12 microprobe thermometer positioned in the dish near the muscle. The p1 muscle is strap-like with an approximate thickness of 1 mm. Given this small thickness and the high temperature conductivity of water, we assume muscle temperature tracked saline temperature with only a small delay.

Temperature, lvn activity, and muscle contraction force were continuously recorded using Spike 2 and a 1401plus (Cambridge Electronic Design). In some preparations, the oxygenated saline was switched to unoxygenated saline, which was normal saline that had been placed in a refrigerator undisturbed for at least 24 hours and then carefully transferred to the perfusion feed flask so as to introduce as little turbulence, and hence atmospheric oxygen, as possible. Oxygen concentrations of the perfusing saline were measured in the dish using a Clarke-type oxygen electrode and a Strathkelvin Model 781 oxygen meter.

Stimulated Muscle Activity

Dissection was performed as above but the lvn was cut immediately distal to its branch point from the dorsal ventricular nerve (which connects the lvn to the stomatogastric ganglion) and pinned out in a Sylgard dish, taking care to maintain p1 muscle innervation. The muscle was then prepared as described above. Bipolar stainless steel pin electrodes were placed on the lvn and insulated from the bath using petroleum jelly. The lvn was stimulated using the 1401plus and a stimulus isolation unit – 10 spikes at 27 Hz, which is the upper end of the physiological range, chosen to obtain large but still physiologically relevant contractions and with a period long enough to allow the muscle to fully relax between stimulations. Stimulation current was gradually increased until further increases in current did not increase contraction amplitude. The muscle was then allowed to rest for approximately 5 minutes. The muscle was then stimulated as before while saline temperature was altered from 9–22°C. Muscle force was recorded using the same transducer as above and the 1401plus. In some experiments 10^{-7} to 10^{-5} M dopamine (Sigma) containing saline was applied to the preparation.

Feeding Experiments

Animals were unfed and acclimated to either 9°C or 15°C for at least 48 hours before feeding. Each animal was hand fed 1 g of fish

or mussel. The animal was returned to its original tank and left undisturbed for 2 hours, after which the stomach was dissected as above. Undigested food was removed and weighed.

Data Analysis

As noted above, the slopes of the warming and cooling phases differed. Furthermore, responses to warming and cooling could intrinsically differ. To ensure that all measurements were made under equivalent conditions, quantitative analysis was performed only on contractions in the warming phase of the temperature variations in the lvn stimulation experiments. Measurements were made on continuously changing temperature gradients occurring over ten to fifteen minutes.

LP neuron phase was calculated by measuring the delay from the beginning of each cycle's PD neuron burst to the beginning of each cycle's LP neuron burst and dividing by that cycle's period, defined as the duration from one PD neuron burst beginning to the beginning of the next.

Linear fits and statistical analyses were performed in Origin (OriginLab) and Kaleidagraph (Synergy Software).

Results

Tang et al. [18] showed that crab (*Cancer borealis*) pyloric network motor neuron output maintained phase across a wide temperature range. We verified that this was also true in lobster in three experiments. Mean pyloric cycle period decreased from 1.38±0.12 s at 9°C to 0.67±0.02 s at 16°C ($p = 0.009$, Student's paired t-test), a 2.1-fold decrease. Mean LP neuron (the neuron innervating the muscle examined here) phase changed over this temperature range only from 0.42±0.04 to 0.58±0.08. Although this phase change was significant ($p = 0.023$, Student's paired t-test), it was much smaller than the shift expected (to a phase of approximately 0.9 rather than the observed 0.58) if LP neuron firing delay after PD neuron burst beginning had not shortened as temperature increased. Thus, although not as perfect as that observed in *Cancer*, lobster pyloric networks also showed substantial phase compensation as temperature changed.

To test whether this phase-compensated motor neuron output would induce temperature invariant neuromuscular responses, we measured (in animals that had been housed in 9–11°C aquaria) p1 muscle force production in response to spontaneous *in vitro* pyloric network activity as saline temperature was varied (Figure 1). Contraction force was much larger at colder temperatures. In Figure 1A, saline temperature (top trace) was initially approximately 16°C and the muscle showed very small or no contractions (middle trace). As the saline was cooled, the muscle began to contract and muscle contractions continually strengthened as saline temperature decreased. Warming the saline again caused the contractions to weaken and eventually nearly stop. This response was repeatable multiple times within single experiments. Eleven animals were used and in every animal contraction force in warm saline was always much smaller than in cold (0.047±0.046 N at 9°C, 0.007±0.01 N at 16°C, different at $p = 0.01$, Student's paired t-test), although in some experiments contraction amplitude did not shrink to near zero as in Figure 1A.

Figures 1B and 1C show expansions of small time windows from Figure 1A. Even though the muscle had nearly ceased contracting in Figure 1C, the LP neuron had not stopped firing, as shown by LP neuron action potentials continuing to be recorded at the extracellular electrode (bottom trace, all three panels). Furthermore, at least some of these action potentials further propagated to reach the muscle during every burst, as expansion of the muscle force trace (inset, Fig. 1C) shows that each motor neuron burst

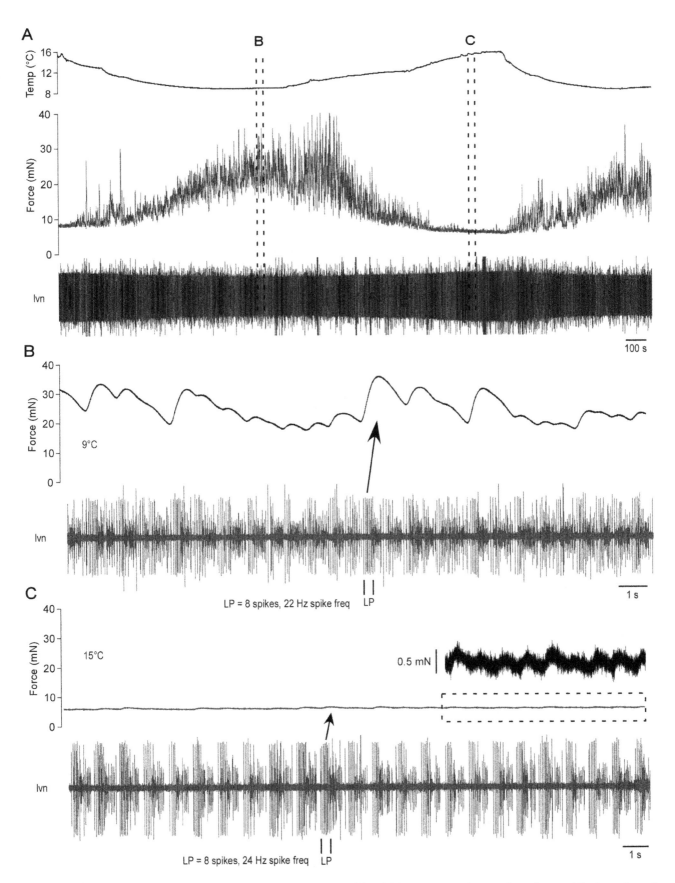

Figure 1. The lobster p1 neuromuscular system is temperature-sensitive. (A) As temperature (top trace) was decreased the force of muscle contraction (middle trace) increased. The activity of the nerve containing the LP neuron input to the muscle is shown in the bottom trace. (B) and (C)

Time expansion from (A) showing muscle force (top trace) and neural input (bottom trace) at 9°C and 15°C. Arrows show that two LP neuron bursts chosen for having essentially identical characteristics induced very different muscle contraction amplitudes at the two temperatures. Inset in (C) is muscle force at an expanded scale to show that even at warm temperatures each motor neuron burst continued to induce (very small) muscle contractions.

continued to induce a (very small) muscle contraction. To make this comparison more explicit, we also identified neuron bursts with nearly identical (each had 8 spikes and 22 or 24 Hz spike frequency) LP motor neuron activity in Figures 1B and 1C. Despite this nearly identical activity at the level of the LP neuron distal axon, the active muscle contraction (the continuous 'baseline' force production is due to passive muscle stretch at rest length) at 15°C was essentially zero, even though the 9°C contraction was the largest in the shown data.

Gas solubility decreases as temperature increases, therefore decreased oxygen availability could affect neuromuscular function. Although all these experiments were performed in oxygenated saline, it was possible that the temperature dependence of neuromuscular function we had observed was caused by temperature-dependent changes in dissolved oxygen. Three lines of evidence show this possibility is unsupported. First, over these relatively small temperature ranges only very small changes in dissolved oxygen would be expected theoretically [19]. Second, direct measurements showed that dissolved oxygen levels in the dish were essentially identical at 10°C (158 mmHg O_2) and 15°C (157 mmHg O_2). Third, we performed experiments (n = 3, animals housed in 9–11°C aquaria) with unoxygenated saline (40 mmHg O_2 at 10°C, 51 mmHg at 15°C). Thus, this saline contained less than one-third of the oxygen, regardless of temperature, of the oxygenated saline. We repeated the experiment shown in Figure 1, but switched to the unoxgenated saline partway through (Figure 2, arrow). The amount of force the muscle produced did not change when the unoxygenated saline was introduced and the muscle remained sensitive to temperature changes. Temperature-dependent changes in dissolved oxygen thus cannot be causing the changes in neuromuscular function shown in Figure 1.

Although pyloric network activity continued at all temperatures, it did change with temperature – in addition to the cycle period and LP neuron phase changes noted above, the LP bursts also became more regular at higher temperatures. In order to ensure that the change in neuromuscular function in response to temperature was not because of these changes in pyloric network activity, we performed experiments in which the lvn connection to the stomatogastric ganglion was cut and we rhythmically stimulated the lvn to provide a completely controlled driving input to the neuromuscular system. Even when receiving this unvarying stimulation, muscle force still strongly decreased in warm saline (Figures 3A1, 3A2). Importantly, and in contrast to the response of the pyloric network to temperature in the crab [18], the animal in Figures 3A1, 3A2 had been acclimated to 15°C for 48 hrs. In 7 out of 8 experiments on animals housed at 15°C the muscles showed much reduced contractions at higher temperatures, including 15°C; 9°C and 15°C contraction amplitudes in these animals (including the one in which contraction amplitude did not decrease with temperature) differed at $p = 0.018$, Student's paired t-test (0.014 ± 0.009 N at 9°C vs. 0.0035 ± 0.005 N at 15°C. Thus, the sensitivity of the neuromuscular system did not depend on the temperature at which the animals were housed.

These observations raised the question of whether animals housed in warm tanks could digest food. We therefore fed lobsters housed in 9°C and 15°C tanks, returned them to the tanks they had been housed in, and measured how much food remained in their stomachs two hours after feeding. Each animal ingested the full 1 g of food and no difference between the two groups was observed (mean food remaining at 9°C, 0.43 ± 0.12 g; at 15°C, 0.35 ± 0.15 g; $p = 0.468$, Student's t-test).

The ability of the lobsters to continue to digest food at temperatures at which, *in vitro*, the muscles nearly stop contracting, shows that some compensation mechanism that maintains neuromuscular function must be present *in vivo*. The stomatogastric neuromuscular system is extensively neuromodulated (neural data review [20]; muscle data [21,22,23,24,25,26,27]). We therefore examined the effects of several neuromodulators on neuromuscular function vs. temperature and found that dopamine increased muscle contraction force in cold saline (Figure 3B1, compare to Figure 3A1) and allowed the neuromuscular system to continue to function even in warm saline (Figure 3B2). In dopamine, in which substantial muscle forces were present at all temperatures, it was also possible to observe an additional effect of increased temperature – it resulted in an increased relaxation rate (compare Figures 3B1 and 3B2). This increased relaxation rate would also help maintain the temporal characteristics of muscle contraction with warming (see Discussion). These effects reversed upon wash (Figures 3C1, 3C2). Figures 3A–C are from a single animal housed at 15°C. Whether dopamine had an effect only on animals housed at 15°C was tested by applying dopamine to one animal housed at 9°C; dopamine similarly maintained contraction amplitude at warm experimental temperatures in this animal(Figures 3D1, 3D2).

Quantitative and grouped data across experiments (all animals housed at 15°C) confirmed the dopamine effects. Figure 4 shows temperature binned (1°C) mean contraction force plots from six lvn-stimulation experiments. Figure 4A shows each experiment's data (matching colors are data from the same experiment); closed circles are control saline and open circles the dopamine treatment (the wash data are not shown to allow for easier viewing of the control saline fits). At all temperatures, mean contraction force production in dopamine was larger than in control saline. Figure 4B shows across-experiment mean data for each temperature bin. A two-way repeated-measures ANOVA on these data was significant ($p < 0.0001$) for both condition (control, dopamine, wash, F = 27.65, 2 degrees of freedom) and temperature (F = 10.46, 6 degrees of freedom). This analysis, however, does not reveal in which condition(s) the temperature dependence is present. We therefore also performed one-way repeated-measures ANOVAs with Tukey's All Pairs Comparisons on each condition's data. These showed that control and wash contraction forces depended on temperature at $p < 0.0001$ for control (F = 15.87, 6 degrees of freedom) and at $p = 0.004$ (F = 4.1, 6 degrees of freedom) for wash, but contraction force in dopamine did not ($p = 0.91$, F = 0.34, 6 degrees of freedom). These analysis thus showed that dopamine not only increased contraction amplitude, but, and more importantly here, removed contraction force's dependence on temperature. With respect to the nature of the dependence on temperature in control and wash conditions, in control saline the dependence appeared to be linear (solid lines in Figure 4A; all fit p values < 0.005). In four of the experiments the linear dependence on temperature returned in the wash; in the other two, the linear fits were no longer significant, although contraction amplitude did decrease with increasing temperature.

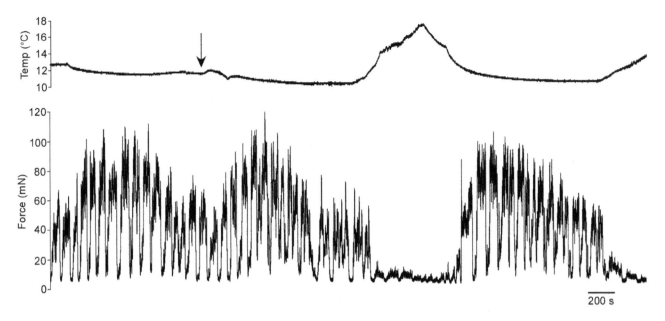

Figure 2. Changing available dissolved oxygen does not affect temperature sensitivity. The preparation was initially perfused with cold, oxygenated saline (top trace) and then switched (arrow) to cold saline containing at least 3 fold less dissolved oxygen. The muscle showed no change in activity (bottom trace) when the reduced oxygen saline was introduced. However, the temperature sensitivity remained and was still reversible despite the much lower oxygen availability. The periodic large decreases in muscle force every 75–100 s are due to the activity of another, much more slowly cycling, stomatogastric network, the gastric mill, which greatly reduces lateral pyloric neuron activity during one phase of gastric mill activity [13,15].

These experiments were all performed with 10^{-5} M dopamine, a very high concentration for a circulating hormone, and there is no evidence of a direct, local dopaminergic innervation of lobster stomach muscles. We therefore examined the threshold concentration for dopamine's effects. 10^{-8} M and less had no effect on muscle contraction (2 experiments). 10^{-7} M had no effect in three experiments and increased muscle contraction in three experiments, but in only one of these three did contractions continue at warm temperatures (6 experiments total). 10^{-6} M caused larger contractions in three experiments, in two of which the contractions also continued at warm temparatures. The threshold for dopamine effects was thus between 10^{-7} and 10^{-6} M.

Discussion

We have shown that pyloric neuromuscular function is highly temperature dependent, decreasing to near zero as temperature rises from 9°C to 16°C. This decrease was not because of decreases in dissolved oxygen and was independent of the temperature at which the animals were housed. However, the lobsters continued to digest food at warm temperatures. Application of a known neuromodulator of the stomatogastric system, dopamine, prevented the decrease in muscle contraction force.

Mechanism Underlying Temperature Dependence

These data give no information as to whether the locus of temperature's action is pre- or post-synaptic. Pyloric muscles are not innervated at a single end plate, but instead by multiple small processes branching from the main motor neuron axon as it courses over the muscle length, each process ending in one or more synaptic boutons. As such, although the continuance of very small one-for-one contractions with each motor neuron burst even at high temperatures shows that at least some of each burst's spikes are reaching the muscle, one explanation for the temperature dependence could be increased action potential failure with

warming where the small processes branch from the main axon. Warming could alternatively be decreasing the amount of transmitter released per action potential, or any of the postsynaptic steps in the process by which the muscle generates force in response to transmitter binding. Dopamine could similarly work at any level in the neuromuscular system, and in particular need not exert its compensatory effects at the same locus that temperature affects.

Comparison to Prior Work

This research was undertaken in part because of work showing that the crab pyloric neural network intrinsically maintains phase as temperature increases, which suggested that the pyloric neuromuscular system might show similar intrinsic temperature compensation. We have shown here that it does not, which raises the question of why not. The neural intrinsic compensation results from the electrically-active membrane proteins that underlie pyloric neuron activity changing in a coordinated fashion and to similar degrees with temperature. An argument could be made that neuromuscular system's failure to compensate lies at the level of the muscles, arising from their requirement to translate electrical activity into force and length changes. This requirement could make them in some way fundamentally more complicated than neurons, which function exclusively in the electrical realm, with this additional complexity preventing intrinsic temperature compensation from evolving in the muscles.

However, from the molecular standpoint no obvious reason exists why it should be more 'difficult' for the set of interacting proteins that transform membrane depolarization to actomyosin head rotation to become temperature resistant than it is for the set of interacting proteins that generate pyloric neuron activity. Regardless, despite the functional disadvantages this dependence would entail for such animals unless they live in temperature invariant environments, strong temperature dependence appears

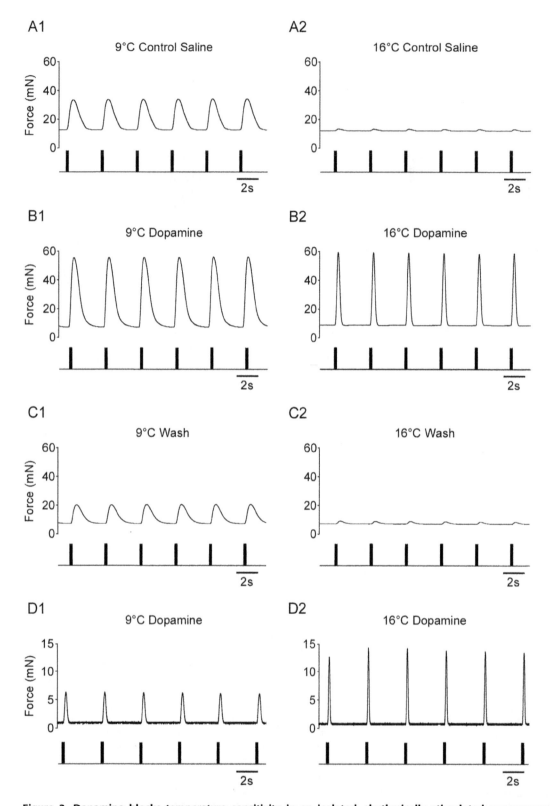

Figure 3. Dopamine blocks temperature sensitivity in an isolated, rhythmically stimulated neuromuscular preparation. (A) A neuromuscular preparation that has been isolated from the spontaneous activity of the pyloric neural network by severing the lvn. Contractions instead elicited by direct motor nerve stimulation with unvarying input (10 spikes at 27 Hz). Muscle contraction amplitude still declined dramatically in warmer saline. This animal had been acclimated to 15°C for 48 hrs, and thus these data also show that neuromuscular temperature sensitivity is independent of animal housing temperature. (B) Adding dopamine (10^{-5}) to the saline increased force generation at colder temperatures and allowed the neuromuscular system to continue functioning at warmer temperatures. (C) The dopamine effect reversed upon wash. (D) Dopamine also maintained contraction amplitude in neuromuscular systems from animals held in 9°C aquaria for 48 hrs before the experiment. Data in panels A, B, C all from same animal.

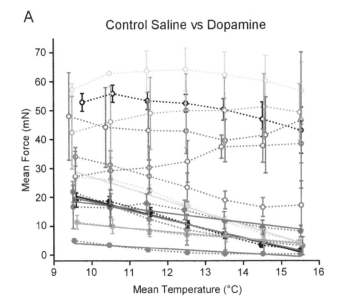

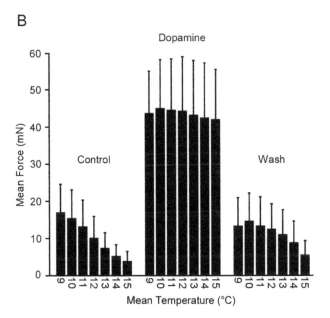

Figure 4. Dopamine allows the neuromuscular system to generate greater force at cold temperatures and continue functioning at warm temperatures. (A) Data from six motor nerve stimulation experiments (closed circles, control saline; open circles, dopamine; matching color lines are data from the same experiment; all animals housed at 15°C). Where present, solid lines show that linear fits to the data were significant. (B) Data for each experiment were binned (1°C) and mean contraction force was determined for each bin. Dopamine differed from control and wash conditions both in amplitude and in temperature sensitivity (present in control and wash, absent in dopamine). See text for statistical details.

to be widely present in crustacean neuromuscular systems (see Introduction). Taken together, these observations suggest that evolving temperature-compensating neuromuscular systems may be more difficult than evolving temperature-compensating neural networks, although why this should be so is unclear.

Maintenance of Motor Function

In the same manner that most invertebrates can continue to make other movements across wide temperature ranges, our feeding experiments showed that lobster stomachs continue to process food even at temperatures at which, *in vitro*, p1 muscle contractions have essentially zero amplitude. The implied presumption is that modulatory influences (presumably hormonal, as no modulatory neuronal input to pyloric muscles is known) maintains neuromuscular function at elevated temperatures, and dopamine indeed restores neuromuscular function at warm temperatures.

This demonstration does not prove that circulating dopamine in the intact animal serves this purpose. Indeed, the relatively high threshold concentration (between 10^{-7} and 10^{-6} M) for dopamine's effects suggests that circulating dopamine is unlikely, acting alone, to be responsible for the ability of intact lobsters to digest food at warm temperatures. However, lobsters have large numbers of neuromodulatory substances, many of them hemolymph borne, that increase pyloric neuromuscular function [24,27]. Dopamine could thus be one of a mixture of circulating hormones that maintains motor function at warm temperatures. More importantly, the demonstration that dopamine can maintain neuromuscular function as temperature changes provides proof of principle that modulators could serve such a role, which was the goal of this portion of this research.

In the presence of dopamine, relaxation rate dramatically increases as temperature increases (compare Figures 3B1 and 3B2). Pyloric muscles relax slowly enough that their contractions summate when driven by physiologically-timed (0.75–2 Hz cycle frequency) motor neuron bursts [11] (the stimulations in Figure 3 were purposefully delivered at a period long enough for full muscle relaxation to occur). Pyloric cycle frequency also strongly increases with increasing temperature in both the lobster (data presented here) and the crab [18]. Even with phase maintenance, this frequency increase, without a change in muscle relaxation rate, would make the muscle contractions become increasingly tonic, displaying only very small rhythmic contractions riding on an underlying large, sustained muscle contraction (e.g., Figure 5 of [11]). As such, if neuromodulators (e.g., dopamine) would allow muscle relaxation rate to increase as temperature increased, such an effect would counteract the temporal summation that would otherwise accompany the increased pyloric rhythm frequency.

Modulation as a Mechanism to Maintain Behaviors

Modulation is often interpreted as a mechanism for altering existing motor patterns (e.g., changing walk cycle frequency) or creating new ones (walking vs. running). However, another role of neuromodulators, particularly in invertebrates which typically regulate internal conditions less well than vertebrates, may be to maintain existing behaviors as their internal conditions change (temperature, hemolymph osmotic strength, pH, dissolved oxygen levels, etc.). With respect to temperature, such compensation is often believed to be mediated via heat shock proteins [28,29]. However, the expression and de-expression of these proteins is presumably metabolically more expensive and slower than neuromodulator release and re-uptake. As such, our data suggest it might be worthwhile to examine the relative importance of modulation vs. heat-shock proteins in temperature responses, and also, given the advantages modulation might confer, if temperature-compensating neuromodulators down-regulate heat-shock protein induction.

Author Contributions

Conceived and designed the experiments: JBT SLH. Performed the experiments: JBT KHH HJB NSS. Analyzed the data: JBT KHH HJB SLH. Wrote the paper: JBT SLH.

References

1. Tang LS, Goeritz ML, Caplan JS, Taylor AL, Fisek M, et al. (2010) Precise temperature compensation of phase in a rhythmic motor pattern. PLoS Biol 8(8): e1000469. doi:10.1371/journal.pbio.1000469.
2. Harri M, Florey E (1977) The effects of temperature on a neuromuscular system of the crayfish, *Astacus leptodactylus*. J Comp Physiol A 117: 47–61.
3. Harri M, Florey E (1979) The effects of acclimation temperature on a neuromuscular system of the crayfish, *Astacus leptodactylus*. J Exp Biol 78: 281–293.
4. Fischer L, Florey E (1981) Temperature effects on neuromuscular transmission (opener muscle of crayfish, *Astacus leptodactylus*). J Exp Biol 94: 251–268.
5. Dipolo R, Latorre R (1972) Effect of temperature on membrane potential and ionic fluxes in intact and dialysed barnacle muscle fibres. J Physiol 225: 255–273.
6. Florey E, Hoyle G (1976) The effects of temperature on a nerve-muscle system of the Hawaiian ghost crab, *Ocypode ceratophthalma* (Pallas). J Comp Physiol A 110: 51–64.
7. Stephens PJ, Atwood HL (1983) Conversion of synaptic performance in crab motor axons by temperature changes. J Comp Physiol A 153: 455–466.
8. Dudel J, Rudel R (1968) Temperature dependence of electro-mechanical coupling in crayfish muscle fibers. Pflugers Arch 301: 16–30.
9. Hoover NJ, Weaver AL, Harness PI, Hooper SL (2002) Combinatorial and cross-fiber averaging transform muscle electrical responses with a large random component into deterministic contractions. J Neurosci 22: 1895–1904.
10. Morris LG, Hooper SL (1997) Muscle response to changing neuronal input in the lobster (*Panulirus interruptus*) stomatogastric system: Spike number vs. spike frequency dependent domains. J Neurosci 17: 5956–5971.
11. Morris LG, Hooper SL (1998) Muscle response to changing neuronal input in the lobster (*Panulirus interruptus*) stomatogastric system: Slow muscle properties can transform rhythmic input into tonic output. J Neurosci 18: 3433–3442.
12. Morris LG, Hooper SL (2001) Mechanisms underlying stabilization of temporally summated muscle contractions in the lobster (*Panulirus interruptus*) pyloric system. J Neurophysiol 85: 254–268.
13. Morris LG, Thuma JB, Hooper SL (2000) Muscles express motor patterns of non-innervating neural networks by filtering broad-band input. Nat Neurosci 3: 245–250.
14. Thuma JB, Hooper SL (2010) Direct evidence that stomatogastric (*Panulirus interruptus*) muscle passive responses are not due to background actomyosin cross-bridges. J Comp Physiol A 196: 649–65.
15. Thuma JB, Morris LG, Weaver AL, Hooper SL (2003) Lobster (*Panulirus interruptus*) pyloric muscles express the motor patterns of three neural networks, only one of which innervates the muscles. J Neurosci 23: 8911–8920.
16. Thuma JB, Harness PI, Koehnle TJ, Morris LG, Hooper SL (2007) Muscle anatomy is a primary determinant of muscle relaxation dynamics in the lobster (*Panulirus interruptus*) stomatogastric system. J Comp Physiol A 193: 1101–1113.
17. Selverston AI, Russell DF, Miller JP, King DG (1976) The stomatogastric nervous system: structure and function of a small neural network. Prog Neurobiol 7: 215–290.
18. Tang LS, Taylor AL, Rinberg A, Marder E (2012) Robustness of a rhythmic circuit to short- and long-term temperature changes. J Neurosci 32: 10075–10085.
19. Miyake Y (1952) On the tables of the saturated vapour pressure of sea water. Oceanogr Mag 4: 95–118.
20. Stein W (2009) Modulation of stomatogastric rhythms. J Comp Physiol A 195: 989–1009.
21. Lingle C (1981) The modulatory action of dopamine on crustacean foregut neuromuscular preparations. J Exp Biol 94: 285–299.
22. Meyrand P, Moulins M (1986) Myogenic oscillatory activity in the pyloric rhythmic motor system of crustacea. J Comp Physiol A 158: 489–503.
23. Meyrand P, Marder E (1991) Matching neural and muscle oscillators: control by FMRFamide-like peptides. J Neurosci 11: 1150–1161.
24. Jorge-Rivera JC, Marder E (1996) TNRNFLRFamide and SDRNFLRFamide modulate muscles of the stomatogastric system of the crab *Cancer borealis*. J Comp Physiol A 179: 741–751.
25. Jorge-Rivera JC, Marder E (1997) Allatostatin decreases stomatogastric neuromuscular transmission in the crab *Cancer borealis*. J Exp Biol 200: 2937–2946.
26. Weimann JM, Skiebe P, Heinzel H-G, Soto C, Kopell N, et al. (1997) Modulation of oscillator interactions in the crab stomatogastric ganglion by crustacean cardioactive peptide. J Neurosci 17: 1748–1760.
27. Jorge-Rivera JC, Sen K, Birmingham JT, Abbott LF, Marder E (1998) Temporal dynamics of convergent modulation at a crustacean neuromuscular junction. J Neurophysiol 80: 2559–2570.
28. Spees JL, Chang SA, Snyder MJ, Chang ES (2002) Thermal acclimation and stress in the American lobster, *Homarus americanus*: equivalent temperature shifts elicit unique gene expression patterns for molecular chaperones and poly-ubiquitin. Cell Stress & Chap 7: 97–106.
29. Lejeusne C, Perez T, Sarrazin V, Chevaldonne P (2006) Baseline expression of heat-shock proteins (HSPs) of a "thermotolerant" Mediterranean marine species largely influenced by natural temperature fluctuations. Can J Fish Aquat Sci 63: 2028–2037.

14

Comparative Biomechanical Modeling of Metatherian and Placental Saber-Tooths: A Different Kind of Bite for an Extreme Pouched Predator

Stephen Wroe[1,2]*, **Uphar Chamoli**[2,3], **William C. H. Parr**[2], **Philip Clausen**[1], **Ryan Ridgely**[4], **Lawrence Witmer**[4]

1 School of Biological, Earth and Environmental Sciences, University of New South Wales, Sydney, NSW, Australia, **2** School of Engineering, University of Newcastle, Callaghan, NSW, Australia, **3** St. George Clinical School, University of New South Wales, Sydney, NSW, Australia, **4** Department of Biomedical Sciences, Heritage College of Osteopathic Medicine, Ohio University, Athens, Ohio, United States of America

Abstract

Questions surrounding the dramatic morphology of saber-tooths, and the presumably deadly purpose to which it was put, have long excited scholarly and popular attention. Among saber-toothed species, the iconic North American placental, *Smilodon fatalis,* and the bizarre South American sparassodont, *Thylacosmilus atrox,* represent extreme forms commonly forwarded as examples of convergent evolution. For *S. fatalis,* some consensus has been reached on the question of killing behaviour, with most researchers accepting the canine-shear bite hypothesis, wherein both head-depressing and jaw closing musculatures played a role in delivery of the fatal bite. However, whether, or to what degree, *T. atrox* may have applied a similar approach remains an open question. Here we apply a three-dimensional computational approach to examine convergence in mechanical performance between the two species. We find that, in many respects, the placental *S. fatalis* (a true felid) was more similar to the metatherian *T. atrox* than to a conical-toothed cat. In modeling of both saber-tooths we found that jaw-adductor-driven bite forces were low, but that simulations invoking neck musculature revealed less cranio-mandibular stress than in a conical-toothed cat. However, our study also revealed differences between the two saber-tooths likely reflected in the *modus operandi* of the kill. Jaw-adductor-driven bite forces were extremely weak in *T. atrox,* and its skull was even better-adapted to resist stress induced by head-depressors. Considered together with the fact that the center of the arc described by the canines was closer to the jaw-joint in *Smilodon,* our results are consistent with both jaw-closing and neck musculature playing a role in prey dispatch for the placental, as has been previously suggested. However, for *T. atrox,* we conclude that the jaw-adductors probably played no major part in the killing bite. We propose that the metatherian presents a more complete commitment to the already extreme saber-tooth 'lifestyle'.

Editor: Alistair Robert Evans, Monash University, Australia

Funding: SW acknowledges support from the Australian Research Council (DP0666374 and DP0987985). LW and RR acknowledge support from the United States National Science Foundation (IOB-0517257, IOS-1050154), Ohio University Heritage College of Osteopathic Medicine, and the Ohio Supercomputer Center. The funders had no role in study design, data collection and analysis, decision to publish, or preparation of the manuscript.

Competing Interests: The authors have declared that no competing interests exist.

* E-mail: s.wroe@unsw.edu.au

Introduction

Saber-tooth morphology has a deep history, having independently evolved at least twice in the Permo-Triassic among non-mammalian cynodonts and at least five times among Cenozoic mammals, i.e., within the creodont, nimravid, barbourofelid and machairodontine placental, and sparassodont metatherian (a sister group to marsupials) clades [1–4]. Consequently, saber-toothed taxa have long figured prominently in analyses and discussions of adaptive convergence.

Of all saber-toothed species, representatives of the felid subfamily Machairodontinae are the best known. There are two widely recognized morphotypes, dirk- and scimitar-tooths. Scimitar-toothed taxa, e.g., *Homotherium serum,* are characterized by shorter, broader upper canines, longer limbs and more gracile physiques. Dirk-tooths, which include the iconic *Smilodon fatalis,* possess longer, more laterally compressed upper canines, and are typically much more robust, with shorter legs and lumbar regions

[5]. A third morphotype based on a single machairodontine species has been proposed, incorporating a combination of features [6].

With its extremely long upper canine teeth, powerful neck and forelimb musculature, short limbs, and short lower back, the Miocene-Pliocene metatherian saber-tooth, *Thylacosmilus atrox* appears most similar to specialized dirk-toothed machairodontines such as *S. fatalis,* although separated by at least 125 million years of evolution [7]. It is generally agreed that the bauplan of both *T. atrox* and *S. fatalis* represents an adaptation to the punishing habit of killing relatively large prey and the two are commonly compared in the context of convergent evolution [1,2,4,5,8–16].

Although most authors have long agreed that the dirk-toothed morphotype evolved to preferentially exploit and rapidly kill relatively large prey, our understanding of precisely how they delivered the fatal bite is the subject of one of palaeontology's longest running debates [4,12,17–19]. Over the last few decades some consensus has been achieved on the question of killing behaviour, at least with respect to *S. fatalis*. It is now widely recognised that the machairodont's jaw-closing muscles were relatively small and that at wide gapes mechanical advantage was reduced (i.e., leverage and hence bite reaction or output force was diminished), and, further that the neck muscles likely played an important role in the insertion of the canine teeth, especially in the initial stages of the bite [2,20,21]. It is thought that the head-depressing muscles were brought into play first, with the role of the jaw musculature increasing as the gape reduced, possibly with the lower jaw being held against the prey [2,11]. This *modus operandi*, the 'canine-shear bite" [11], is essentially an extension of the killing bite applied by living big cats.

Regarding *T. atrox*, however, our understanding of the anatomy of the kill is less clear. Qualitative assessment based on the detailed examination of origin and insertion sites of the primary head-depressors has led to the inference that its neck musculature was relatively even more powerful than that of other saber-tooths, including *S. fatalis* [16]. The same author concluded that the metatherian's jaws and associated musculature were relatively weaker still. On the other hand, it has also been argued that *T. atrox* may have been capable of a relatively powerful bite [22]. Although it has been suggested that *T. atrox* may have been more specialized than *S. fatalis* on the basis of geometric morphometric studies [23], results from other work based on 2D mandibular force profiling has been interpreted as evidence that the metatherian's killing behaviour was very similar to that of placental dirk-tooths [22].

In the present study we aim to determine the degree to which killing behaviour may have converged in *Thylacosmilus atrox* and *Smilodon fatalis* through the application of virtual reconstruction techniques and a 3D biomechanical modelling approach known as Finite Element Analysis (FEA). FEA is a powerful non-destructive engineering tool, originally developed for the aerospace industry, but now increasingly used in comparative analyses to predict relative performance in living and fossil taxa, as well as in biomedicine [24–36]. Importantly, in addition to facilitating more accurate estimates of reaction forces, such as bite force, with FEA it is also possible to predict, within relative contexts, whether structures are well-adapted to resist hypothesized loads (i.e., simulated behaviors) [35].

This approach has previously been applied in a comparison of biomechanical performance in the crania of *S. fatalis* and a living conical-toothed felid [4], but no FEA-based investigation has included *T. atrox*, or, for that matter, any two saber-toothed species. Our analysis represents a further advance on this earlier work in that we simulate the head-depressing musculature in more detail, estimate maximum gape angles using a new 3D virtual approach, and predict differences in bite force and cranio-mandibular stress at different gapes.

Materials and Methods

We note that the name *Thylacosmilus atrox* may be a junior synonym of *Achlysictis lelongi* [37] but retain use of the more familiar name until or unless the synonymy becomes more widely accepted. Specimens of *Smilodon fatalis* (FMNH P12418) and *Thylacosmilus atrox* (FMNH P14531, FMNH P14344) were scanned at O'Bleness Memorial Hospital in Athens, OH, USA, using a General Electric LightSpeed Ultra MultiSlice CT scanner with a slice thickness of 625 µm at 120 kV and 200 mA with Extended Hounsfield engaged and bone-reconstruction algorithm. Data were resampled to 300 µm isotropic voxels. For comparative purposes an extant conical-toothed felid, *Panthera pardus* (MM149),

was also scanned and modelled. Scanning for this specimen was conducted at the Mater Hospital (Newcastle, Australia) using a Toshiba Aquilion 16 scanner with a slice thickness of 500 µm at 120 kV and 140 mA.

Specimens of both *T. atrox* and *S. fatalis* each retained a single complete upper canine including tooth roots. A complete upper left canine (*T. atrox*) and complete upper right canine (*S. fatalis*), including the tooth roots, were segmented out from the remainder of the crania for both. These were mirrored in Mimics (vers. 13.02) to provide complete upper canines on the opposing sides. For *T. atrox* the cranium was well-preserved in FMNH P14531, but not the dentary, which was taken from P14344. Altogether, for *T. atrox* most of the right upper 3rd premolar, M3 and M4 of FMNH P14531 were missing, and, P14344 comprised a left dentary only. The same mirroring process was applied to reconstruct a complete cranium and mandible. The reconstructed mandible was scaled to fit the slightly larger cranium in Mimics. Upper canines, including tooth roots, were similarly segmented out for *P. pardus*.

3D Finite Element Models (FEMs) for skulls of *S. fatalis*, *T. atrox*, and the extant conical-toothed felid *Panthera pardus* (leopard) were generated in Mimics with the upper canine teeth and their roots meshed separately so that distinct material properties could be assigned (see Figures 1, 2, 3, 4). External parts of the canines were attached using rigid links [4,38] and assigned properties for dentine with surface elements assigned properties for enamel [4]. The remainder of the skull was assigned properties for cortical bone [4]. Jaw adducting musculature was assembled using pre-tensioned 'truss' elements following previously established proto-

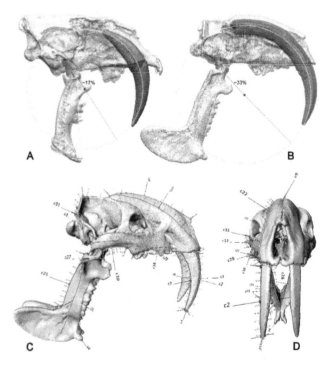

Figure 1. Centres of arcs described by the upper canine teeth. (A) *Smilodon fatalis* and (B) *Thylacosmilus atrox*. The distance of the centre from the jaw joint in *Thylacosmilus atrox* suggests that considerable translation as well as rotation was involved in the insertion of the canine teeth. Landmark positions shown on *Thylacosmilus atrox*. (C) lateral and (D) frontal views of right hand side landmarks. Curves shown in colour relate to Landmark point Von Mises mean stresses. Right hand side landmarks only shown.

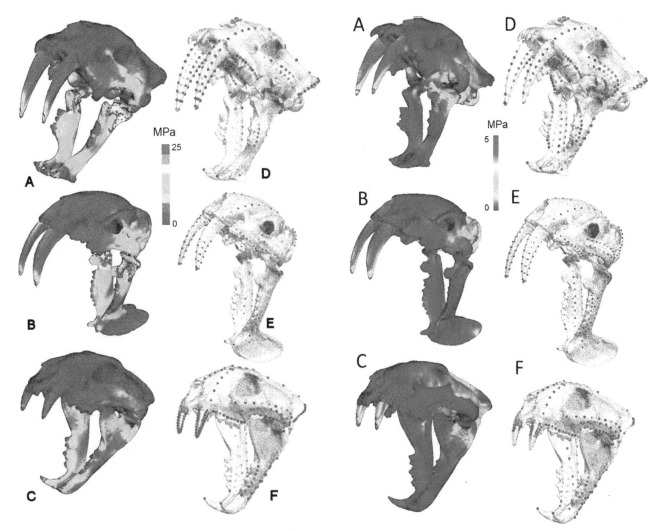

Figure 2. Stress distributions in scaled models for jaw adductor driven bites. Von Mises stress distributions and mean landmark point VM stresses given respectively for (A & D) *Smilodon fatalis*, (B & E) *Thylacosmilus atrox*, (C & F) *Panthera pardus*. MPa = Megapascals. Muscle forces scaled to bite reaction forces predicted on the basis of body mass.

Figure 3. Stress distributions in scaled models for neck muscle driven bites. Von Mises (VM) stress distributions and mean landmark point VM stresses given respectively for (A & D) *Smilodon fatalis*, (B & E) *Thylacosmilus atrox*, (C & F) *Panthera pardus*. MPa = Megapascals. Muscle forces scaled to bite reaction forces predicted on the basis of body mass.

cols [4]. Muscle force estimation also largely followed previous methods (Figure 4) and see below for more detail.

All volumetric meshes comprised four-noded (tet4) 'brick' elements and model size was maintained at between 1.63 and 1.65 million 'bricks' for each FEM (see Tables S1, S2, S3 in File S1). Volumetric models were imported into Strand7 (vers. 2.4) Finite Element Analysis software. Inputs are given in Tables S1, S2, S3 in File S1. Protocols largely followed those described in recent works [4,39].

We modelled the head depressing musculature with multiple pre-tensioned trusses and introduced 'hinges' to more realistically model muscle action (and see Tables S1, S2, S3 in File S1). These models served as bases for comparative investigations into the influence of gape on bite force and to assess their capacities to sustain loads applied by jaw-closing as opposed to head-depressing muscles.

Muscle forces for the jaw adductors were predicted using the 'dry-skull' method for approximating muscle cross-sectional areas [15,40,41] following previously applied protocols [4] and see

Supporting Information (File S1). This approach does not allow for additional force that might be generated as a consequence of pennation and is thus likely to underestimate actual maximal bite forces [4,40]. We stress that our primary objective here is to compare relative performance [4,42]. We do not apply a scaling factor for pennation which would introduce additional assumptions. Muscle origin and insertion areas were approximated on the basis of previous works [16,43].

For simulations wherein jaw adductors only were recruited constraints were applied at the occipital condyle and the tips of each canine [4,42]. Previous studies have used a variety of techniques to model the jaw mechanism including constraining a single node against displacement at each temporomandibular joint (TMJ), effectively creating an axis of rotation for the skull [26,44,45]. Such techniques have their own implications as the mandible and cranium are not modelled as an articulating structure, and the model therefore does not account for the effect of jaw movement. To overcome the problem of joint articulation,

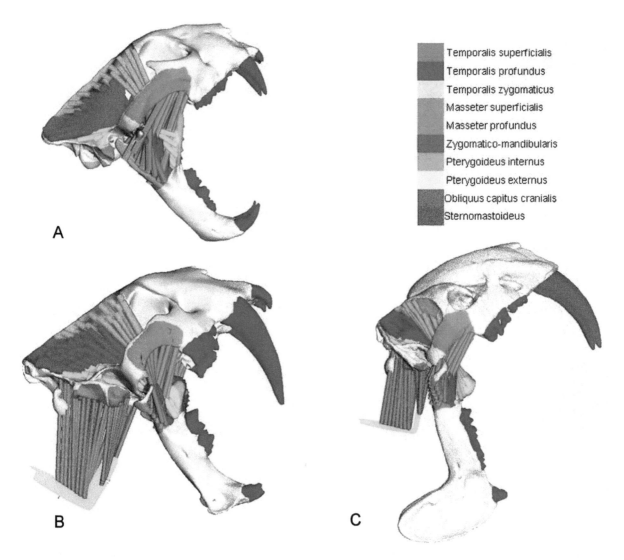

A

B

C

	Temporalis superficialis
	Temporalis profundus
	Temporalis zygomaticus
	Masseter superficialis
	Masseter profundus
	Zygomatico-mandibularis
	Pterygoideus internus
	Pterygoideus externus
	Obliquus capitus cranialis
	Sternomastoideus

Figure 4. Muscle simulations. (A) jaw-adducting muscles in *Panthera pardus*, (B) head depressing and jaw-adducting muscles in *Smilodon fatalis*, and (C) head-depressing and jaw-adducting muscles in *Thylacosmilus atrox*.

a hinge mechanism was used to simulate jaw operation [4,36,39]. Surface plates in the condyle and cotyle region were first selected and tessellated to create a network of fine beams. This was done to minimize stress singularities at the points of attachment of the jaw hinge. The jaw hinge mechanism used rigid links and beams to connect the cranium and mandible, providing a stiff connection between the articulating surfaces and a point on the axis of rotation to which the hinge beam was connected. The beam provided the pivot or hinge in the joint.

The length-tension relationship is a basic property of muscle fibers. Typically, maximum force is generated when fibers are only moderately stretched, and maximizing gape will theoretically compromise bite forces. However, the musculoskeletal configuration of saber-tooths may have allowed them to operate within a more favorable portion of the length–tension curve at larger gapes, as has been demonstrated in some other mammalian taxa [46]. Among living felids there is evidence for increased fiber length in the jaw adductors of species that have wider gapes and that take relatively large prey [47]. This may suggest some mitigation of the tendency to lose muscle force at wide gapes in these species. Our arrangement of truss elements broadly accounts for musculoskel-

etal features that may have improved performance at wide gapes in saber-tooths [2]. No experimentally derived data is available for the length-tension relationship of the masticatory muscles in large felid or marsupial carnivores and, rather than introduce further assumptions, our modeling effectively accepts that muscle tensions do not decrease with increasing gape. Thus our modeling assumes maximal performance at maximal gapes for jaw closing muscles and we consider it likely that this will result in at least some overestimation of jaw-muscle-driven bite force at wide gapes.

The two major head depressors, M. obliquus capitis and M. sternomastoideus and their origin and insertion points were reconstructed in the FEMs of *S. fatalis*, *T. atrox* and *P. pardus* based on known mastoid anatomy [1,10,48]. Crania and mandibles were first rotated about the TMJ to the theoretical maximal gape angle (see below). Rigid links were then used to create an ellipse (major and minor axis in mm: 40 and 26 for *S. fatalis*, 36 and 25 for *T. atrox*, and 30 and 20 for *P. pardus*) and a circle (radius in mm: 30 for *S. fatalis*, 26 for *T. atrox*, and 23 for *P. pardus*) that served as attachment 'webs' for the head-flexors. The circular and elliptical webs were kept perpendicular to each other, and their dimensions were proportional to skull length. The centre node in each was fixed in all six degrees of freedom.

Forty truss elements were used to simulate the action of the sternomastoideus muscles and thirty elements were used for the obliquus capitis. In *S. fatalis* each head-depressing truss element was assigned a pretension of 25N. Body mass scaled canine bite force output was then estimated for *T. atrox* and *P. pardus* using *S. fatalis* as reference [4,15]. Head-flexor muscle recruitment needed to generate this bite force was deduced from the finite element solves for *T. atrox* and *P. pardus*. Jaw adductors were not recruited in these simulations.

Maximum gape angles were predicted on the basis of surface meshes generated from the FEMs. A surface model (in stl format) was exported from the solid model for each specimen. The articulating surfaces of the cranium and mandible were extruded by 1 mm to simulate cartilage covering of the joint. No data is available for articular cartilage thickness in large felids or metatherians and here we use a median value reported for canids [49]. An Iterative Closest Point registration process was then used to fit the cartilage surfaces together [50]. By selecting the regions of the cartilage layers that were in contact when the jaw is opened wide, the rough maximum gape angle can be determined. However, at this point the cartilage layers still overlap considerably. The mandible was then moved until the cartilage layers just touched. A point was placed where cartilage contacted between the mandible and cranium for each TMJ. When connected, these points formed the rotational axis of mandible movement. For each model the mandible was then rotated around this axis until bone-bone contact was achieved at the articulating surfaces of the TMJ. The mandible was then rotated back away from contact with the cranium to account for soft tissue between the angular process on the mandible and the temporal bone to give the final maximum gape angle.

We assessed relative mechanical performance on the basis of visual output of the post-processing software, mean brick stress for selected regions [38], and mean landmark point data [27]. The application of landmarks to reveal mean landmark point VM stresses allows comparisons of values at homologous points in different FEMs [27,31,51], thus integrating shape and Finite Element Analyses. We used von Mises (VM) stress because it is a good predictor of material failure in relatively ductile material such as bone [52]. We note, however, that we do not expect to predict actual material failure in these models. Safety factors in mammalian bone can exceed 1000% [53] and, as observed above, our muscle force estimates are likely to be underestimates. Importantly, the approach followed in the present study, like that followed in most similar analyses, is strictly comparative [26,54–57], and it is not actual stress values, but their values and distributions relative to those in other specimens that are of interest [57]. We further observe that we have compared two independently evolved, but at least broadly convergent extremes and have not attempted to compare them in full phylogenetic contexts. This is because there are no living close relatives known for *Thylacosmilus atrox*.

Results and Discussion

Determining maximal gape is critical to understanding functional adaptation in saber-tooths [32,58]. Maximal 2D gape angles measured between the upper mesial incisor, jaw-joint, and lower mesial incisor were 87.1° for *S. fatalis*, 105.8° for *T. atrox*, and 72.6° for *P. pardus*. Respectively, these results were 2.5–12.5° less than determined in previous studies for *S. fatalis* [21,58], slightly higher than the figure of 102° previously suggested for *T. atrox* [9], and,

within the 65–70° range predicted for extant felids for *P. pardus* [58].

We found that the center of the arc described by the upper canines (saber-teeth) was considerably closer to the jaw-joint in *S. fatalis* (~17% of the distance of a line from the fulcrum to the circumference intersecting the center of the arc) as opposed to a value of ~33% in *T. atrox* for the same measurements. This is more consistent with the canine-shear bite hypothesis in *S. fatalis* than in *T. atrox*, as it means that the canines of the machairodont could have been inserted along a path of less (but not least) resistance, with the mandible rotated about the hinge throughout a killing bite. The far more ventral and anterior position of the center described by the arc of the canines in *T. atrox* means that, for minimal resistance to be maintained, more translation, and hence more input from the cervical musculature, would be necessary while the canines were driven into the prey (Figure 1). However, our findings here suggest that neither species is fully 'optimized' in this respect, further supporting the argument that at least some input from the head-depressors was characteristic of the killing bite in both.

Simulations of biting at the canine teeth at maximum gape angles using muscle forces derived on the basis of estimated cross-sectional area [40] gave bite reaction forces of 519 Newtons (N) for *S. fatalis*, 484 N for *P. pardus*, and 38 N for *T. atrox* (Table 1). Estimates of body mass were 259 kg, 68 kg, and 82 kg, respectively. For the fossil taxa these are based on proximal limb data. This was not possible for the leopard as the specimen was represented by the skull only (see Text S1 in File S1).

Relative to the conical-toothed cat, jaw-muscle-driven bite forces at wide gapes were relatively weak for *S. fatalis* and extremely weak for *T. atrox*, this despite the fact that our simulations assumed a constant length-tension relationship for muscle fibers at wider gapes. We further note that the estimate for body mass in *T. atrox* used in the present study is conservative and that some authors have predicted figures approaching 120 kg [59,60], which would make relative jaw-muscle-driven bite force weaker still in the metatherian. *Panthera pardus* was more efficient in converting jaw muscle force to bite reaction force at all gape angles than either saber-tooth. This differential became less marked with decreasing gape, but was still pronounced at smaller angles (see Figure S1 in File S1). At near optimal gape angles of 15° for achieving maximal jaw-muscle-driven bite force, reaction forces at the canines were 1408 N for *S. fatalis*, 1222 N for *P. pardus*, and 585 N for *T. atrox*. The result for this specimen of *S. fatalis* was higher than the 1100 N predicted for a smaller specimen previously modeled using a 3D approach [4], but still very low relative to that predicted for an extant large cat of comparable size, i.e., ~2906 N for a large male African lion [42].

Although few experimental data are available, and none for large felid or metatherian carnivores, the relationship between vertebrate body mass and bite force is thought to be allometric [15,61]. All else being equal, the expected relationship between bite reaction force and body mass should be a power function of $^{2/3}$ because muscle force is proportional to area and body mass is proportional to volume [62]. To account for differences in size between the three species, further simulations were performed with jaw muscle forces scaled to achieve the bite force expected on the basis of size (i.e., assuming a 2/3 power relationship). Under these inputs, our results showed that, relative to *P. pardus*, the crania and mandibles of both saber-tooths would have developed much higher stresses at maximal gapes in jaw-adductor-driven biting, with mean landmark point VM stresses consistently higher for both saber-tooths than for *P. pardus*. This was especially so for *T. atrox*, which recorded values more than four times greater than

Table 1. Body-mass-adjusted canine bite-force results and mean brick VM stresses for selected regions in a jaw-adductor-driven bite at maximum gape.

	Body mass estimate (kg)	Jaw muscle recruitment force (N)	Canine bite force (N)- 2/3rd power rule	Mean VM stress (MPa)		
				Tooth root	Canine-crowns	Rest of the Cranium
S. fatalis	259	3785*	519	0.552	2.593	1.074
T. atrox	82	24010*	241	0.486	2.311	1.577
P. pardus	68	1658*	212	0.397	1.848	0.584

*Muscle forces were back-calculated from FE models that gave the body-mass-scaled bite-force output at canines assuming a 2/3 power relationship. The choice of reference taxon is immaterial in this context and *S. fatalis* was arbitrarily chosen here. kg = kilograms; N = Newtons.

the leopard in the zygomatic arch. Similarly, mean 'brick' element stresses in the cranium were 1.8 times those of *P. pardus* in *S. fatalis* and 2.7 those of *P. pardus* in *T. atrox* (Figure 2, Table 2 and Table S4 in File S1).

Our analysis further shows that in order to achieve bite forces consistent with a 2/3 power relationship at maximum gape, *S. fatalis* would need to recruit 2.3 times the jaw adductor muscle force of *P. pardus*. At maximum gape, *Thylacosmilus atrox* would need to generate 14.5 times the jaw adductor muscle force of *P. pardus* in order to achieve a bite force consistent with its body mass. In contrast, when neck muscle forces only were applied, assuming a 2/3 power relationship between body mass and reaction force at the canines, mean VM landmark point stresses and mean 'brick' element stresses were comparable between *S. fatalis* and *P. pardus* and relatively low in *T. atrox* (Figure 3 and Table S5 in File S1).

Although our results are arguably consistent with the canine-shear bite hypothesis for *S. fatalis* [8], the extremely low jaw-adductor-driven bite forces predicted at all gape angles for *T. atrox* suggest that the jaw muscles played an insignificant role in the dispatch of prey by the metatherian. Moreover, our findings suggest that in order to minimize stress on the canine teeth and resistance as the canines were inserted, *T. atrox* needed to move its head considerably further forward and downward relative to the position of the jaw-joint than would *S. fatalis*. This could not be achieved simply through rotation about the jaw-joint and would have required manipulation by cervical and/or other postcranial muscles. The relatively low VM stresses predicted for *T. atrox* in scaled modelling of a neck-muscle-driven bite further support this interpretation.

As has been argued for a range of cranial and postcranial character systems, our simulations provide further evidence for convergence in these two highly derived mammalian predators with respect to the mechanics of the killing bite. At wide gapes, in both species, jaw-muscle-driven bite forces are low, and predicted stress magnitudes and distributions suggest that their crania are less well-adapted to resist high jaw-muscle-driven bite forces, but well-adapted to dissipate loads applied by powerful cervical musculature.

Fewer studies have offered interpretations of hunting and killing behaviour for *T. atrox* than for *S. fatalis*, but a considerable range of possibilities have been forwarded nonetheless. A majority of previous assessments have concluded that *T. atrox* was most likely an ambush predator, however, recent application of geometric morphometric and phylogenetic comparative methods to postcranial data leaves open the possibility that it was capable of sustained; albeit not rapid pursuit [63]. A number of studies have commented on the apparent lack of retractile claws in *T. atrox* and possible limits imposed thereby on its ability to capture and secure prey, leading to speculation that it may have used its head to knock prey over [64]. It has also been argued that the wide gape of *T. atrox* may have allowed it to stab prey at nearly right angles to its body without first needing to restrain it with its claws [9]. Our analyses do not directly assess the likelihood of these suggestions, but we note that the laterally compressed morphology of the canines may have left them vulnerable to breakage in stabbing unsecured prey and that at least some extant ursids are known to capture and immobilize relatively large animals without retractile claws [65]. Among felid, nimravid and barbourofelid saber-tooths there is strong correlation between upper canine length and

Table 2. Body-mass-scaled bite-force results and mean brick VM stresses for selected regions in for a cervical-musculature-driven bite.

	Body mass (kg)	Head depressing muscle force (N)	Canine bite force (N)	Mean VM stress (MPa)		
				Tooth root	Canine-crowns	Rest of the cranium
S. fatalis	259	1750 *	269	0.193	0.585	0.446
T. atrox	82	1547*	125	0.19	0.44	0.45
P. pardus	68	1076*	110	0.269	0.969	0.574

*Muscle forces were back-calculated from FE models that gave the body-mass-scaled bite-force output at canines assuming a 2/3 power relationship. *S. fatalis* was arbitrarily used as a reference and head-depressing muscle force used in the model was a hypothetical value. The choice of taxon or value for the reference taxon is immaterial in this context. kg = kilograms; N = Newtons.

forelimb robusticity, indicating that powerful forelimbs may be a prerequisite needed to immobilise prey in placental saber-tooths and that this becomes increasingly important as canines become longer and more fragile [66]. Although *T. atrox* was not included in that study there is no doubt that its canines were particularly long and laterally compressed and that its forelimbs were very robust [10,58].

Analyses based on beam theory have alternatively suggested that *T. atrox* had a weak or powerful jaw-adductor-driven bite [15,22]. A number of previous authors have suggested that jaw-adductor-driven bite forces may have been particularly weak and that head depressors were especially well-developed, asserting that the head-depressors may have played a particularly important role in driving the canines into prey for the saber-toothed metatherian [9,10]. Results tendered in the present study provide strong quantitative support for these latter interpretations.

Our findings further suggest that cranio-dental adaptation in *T. atrox* was more specialized than in the machairodontine *S. fatalis*, but the possibility remains open that the metatherian may have converged more completely on other placental saber-tooths not included in the present study. Among these, perhaps the closest in terms of overall cranio-dental and postcranial morphology may have been *Barbourofelis fricki*. Some previous authors have alluded to specific similarities between *T. atrox* and this derived barbour-ofelid, including possession of a postorbital bar, very long canines, a particularly wide gape, mandibular flanges, and relatively short front and hind limbs [58,67]. Inclusion of *B. fricki* in future 3D biomechanical analyses could be very informative.

Among placental saber-tooth clades, the evidence now points to independently derived trends toward decreasing jaw-adductor-driven bite force, increasing reliance on head-depressing-muscu-lature, and increasing canine length and forelimb robusticity (i.e., for nimravids, barbourofelids and machairodontines) [2,4,66,68]. A majority of authors have concluded that this suite of features are associated with strong selective pressure for a rapid kill facilitated by precisely directed deep bites into soft tissue that first require effective immobilisation of the prey to limit the risk of damage to the laterally compressed upper canines [4,66,68].

Regarding those performance indicators considered in the present study, the very weak jaw-adductor-driven bite forces, cranio-dental anatomy inconsistent with jaw-adductor-driven insertion of the canines along a line of least resistance, and adaptation in the cranium to resist powerful neck-driven-forces present in *T. atrox*, suggest extreme specialization. Whether the metatherian ambushed or ran down its prey, we consider it likely that it was immobilized and secured first because the particularly long and laterally compressed canines would have been especially vulnerable to breakage. This is consistent with evidence for powerful and flexible forelimb musculature, together with other postcranial adaptations for stability [10].

A final point to be considered here is that the flattened canines of *T. atrox* may have required less force to insert than did those of *S. fatalis*. On this basis it could reasonably be argued that the jaw adductors may still have played a significant role in the kill. We would maintain, however, that both our biomechanical evidence suggesting that the cranium was much better adapted to resist forces incurred by a neck-driven-bite, together with that showing that canine morphology was not 'optimized' for a jaw-adductor-driven bite, remains inconsistent with a significant role for the jaw adductors in the kill.

The fossil record evidencing distinct structural intermediates between more generalized sparassodonts and *T. atrox* remains poor, despite the recent discovery of new material [69]. However, regardless of the process through which the distinctive morphology of *T. atrox* was derived, we suggest that in the craniodental mechanics of the killing bite that define the dirk-toothed morphotype, the metatherian represents a further extreme in functional adaptation relative to that of *S. fatalis*. Our results further support the contention that despite far lower species richness and greater geographic restriction over time relative to their placental counterparts, metatherian carnivores achieved broadly comparable diversity in terms of behaviour and craniodental morphology [14,23].

Supporting Information

File S1   Text S1, Body mass estimates. **Figure S1,** Variations in canine bite reaction force (BF) and jaw muscle recruitment (MR) with changing gape angle. **Table S1,** Inputs for Finite Element Model of Smilodon fatalis. **Table S2,** Inputs for Finite Element Model of *Thylacosmilus atrox*. **Table S3,** Inputs for Finite Element Model of *Panthera pardus*. **Table S4,** Mean landmark point Von Mises stresses for jaw-muscle-driven bite scaled to body mass. **Table S5,** Mean landmark point Von Mises stresses for neck-muscle-driven bite scaled to body mass.

Acknowledgments

For loan of specimens, we thank W. F. Simpson, P. J. Makovicky, and the Field Museum of Natural History, Chicago. For CT scanning, we thank E. Cunningham, CT Unit, Mater Hospital, Newcastle, NSW and H. Rockhold and O'Bleness Memorial Hospital, Athens, OH. For discussion and assistance, we thank D. Croft.

Author Contributions

Conceived and designed the experiments: SW UC PC LW. Performed the experiments: SW UC RR WP. Analyzed the data: SW. Contributed reagents/materials/analysis tools: WP RR. Wrote the paper: SW UC WP PC RR LW.

References

1. Argot C (2004) Evolution of South American mammalian predators (Borhyae-noidea): anatomical and palaeobiological implications. Zoological Journal of the Linnean Society 140: 487–521.
2. Christiansen P (2011) A dynamic model for the evolution of sabrecat predatory bite mechanics. Zoological Journal of the Linnean Society 162: 220–242.
3. Van Valkenburgh B, Jenkins I (2002) Evolutionary patterns in the history of Permo-Triassic and Cenozoic synapsid predators. Paleontological Society Papers 8: 267–288.
4. McHenry CR, Wroe S, Clausen PD, Moreno K, Cunningham E (2007) Supermodeled sabercat, predatory behavior in *Smilodon fatalis* revealed by high-resolution 3D computer simulation. Proceedings of the National Academy of Sciences (USA) 104: 16010–16015.
5. Wroe S, Lowry MB, Anton M (2008) How to build a mammalian super-predator. Zoology 111: 196–203.
6. Martin LD, Babiarz JP, Naples VL, Hearst J (2000) Three Ways To Be a Saber-Toothed Cat. Naturwissenschaften 87: 41–44.
7. Luo Z-X, Qiang J, Wible JR, Yuan C-X (2003) An Early Cretaceous Tribosphenic Mammal and Metatherian Evolution. Science 302: 1934–1940.
8. Christiansen P, Harris JM (2005) Body size of *Smilodon* (Mammalia: Felidae). Journal of Morphology 266: 369–384.
9. Churcher CS (1985) Dental functional morphology in the marsupial sabre-tooth Thylacosmilus atrox (Thylacosmilidae) compared to that of felid sabre-tooths. Australian Mammalogy 8: 201–220.
10. Argot C (2004) Functional-adaptive features and palaeobiologic implications of the postcranial skeleton of the late Miocene sabretooth borhyaenoid *Thylacosmilus atrox* (Metatheria). Alcheringa 28: 229–266.
11. Akersten W (1985) Canine function in *Smilodon* (Mammalia, Felidae, Machair-odontinae). Los Angeles County Museum Contributions in Science 356: 1–22.

12. Christiansen P (2007) Comparative bite forces and canine bending strength in feline and sabretooth felids: implications for predatory ecology. Zoological Journal of the Linnean Society 151: 423–437.

13. Marshall LG (1976) Evolution of the Thylacosmilidae, extinct saber-toothed marsupials of South America. Paleobios 23: 1–30.

14. Wroe S, Milne N (2007) Convergence and remarkably consistent constraint in the evolution of carnivore skull shape. Evolution 61: 1251–1260.

15. Wroe S, McHenry C, Thomason J (2005) Bite club: comparative bite force in big biting mammals and the prediction of predatory behaviour in fossil taxa. Proceedings of the Royal Society of London, Series B 272: 619–625.

16. Turnbull WD (1976) Restoration of the masticatory musculature of Thylacosmilus. In: Churcher CS, editor. Essays on Palaeontology in honour of Loris Shanno Russel. Ontario: Royal Ontario Museum. 169–185.

17. Warren JC (1853) Remarks on Felis smylodon. Proceedings of the Boston Society of Natural History 4: 256–258.

18. Matthews WD (1910) The phylogeny of the Felidae. Bulletin of the American Museum of Natural History 28: 289–316.

19. Slater GJ, Van Valkenburgh B (2008) Long in the tooth: evolution of sabertooth cat cranial shape. Paleobiology 34: 403–419.

20. Kurtén B (1954) The Chinese Hipparion Fauna: A quantitative survey with comments on the ecology of machairodonts and hyaenids and the taxonomy of the gazelles. Commentationes Biologicae Societas Scientiarum Fennica 13: 1–82.

21. Bryant HN (1996) Force generation by the jaw adductor musculature at different gapes in the Pleistocene saber-toothed felid Smilodon. In: Steward KM, Seymour KL, editors. Paleoecology and Paleoenvironments of Late Cenozoic Mammals. Toronto: University of Toronto Press. 283–299.

22. Therrien F (2005) Feeding behaviour and bite force of sabretoothed predators. Zoological Journal of the Linnean Society 145: 393–426.

23. Goswami A, Milne N, Wroe S (2011) Biting through constraints: cranial morphology, disparity and convergence across living and fossil carnivorous mammals. Proceedings of the Royal Society B: Biological Sciences 278: 1831–1839.

24. Rayfield EJ, Norman DB, Horner CC, Horner JR, Smith PM, et al. (2001) Cranial design and function in a large theropod dinosaur. Nature 409: 1033–1037.

25. Strait DS, Grosse IR, Dechow PC, Smith AL, Wang Q, et al. (2010) The Structural Rigidity of the Cranium of Australopithecus africanus: Implications for Diet, Dietary Adaptations, and the Allometry of Feeding Biomechanics. The Anatomical Record: Advances in Integrative Anatomy and Evolutionary Biology 293: 583–593.

26. Strait DS, Weber GW, Neubauer S, Chalk J, Richmond BG, et al. (2009) The feeding biomechanics and dietary ecology of Australopithecus africanus. Proceedings of the National Academy of Sciences USA 106: 2124–2129.

27. Parr W, Wroe S, Chamoli U, Richards HS, McCurry M, et al. (2012) Toward integration of geometric morphometrics and computational biomechanics: New methods for 3D virtual reconstruction and quantitative analysis of Finite Element Models. Journal of Theoretical Biology 301: 1–14.

28. Rayfield EJ (2007) Finite Element Analysis and Understanding the Biomechanics and Evolution of Living and Fossil Organisms. Annual Review of Earth and Planetary Sciences 35: 541–576.

29. Fry BG, Wroe S, Teeuwisse W, van Osch MJP, Moreno K, et al. (2009) A central role for venom in predation by Varanus komodoensis (Komodo Dragon) and the extinct giant Varanus (Megalania) priscus. Proceedings of the National Academy of Sciences of the United States of America 106: 8969–8974.

30. Moazen M, Curtis N, O'Higgins P, Evans SE, Fagan MJ (2009) Biomechanical assessment of evolutionary changes in the lepidosaurian skull. Proceedings of the National Academy of Sciences (USA) 106: 8273–8277.

31. Evans SP, Parr WCH, Clausen PD, Jones A, Wroe S (2012) Finite element analysis of a micromechanical model of bone and a new 3D approach to validation. Journal of Biomechanics 45: 2702–2705.

32. O'Higgins P, Cobb SN, Fitton LC, Groning F, Phillips R, et al. (2011) Combining geometric morphometrics and functional simulation: an emerging toolkit for virtual functional analyses. Journal of Anatomy 218: 3–15.

33. Bourke J, Wroe S, Moreno K, McHenry C, Clausen P (2008) Effects of gape and tooth position on bite force and skull stress in the Dingo (Canis lupus dingo) using a 3-Dimensional Finite Element Approach. PLoS ONE 3 (e2200).

34. Degrange FJ, Tambussi CP, Moreno K, Witmer LM, Wroe S (2010) Mechanical Analysis of Feeding Behavior in the Extinct Terror Bird Andalgalornis steulleti (Gruiformes: Phorusrhacidae). PLoS ONE 5: e11856.

35. Wroe S, Ferrara TL, McHenry CR, Curnoe D, Chamoli U (2010) The craniomandibular mechanics of being human. Proceedings of the Royal Society B: Biological Sciences 277: 3579–3586.

36. Wroe S, Clausen P, McHenry C, Moreno K, Cunningham E (2007) Computer simulation of feeding behaviour in the thylacine and dingo as a novel test for convergence and niche overlap. Proceedings of the Royal Society of London, Series B 274: 2819–2828.

37. Goin FJ (1997) In:Kay RF, Madden RH, Cifelli RL, Flynn J, editors. A History of the Neotropical fauna Vertebrate paleobiology of the Miocene in Colombia: Smithsonian Institution Press. 185–204.

38. Chamoli U, Wroe S (2011) Allometry in the distribution of material properties and geometry of the felid skull: Why larger species may need to change and how they may achieve it. Journal of Theoretical Biology 283: 217–226.

39. Oldfield C, McHenry C, Clausen P, Chamoli U, Parr WCH, et al. (2012) Finite Element Analysis of ursid cranial mechanics and the prediction of feeding behaviour in the extinct giant Agriotherium africanum: the bare facts. Journal of Zoology 286: 163–170.

40. Thomason JJ (1991) Cranial strength in relation to estimated biting forces in some mammals. Canadian Journal of Zoology 69: 2326–2333.

41. Christiansen P, Wroe S (2007) Bite forces and evolutionary adaptations to feeding ecology in carnivores. Ecology 88: 347–358.

42. Wroe S (2008) Cranial mechanics compared in extinct marsupial and extant African lions using a finite-element approach. Journal of Zoology (London) 274: 332–339.

43. Turnbull WD (1970) Mammalian masticatory apparatus. Fieldiana: Geology 18: 149–356.

44. Strait DS, Wang Q, Dechow PC, Ross CF, Richmond BG, et al. (2005) Modeling elastic properties in finite-element analysis: How much precision Is needed to produce an accurate model? The Anatomical Record, Part A 283A: 275–287.

45. Slater GJ, van Valkenburgh B (2009) Allometry and performance: the evolution of skull form and function in felids. Journal of Evolutionary Biology 22: 2278–2287.

46. Eng CM, Ward SR, Vinyard CJ, Taylor AB (2009) The morphology of the masticatory apparatus facilitates muscle force production at wide jaw gapes in tree-gouging common marmosets (Callithrix jacchus). The Journal of Experimental Biology 212, 4040–4055 212: 4040–4055.

47. Hartstone-Rose A, Perry JMG, Morrow CJ (2012) Bite Force Estimation and the Fiber Architecture of Felid Masticatory Muscles. The Anatomical Record: Advances in Integrative Anatomy and Evolutionary Biology 295: 1336–1351.

48. Anton M, Salesa MJ, Pastor JF, Sanchez IM, Fraile S, et al. (2004) Implications of the mastoid anatomy of larger extant felids for the evolution and predatory behaviour of sabretoothed cats (Mammalia, Carnivora, Felidae). Zoological Journal of the Linnean Society 140: 207–221.

49. Frisbie DD, Cross MW, McIlwraith CW (2008) A comparative study of articular cartilage thickness in the stifle of animal species used in human pre-clinical studies compared to articular cartilage thickness in the human knee. Veterinary and Comparative Orthopaedics and Traumatology 19: 142–146.

50. Besl PJ, Mckay ND (1992) A method for registration of 3-D shapes. IEEE Transactions on Pattern Analysis and Machine Intelligence 14 239–256.

51. Parr WCH, Chamoli U, Jones A, Walsh WR, Wroe S (2013) Finite element micro-modelling of a human ankle bone reveals the importance of the trabecular network to mechanical performance: New methods for the generation and comparison of 3D models. Journal of Biomechanics 46: 200–205.

52. Tsafnat N, Wroe S (2011) An experimentally validated micromechanical model of a rat vertebra under compressive loading. Journal of Anatomy 218: 40–46.

53. Thomason JJ, Russell AP (1986) Mechanical factors in the evolution of the mammalian secondary palate: A theoretical analysis. Journal of Morphology 189: 199–213.

54. Slater GJ, Figueirido B, Louis L, Yang P, Van Valkenburgh B (2010) Biomechanical Consequences of Rapid Evolution in the Polar Bear Lineage. PLoS ONE 5: e13870.

55. Tseng ZJ, Wang X (2010) Cranial functional morphology of fossil dogs and adaptation for durophagy in Borophagus and Epicyon (Carnivora, Mammalia). Journal of Morphology 271: 1386–1398.

56. Rayfield EJ (2005) Using finite-element analysis to investigate suture morphology: A case study using large carnivorous dinosaurs. Anatomical Record, Part B 283A: 349–365.

57. Wroe S (2010) Cranial mechanics of mammalian carnivores: Recent advances using a Finite Element approach. In: Goswami A, editor. New Views on Phylogeny, Form, and Function. Cambridge: Cambridge University Press. 466–485.

58. Emerson SB, Radinsky L (1980) Functional analysis of sabertooth cranial morphology. Paleobiology 6: 295–312.

59. Ercoli MD, Prevosti FJ (2011) Estimacion de masa de las especies de Sparassodontia (Mammalia, Metatheria) de Edad Santacucense (Mioceno Temprano) a partir del tamano del centroide de los elementos apendiculares: Inferencias. Armeghiniana 48: 462–479.

60. Wroe S, Myers TJ, Wells RT, Gillespie A (1999) Estimating the weight of the Pleistocene marsupial lion, Thylacoleo carnifex (Thylacoleonidae: Marsupialia): Implications for the ecomorphology of a marsupial super-predator and hypotheses of impoverishment of Australian marsupial carnivore faunas. Australian Journal of Zoology 47: 489–498.

61. Huber DR, Eason TG, Hueter RE, Motta PJ (2005) Analysis of the bite force and mechanical design of the feeding mechanism of the durophagous horn shark Heterodontus francisci. The Journal of Experimental Biology 208: 3553–3571.

62. Wroe S, Huber D, Lowry M, McHenry C, Moreno K, et al. (2008) Three-dimensional computer analysis of white shark jaw mechanics: how hard can a great white bite? Journal of Zoology (London) 276: 336–342.

63. Ercoli MD, Prevosti FJ, ÁLvarez A (2012) Form and function within a phylogenetic framework: locomotory habits of extant predators and some Miocene Sparassodonta (Metatheria). Zoological Journal of the Linnean Society 165: 224–251.

64. Goin FG, Pascual R (1987) News on the biology and taphonomy of the marsupials Thylacosmilidae (Late Tertiary of Argentina). Anales de la Academia Nacional de Ciencias Exactas, Fisicas y Naturales 39: 219–246.

65. Martin LD (1980) Functional morphology and the evolution of cats. Transactions of the Nebraska Academy of Sciences 8: 141–154.

66. Meachen-Samuels JA (2012) Morphological convergence of the prey-killing arsenal of sabertooth predators. Paleobiology 38: 1–14.

67. Prevosti FJ, Turazzini GF, Ercoli MD, Hingst-Zaher E (2012) Mandible shape in marsupial and placental carnivorous mammals: a morphological comparative study using geometric morphometrics. Zoological Journal of the Linnean Society 164: 836–855.

68. Christiansen P (2008) Evolution of Skull and Mandible Shape in Cats (Carnivora: Felidae). PLoS ONE 3: e2807.

69. Forasiepi AM, Carlini AA (2010) A new thylacosmilid (Mammalia, Metatheria, Sparassodonta) from the Miocene of Patagonia, Argentina. Zootaxa 2552: 55–68.

15

Neurogenic Detrusor Overactivity Is Associated with Decreased Expression and Function of the Large Conductance Voltage- and Ca^{2+}-Activated K^{+} Channels

Kiril L. Hristov[1], Serge A. Y. Afeli[1], Shankar P. Parajuli[1], Qiuping Cheng[1], Eric S. Rovner[2], Georgi V. Petkov[1,2]*

1 Department of Drug Discovery and Biomedical Sciences, South Carolina College of Pharmacy, University of South Carolina, Columbia, South Carolina, United States of America, **2** Medical University of South Carolina, Charleston, South Carolina, United States of America

Abstract

Patients suffering from a variety of neurological diseases such as spinal cord injury, Parkinson's disease, and multiple sclerosis often develop neurogenic detrusor overactivity (NDO), which currently lacks a universally effective therapy. Here, we tested the hypothesis that NDO is associated with changes in detrusor smooth muscle (DSM) large conductance Ca^{2+}-activated K^{+} (BK) channel expression and function. DSM tissue samples from 33 patients were obtained during open bladder surgeries. NDO patients were clinically characterized preoperatively with pressure-flow urodynamics demonstrating detrusor overactivity, in the setting of a clinically relevant neurological condition. Control patients did not have overactive bladder and did not have a clinically relevant neurological disease. We conducted quantitative polymerase chain reactions (qPCR), perforated patch-clamp electrophysiology on freshly-isolated DSM cells, and functional studies on DSM contractility. qPCR experiments revealed that DSM samples from NDO patients showed decreased BK channel mRNA expression in comparison to controls. Patch-clamp experiments demonstrated reduced whole cell and transient BK currents (TBKCs) in freshly-isolated DSM cells from NDO patients. Functional studies on DSM contractility showed that spontaneous phasic contractions had a decreased sensitivity to iberiotoxin, a selective BK channel inhibitor, in DSM strips isolated from NDO patients. These results reveal the novel finding that NDO is associated with decreased DSM BK channel expression and function leading to increased DSM excitability and contractility. BK channel openers or BK channel gene transfer could be an alternative strategy to control NDO. Future clinical trials are needed to evaluate the value of BK channel opening drugs or gene therapies for NDO treatment and to identify any possible adverse effects.

Editor: Steven Barnes, Dalhousie University, Canada

Funding: This study was supported by the National Institutes of Health DK084284 grant to GVP. The funders had no role in study design, data collection and analysis, decision to publish, or preparation of the manuscript.

Competing Interests: The authors have declared that no competing interests exist.

* E-mail: petkov@cop.sc.edu

Introduction

Overactive bladder (OAB) is described as urgency, with or without incontinence, usually associated with frequency and nocturia [1]. Patients with various neurological diseases often develop voiding dysfunction which presents clinically as OAB [2]. These OAB symptoms are often caused by dysfunction of the neurological control mechanisms subserving bladder function. When such a condition is the result of urodynamically demonstrable involuntary bladder contractions, it is termed neurogenic detrusor overactivity (NDO). The pathology of NDO is often associated with alteration of the electromechanical properties of the detrusor smooth muscle (DSM), including increased DSM excitability [2]. Aside from the clinical symptoms of frequency, urgency and incontinence, high pressure involuntary contractions of DSM in patients with NDO may eventually lead to irreversible changes in DSM. Such changes may result in decreased bladder compliance with associated high intravesical pressure during the bladder filling phase, and if left untreated may lead to deterioration of the upper urinary tract [3–5].

Currently, there is not an optimal pharmacological agent to treat NDO [6]. Antimuscarinics are used to treat NDO but these agents have limited effectiveness and, due to a lack of specificity for the lower urinary tract, are associated with collateral undesirable adverse effects elsewhere in the body [7–12]. The selective β3-adrenoceptor agonist mirabegron [13,14] has been recently proposed to treat OAB, however its effectiveness in patients with NDO remains uncertain. Newer therapies such as intravesical botulinum toxin [3,15] are not only invasive and expensive but are also associated with safety concerns [3,6,16]. Therefore, novel approaches to treat NDO are urgently needed. A critical step for the development of a new, safe, and more effective therapy for NDO is developing a better understanding of the etiology of NDO and the basic mechanisms that control DSM excitability and contractility in NDO patients.

NDO is characterized by increased spontaneous phasic DSM contractions during the filling phase of urodynamics in an individual with a clinically relevant neurological condition [17,18]. The underlying basis of these spontaneous phasic DSM contractions is the spontaneous action potentials [19]. A number

Table 1. qPCR primers for BKα, BKβ1, BKβ4 subunits and GAPDH.

	Sense	Anti-sense	Product (bp)	Accession Number
BKα	TGCCTAAAGCATGATTTG	GCCGACATGCTAAATAAATTAG	400	NG012270
BKβ1	TGCCACCTGATTGAGACC	TGCGGAGAAGCAGTAGAAG	258	NM004137
BKβ4	CATTTGTGGTGGGCTTTCT	ACATGTTCCGCAGGTGG	168	NM170782
GAPDH	GGATTTGGTCGTATTGGG	GGAAGATGGTGATGGGATT	205	NM002046

bp – base pairs.

of different types of K^+ channels control DSM action potential generation [20]. The large conductance voltage- and Ca^{2+}-activated K^+ (BK) channel is arguably the most important physiologically relevant K^+ channel involved in the regulation of the DSM action potential, the resting membrane potential, and DSM contractility [20–32]. Iberiotoxin, a selective blocker of the BK channel, inhibits the majority of the whole cell outward K^+ current, depolarizes the DSM cell resting membrane potential, and increases the contractility of human isolated DSM strips [29]. Because of their prominent physiological role in DSM excitability and contractility, BK channels have been identified as a valid target for the pharmacological or genetic control of OAB [18,21,27,29,31,33–37].

The absence of pore-forming BKα subunits or regulatory BKβ1 subunits significantly increases DSM contractility and urination frequency in association with detrusor overactivity (DO) [24,26,30,38]. In a rat model of partial urethral obstruction, there was a significant decrease in whole cell BK channel current associated with over a 2-fold reduction in BKα subunit mRNA and protein expression [39]. Recent studies also demonstrated direct involvement of BK channels in the etiology of OAB in patients with benign prostatic hyperplasia (BPH) and DO [33] as well as NDO [18]. These results reinforce the notion of a significant role for the BK channel in DSM function and dysfunction, and suggest that BK channel dysfunction can lead to the OAB phenotype. However, the role of the BK channel in the pathophysiology of NDO has not been investigated.

Here, we used a multidisciplinary experimental approach utilizing qPCR and patch-clamp electrophysiology on freshly-isolated human DSM cells, functional studies on human DSM tissue strip contractility, as well as pharmacological protocols to evaluate if NDO is associated with changes in the DSM BK channel expression and function.

Materials and Methods

Human DSM Tissue Collection

All procedures for human DSM tissue collection were reviewed and approved by the Institutional Review Board of the Medical University of South Carolina (MUSC) under the protocol HR 16918. According to this protocol, human DSM tissues were collected upon written informed consent to participate in this study. Human DSM tissue samples from control and NDO patients were obtained during open bladder surgeries performed for a variety of indications such as bladder cancer, urothelial carcinoma, and ureteral reimplantation for repair of urinary fistula. NDO patients were clinically characterized preoperatively with pressure-flow urodynamics demonstrating DO in the setting of a clinically relevant neurological condition such as spina bifida, cerebral palsy, and spinal cord injury; with or without an American Urological Association (AUA) symptom score >7.

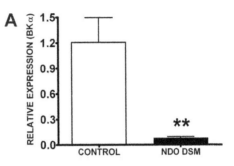

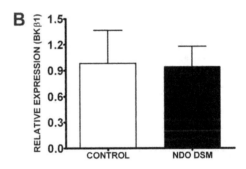

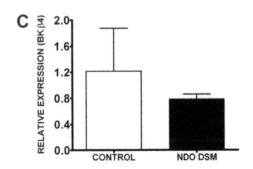

Figure 1. Patients with NDO have decreased BKα subunit mRNA expression in DSM. qPCR analyses showing 15.8-fold, 1.1-fold, and 1.6-fold decreases in BKα (**A**), BKβ1 (**B**), and BKβ4 subunits (**C**) mRNA expression in NDO DSM tissue (n = 3, N = 3) compared to controls (n = 7, N = 7; **P<0.01). Data are shown as relative mRNA expression normalized to GAPDH.

Control patients did not have OAB (defined as an AUA symptom score <8) and did not have a clinically relevant neurological disease. In this study, 33 patients (19 males and 14 females; 26 Caucasians and 7 African-Americans; 62.4±2.8 years average age) were used. From those 33 patients, 4 were with clinically confirmed NDO (4 females; 2 Caucasians and 2 African-Americans; 46.5±14.8 years average age), and 29 patients (19 males and 10 females; 24 Caucasians and 5 African-Americans; 64.6 ± 2.4 years average age) were without NDO and were used as controls. The DSM specimens were obtained from tumor free regions of the bladder dome, posterior or anterior bladder wall. Two types of DSM samples were collected from each patient. The first sample was stored in ice-cold Ca^{2+}-free N-2-hydroxyethylpi-perazine-N-2-ethanesulphonic acid (HEPES)-buffered dissection solution (§**Solutions and Drugs**) and was used to conduct patch-clamp and functional studies on DSM contractility. The second sample was kept in RNAlater solution (QIAGEN GmbH, Hilden Germany) and was used for qPCR experiments. Both samples were transported under controlled conditions to the laboratory after surgery.

DSM Cell Isolation for Patch-clamp Experiments

Human DSM cells for patch-clamp electrophysiological experiments were enzymatically isolated as previously described [21,29,40].

Quantification of BK Channel Subunits mRNA Message by qPCR

Total RNA was extracted from both control and NDO DSM tissue using the RNeasy Mini Kit (Qiagen, Hilden, Germany), then reverse-transcribed into cDNA using oligo d(T) primers (Promega, WI, USA), M-MLV Reverse Transcriptase (Promega, WI, USA), dNTP mix (Fermentas Life Sciences, ME, USA) and RNase inhibitor (Applied Biosystems, USA) as previously described [21,29,40]. Specific primers for BKα, BKβ1, BKβ4 subunits, and GAPDH were designed based on the cDNA complete sequences of human genes in Genbank and synthesized by Integrated DNA Technologies (IDT, Coralville, Iowa, USA) (**Table 1**). qPCR experiments followed a two-step amplification plus melting curve protocol using the $IQ^{TM}5$ Thermo Cycler system (Bio-Rad, California, USA). qPCR experiments were carried out on human DSM tissue cDNA (0.5 µg/µL) using IQ SYBR Green Supermix (Bio-Rad, California, USA). GAPDH was chosen as an internal control gene to analyze BKα, BKβ1, and BKβ4 subunits mRNA relative expression and each sample was run in triplicate. The parameters of the qPCR experiments were as follows: Cycle 1, 95°C for 3 min; cycle 2, 95°C for 10 s, then 61°C for 30 s (repeated 40 times). The melting curve analysis was then run between 61°C and 101°C with 0.5°C increments every 10 s. qPCR products were purified using the GenElute^{TM} PCR Clean-Up Kit (Sigma-Aldrich Co., St. Louis, MO, USA) and sequenced at the University of South Carolina Environmental Genomics Core Facility to confirm their identity.

Electrophysiological (Patch-clamp) Recordings

The amphotericin-B perforated whole cell configuration of the patch-clamp technique was used [41,42]. This approach allows the preservation of the native physiological environment of human DSM cells. Whole cell currents were recorded using an Axopatch 200B amplifier, Digidata 1440A, and pCLAMP version 10.2 software (Molecular Devices, Union City, CA). The signals were filtered by an eight-pole Bessel filter 900CT/9L8L (Frequency Devices). The patch-clamp pipettes were made from borosilicate glass (Sutter Instruments, Novato, CA), coated with dental wax to reduce capacitance, and polished with a Micro Forge MF-830 fire polisher (Narishige Group, Tokyo, Japan) to give a final tip resistance of 4–6 MΩ. All electrophysiological experiments were conducted at room temperature (22–23°C).

Isometric DSM Tension Recordings

5–7 mm long and 1–2 mm wide mucosa-free DSM strips were excised from human DSM tissue for functional studies as previously described [21,29,40]. Briefly, human DSM isolated strips were secured between clips and mounted between a force displacement transducer and a stationary hook. The strips were then submerged in thermostatically controlled tissue baths with Ca^{2+}-containing physiological saline solution (PSS) at 37°C and aerated with 95% O_2/5% CO_2. Next, the DSM strips were stretched to approximately 1.0 g force and were allowed to equilibrate for 1 h. During this equilibration period, strips were washed out with fresh PSS every 15 min.

Solutions and Drugs

The Ca^{2+}-free dissection solution had the following composition (in mM): 80 monosodium glutamate, 55 NaCl, 6 KCl, 10 glucose, 10 HEPES, 2 $MgCl_2$, and pH 7.3 adjusted with NaOH. The Ca^{2+}-containing PSS used in DSM tension recording experiments was prepared daily and contained (in mM): 119 NaCl, 4.7 KCl, 24 $NaHCO_3$, 1.2 KH_2PO_4, 2.5 $CaCl_2$, 1.2 $MgSO_4$ and 11 glucose, and aerated with 95% O_2/5% CO_2 to obtain pH 7.4. The extracellular (bath) solution used in the patch-clamp experiments had the following composition (in mM): 134 NaCl, 6 KCl, 1 $MgCl_2$, 2 $CaCl_2$, 10 glucose, and 10 HEPES, pH adjusted to 7.4 with NaOH. The pipette solution used in the patch-clamp experiments contained (in mM): 110 potassium aspartate, 30 KCl, 10 NaCl, 1 $MgCl_2$, 10 HEPES, and 0.05 EGTA, pH adjusted to 7.2 with NaOH and supplemented with freshly dissolved (every 1–2 h) 200 µg/ml amphotericin-B. Iberiotoxin and tetrodotoxin (TTX) were purchased from Sigma-Aldrich Co.

Data Analysis and Statistics

mRNA relative expression was analyzed using the comparative threshold (Ct) method ($\Delta\Delta$Ct, delta-delta Ct) [43] after determining the Ct values for reference (GAPDH) and target genes (BKα, BKβ1, and BKβ4 subunits) for each sample. Fold-changes in target mRNA expression level were calculated after normalization to GAPDH. MiniAnalysis (Synaptosoft, Inc., Decatur, GA) software version 6.0.7 was used to analyze data and GraphPad Prism 4.03 software (GraphPad Software Inc., San Diego, CA) was used for further statistical analysis. To compare the phasic contraction parameters, data were normalized to the control spontaneous contractions (100%) prior to addition of iberiotoxin and expressed as percentages. Clampfit 10.2 software (Molecular Devices, Inc.) was used for the data analysis of the patch-clamp experiments. The data and original recordings were illustrated using GraphPad Prism and CorelDraw Graphic Suite X3 (Corel Co., Ottawa, Canada) software. Results are summarized as mean$\pm$SE where **N** represents the number of patients, **n** represents the number of human DSM isolated strips, PCR samples, or human DSM cells. Data were compared using two-tailed paired or unpaired Student's t-test. A P-value <0.05 was considered statistically significant.

Results

The Relative Expression Levels of BKα Subunit mRNA is Significantly Decreased in NDO DSM

Recently, we established that human DSM cells express BKα, BKβ1, and BKβ4 subunits at both mRNA and protein levels [29]. Here, we revealed that in patients with NDO, the BKα, BKβ1, and BKβ4 subunit mRNA expression was lower compared to control patients (Fig. 1). There was a 15.8-fold decrease in BKα

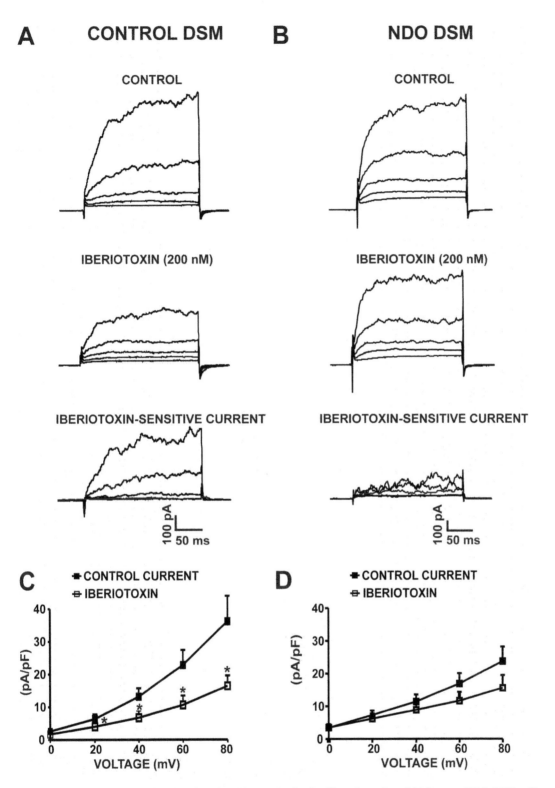

Figure 2. Iberiotoxin-sensitive steady-state BK current is significantly reduced in human NDO DSM cells compared to controls. Original recordings illustrating the effect of 200 nM iberiotoxin on the voltage-dependent steady-state whole cell current in a control DSM cell (**A**) and in an NDO DSM cell (**B**). Current-voltage relationships illustrating the differences in whole cell current density in the absence or presence of 200 nM iberiotoxin in control DSM cells (n = 9, N = 9; *P<0.05) (**C**) and NDO DSM cells (n = 8, N = 4; P>0.05) (**D**).

subunit mRNA relative expression in NDO DSM (n = 3, N = 3) compared to controls (n = 7, N = 7; P<0.01; Fig. 1). The changes in BKβ1 and BKβ4 subunits in NDO DSM compared to controls were not statistically significant and were evaluated at 1.1-fold and 1.6-fold decrease, respectively (P>0.05; Fig. 1). Glyceraldehyde-3-phosphate dehydrogenase (GAPDH) was used as an internal

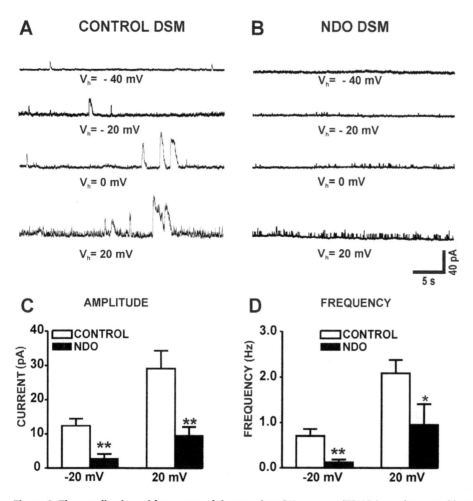

Figure 3. The amplitude and frequency of the transient BK currents (TBKCs) are decreased in NDO DSM cells compared to controls. Original recordings of TBKCs in a control DSM cell (**A**) and an NDO DSM cell (**B**) recorded at different holding potentials. Summary data showing that TBKCs's amplitude (**C**) and frequency (**D**) were significantly decreased in NDO DSM cells (n = 9, N = 3), compared to control DSM cells (n = 12, N = 10; *P<0.05, **P<0.01).

control and did not vary significantly between DSM samples from control and NDO patients. These data suggest that in patients suffering from NDO, there is a statistically significant decrease in BKα subunit expression but not in BKβ1 and BKβ4 subunit expression.

Iberiotoxin-sensitive Whole Cell BK Current is Decreased in NDO DSM Cells

We recently showed that the BK channel is the major regulator of human DSM excitability [21,29]. Here, we examined whether DSM BK channel activity changes during NDO. The average human DSM cell capacitance was 24.4±2.7 pF in NDO DSM cells (n = 16, N = 4), and 20.6±2.2 pF in control DSM cells (n = 20, N = 13; P>0.05). Human DSM cells were held at −70 mV and then stepped from 0 mV to +80 mV in 20 mV increments with 200 ms duration. The cells responded with a gradual increase of the whole cell current with each depolarization step (**Fig. 2**). Application of the selective BK channel inhibitor, iberiotoxin (200 nM), significantly decreased the whole cell current in DSM cells from control patients (n = 9, N = 9; P<0.05; **Fig. 2A**). **Figure 2** illustrates that the iberiotoxin-sensitive BK current represented more than 50% of the total outward current in DSM cells from control patients. However,

iberiotoxin (200 nM) did not significantly affect the amplitude of the whole cell outward current in DSM cells from NDO patients (**Fig. 2B**). **Figure 2** also illustrates that the iberiotoxin-sensitive BK current represented a very small portion of the total whole cell current in NDO DSM cells, whereas iberiotoxin (200 nM) significantly reduced the whole cell outward current in DSM cells from control patients (**Fig. 2C**). There was no significant difference in the current density before and after application of 200 nM iberiotoxin in NDO DSM cells (n = 8, N = 4; P>0.05; **Fig. 2D**). These data showed that the iberiotoxin-sensitive BK current was significantly reduced in NDO DSM cells.

Transient BK Currents (TBKCs) Amplitude and Frequency are Decreased in NDO DSM Cells

Recently, we provided the first electrophysiological evidence for the presence of TBKCs in human DSM cells [29]. Here, we examined if the activity of TBKCs in DSM cells changes under pathological conditions of NDO. TBKCs' amplitude and frequency were significantly reduced in DSM cells in patients with NDO (n = 9, N = 3) compared to the control group (n = 12, N = 10; P<0.05; **Fig. 3**). The results indicate that TBKC activity was significantly reduced in NDO DSM cells.

A

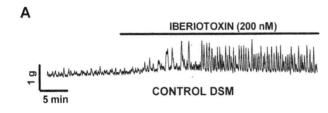

B

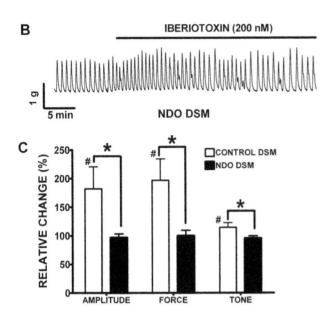

Figure 4. Inhibition of the BK channel with iberiotoxin causes a significant increase in spontaneous phasic and tonic contractions in control DSM but not in NDO DSM isolated strips. Original DSM tension recordings illustrating iberiotoxin (200 nM) effects on spontaneous phasic contractions in control (**A**) and NDO (**B**) DSM isolated strips. (**C**) Summary data showing a statistically significant increase in spontaneous phasic contraction amplitude, muscle force integral, and muscle tone of control DSM strips (n = 12, N = 7; P<0.05), and a lack of significant iberiotoxin effects in NDO DSM strips (n = 13, N = 7; P>0.05). #P<0.05 for control vs. iberiotoxin and *P<0.05 for control vs. NDO.

Pharmacological Inhibition of the BK Channels with Iberiotoxin has a Reduced Effect on the Contractility of DSM Strips Isolated from Patients with NDO

To restrain neuronal activity, TTX (1 µM), a selective voltage-gated Na^+ channel blocker, was added to the bath in the beginning of all experiments. In DSM strips isolated from control patients, iberiotoxin (200 nM) considerably increased the phasic contraction amplitude, muscle force integral, and muscle tone by 81.9±38.7%, 96.9±37.7%, and 14.4±8.3%, respectively (n = 12, N = 7; P<0.05; **Fig. 4A, C**). However, in DSM strips isolated from patients with NDO, iberiotoxin (200 nM) had no significant effects on any of the parameters of DSM contractility, including phasic contraction amplitude, muscle force integral, and muscle tone (n = 13, N = 3; P>0.05; **Fig. 4B, C**). Collectively, these results suggest a decrease in BK channel activity in DSM from patients with NDO, which contributes to the increase in the spontaneous phasic contractions.

Discussion

In the present study, we found significant physiological differences between control and NDO human tissues and cells that reveal important insights into the etiology of NDO. Using a combined multidisciplinary approach, we provide evidence for a critical role of the BK channel in the pathophysiology of NDO and demonstrate a significant decrease in the function of the BK channels in the DSM of such patients. Based on our experimental data, we have noted three important key results. First, mRNA expression of the pore-forming BKα subunit was significantly decreased in NDO DSM compared to controls. Secondly, whole cell BK current and TBKCs were both significantly decreased in NDO DSM cells compared to controls. Thirdly, inhibition of the BK channels with iberiotoxin did not significantly affect the spontaneous NDO DSM contractions, but did so in control DSM tissues, supporting the concept that NDO tissue is fundamentally biologically altered.

Recently, we provided molecular evidence for the expression of the BKα, BKβ1, and BKβ4 subunits in human DSM cells at both the mRNA and protein levels [29]. Here, we investigated whether the expression of BK channel subunits was altered in DSM from NDO patients. The results showed a 15.8-fold decrease of mRNA expression of the pore-forming BKα subunit but no statistical changes in BKβ1 and BKβ4 subunit mRNA expression in NDO DSM as compared to control DSM (**Fig. 1**). This is the first molecular evidence for decreased BK channel expression in DSM from NDO patients. The BKα subunit plays a critical role in DSM function, since it forms the functional pore of the BK channel [24,28,30], whereas the DSM BKβ1 subunits have a regulatory role by increasing BK channel Ca^{2+} sensitivity and modifying BK current activity [20,26]. The functional role of BKβ4 subunit in DSM is still unclear [29]. Therefore, any changes in the BKα or BKβ1 subunits' molecular expression could significantly impact DSM excitability and contractility. This has been well demonstrated in studies with genetically modified mice [24,26,28,30,38]. Deletion of the BKα subunit depolarizes DSM cell membrane potential [24,28], increases DSM contractility [24,30], and results in a phenotype consistent with DO [24,30,38]. The absence of the smooth muscle specific BKβ1 subunit causes an increase in DSM contractility in mice, which suggests that BKβ1 subunit is also an important regulator of DSM function [26]. Decreased mRNA expression of BKα and BKβ1 subunits was observed in animal models of partial urethral outlet obstruction [33,39,44]. Furthermore, patients with BPH and associated DO had a significantly reduced mRNA and protein expression of BKα and BKβ subunits [33]. Our results are consistent with the above study, as we demonstrated that in NDO patients, the mRNA expression of BKα subunit is significantly decreased. These studies support the concept that the NDO phenotype is associated with decreased BK channel expression in DSM.

Recently, we demonstrated that in DSM cells from patients with no history of OAB symptoms, the BK channels carry the majority of the steady-state whole cell current and are responsible for the generation of TBKCs [21,29]. Here, we sought to investigate the role of BK channels in NDO. BK channel function has not previously been investigated in NDO DSM using the perforated patch-clamp technique, which is the only method that can directly access ion channel activity while preserving intracellular signaling mechanisms. Our patch-clamp data showed that the iberiotoxin-sensitive BK current was significantly reduced in DSM cells from NDO patients compared to control patients. Furthermore, TBKCs's amplitude and frequency were significantly decreased in DSM cells from patients with NDO compared to controls

(**Fig. 3**). The patch-clamp results are consistent with our qPCR data, and illustrate that BK channel function is significantly reduced in NDO DSM compared to control DSM.

In patients without symptoms of OAB, the BK channel is also a major regulator of DSM contractility [29]. In the present study, we investigated how the decreased activity of the BK channel affects DSM phasic contractions in NDO patients. Unlike control DSM, inhibition of the BK channel with iberiotoxin did not significantly affect any of the parameters of spontaneous DSM contractility in NDO DSM isolated strips (**Fig. 4**). These results are supported by a recent study reporting no effect of iberiotoxin or NS1619, a BK channel opener on DSM phasic contractions in patients with NDO [18]. The results from our functional studies support the concept that BK channel activity is decreased in NDO DSM.

The complex etiology of NDO is not completely understood. Our results provide strong evidence that decreased BK channel activity is associated with NDO. Teleologically, this may be a consequence of a compensatory or adaptive mechanism in neurologically affected individuals that leads to increased DSM contractility allowing optimization of bladder emptying in the absence of normal innervation. Similar decreases in BK channel expression and activity have been reported in DSM from patients with BPH and DO, which is a condition with a different etiology than NDO [33]. One of the possible explanations for these similarities is that both conditions, regardless of their etiology, utilize similar compensatory mechanisms to decrease the expression of BK channels in DSM, and thus to alter DSM contractility.

Recently, we found that the selective BK channel opener NS1619 significantly decreased human DSM excitability and contractility [21]. We expect that a selective BK channel opener would be a highly effective treatment for NDO. However, currently available agents are not selective for DSM tissue resulting in collateral effects elsewhere in the body. Nevertheless, there is an ongoing effort to develop a new class of more potent and selective BK channel openers [45]. A genetic approach to enhance BK channel expression could also be a successful therapeutic strategy. Injection of BK channel naked DNA has been shown to eliminate bladder overactivity caused by partial urethral outlet obstruction in rats [35]. A clinical Phase I safety trial of plasmid based gene therapy using BK channel *hSlo cDNA* has been completed for erectile dysfunction and a future clinical trial is planned for the treatment of patients with OAB [36,37].

In conclusion, this study provides a significant contribution to our basic understanding of the key functional role of the BK channels in NDO. We demonstrated a decrease in the mRNA expression level of the pore-forming BKα subunit in DSM from NDO patients. Furthermore, we provided evidence for BK channel activity in NDO DSM by using the perforated patch-clamp approach, and revealed decreased whole cell BK currents and TBKCs in the DSM cells from NDO patients. These results are consistent with our functional studies showing a lack of an effect of iberiotoxin on spontaneous contractility in NDO DSM isolated strips. These findings support the pursuit and investigation of novel treatments for NDO which target the BK channel. Our results support the concept that BK channel openers and BK channel gene transfer could be an alternative strategy to control NDO as compared to currently prescribed antimuscarinics.

Acknowledgments

We would like to thank MUSC Urology staff surgeons: Drs. Thomas Keane, Harry Clarke, Stephen Savage, Ross Rames and Jonathan Picard, and Ahmed M. El-Zawahry, as well as the MUSC Urology Residents: Avi C. Weiss, Gary W. Bong, Kelly Doyle, Matthew McIntyre, Matt Eskridge, Jonathan N. Hamilton, Robin Bhavsar, Timothy R. Yoost, Vinh Q. Trang, Lydia Labocetta, Elizabeth Peacock, Matthew Young, Erin Burns, Vaughan Taylor, and Samuel Walker Nickles for their help with human tissue collection; Ms. Whitney F. Kellett for her help with some of the experiments; and Drs. John Malysz, Wenkuan Xin, Rupal Soder, and Ms. Amy Smith for the critical evaluation of the manuscript.

Author Contributions

Conceived and designed the experiments: GVP. Performed the experiments: KLH SAYA SPP QC GVP. Analyzed the data: KLH SAYA SPP QC GVP. Wrote the paper: KLH SAYA ESR GVP.

References

1. Abrams P, Cardozo L, Fall M, Griffiths D, Rosier P, et al. (2003) The standardisation of terminology in lower urinary tract function: report from the standardisation sub-committee of the International Continence Society. Urology 61: 37–49.

2. Andersson KE, Wein AJ (2004) Pharmacology of the lower urinary tract: basis for current and future treatments of urinary incontinence. Pharmacol Rev 56: 581–631.

3. Kuo YC, Kuo HC (2013) Botulinum toxin injection for lower urinary tract dysfunction. Int J Urol 20: 40–55.

4. Stewart WF, Van Rooyen JB, Cundiff GW, Abrams P, Herzog AR, et al. (2003) Prevalence and burden of overactive bladder in the United States. World J Urol 20: 327–336.

5. Cardenas DD, Mayo ME, Turner LR (1995) Lower urinary changes over time in suprasacral spinal cord injury. Paraplegia 33: 326–329.

6. Brubaker L, Richter HE, Visco A, Mahajan S, Nygaard I, et al. (2008) Refractory idiopathic urge urinary incontinence and botulinum A injection. J Urol 180: 217–222.

7. Nitti VW, Dmochowski R, Sand PK, Forst HT, Haag-Molkenteller C, et al. (2007) Efficacy, safety and tolerability of fesoterodine for overactive bladder syndrome. J Urol 178: 2488–2494.

8. Wagg A, Wyndaele JJ, Sieber P (2006) Efficacy and tolerability of solifenacin in elderly subjects with overactive bladder syndrome: a pooled analysis. Am J Geriatr Pharmacother 4: 14–24.

9. Zinner N, Susset J, Gittelman M, Arguinzoniz M, Rekeda L, et al. (2006) Efficacy, tolerability and safety of darifenacin, an M(3) selective receptor antagonist: an investigation of warning time in patients with OAB. Int J Clin Pract 60: 119–126.

10. Staskin DR, Dmochowski RR, Sand PK, Macdiarmid SA, Caramelli KE, et al. (2009) Efficacy and safety of oxybutynin chloride topical gel for overactive bladder: a randomized, double-blind, placebo controlled, multicenter study. J Urol 181: 1764–1772.

11. Armstrong RB, Dmochowski RR, Sand PK, Macdiarmid S (2007) Safety and tolerability of extended-release oxybutynin once daily in urinary incontinence: combined results from two phase 4 controlled clinical trials. Int Urol Nephrol 39: 1069–1077.

12. Oefelein MG (2011) Safety and tolerability profiles of anticholinergic agents used for the treatment of overactive bladder. Drug Saf 34: 733–754.

13. Gras J (2012) Mirabegron for the treatment of overactive bladder. Drugs Today (Barc) 48: 25–32.

14. Tyagi P, Tyagi V (2010) Mirabegron, a beta(3)-adrenoceptor agonist for the potential treatment of urinary frequency, urinary incontinence or urgency associated with overactive bladder. IDrugs 13: 713–722.

15. Conte A, Giannantoni A, Proietti S, Giovannozzi S, Fabbrini G, et al. (2012) Botulinum toxin A modulates afferent fibers in neurogenic detrusor overactivity. Eur J Neurol 19: 725–732.

16. Kuo HC, Liao CH, Chung SD (2010) Adverse events of intravesical botulinum toxin a injections for idiopathic detrusor overactivity: risk factors and influence on treatment outcome. Eur Urol 58: 919–926.

17. Brading AF (1997) A myogenic basis for the overactive bladder. Urology 50: 57–67; discussion 68–73.

18. Oger S, Behr-Roussel D, Gorny D, Bernabe J, Comperat E, et al. (2011) Effects of potassium channel modulators on myogenic spontaneous phasic contractile activity in human detrusor from neurogenic patients. BJU Int 108: 604–611.

19. Hashitani H, Brading AF, Suzuki H (2004) Correlation between spontaneous electrical, calcium and mechanical activity in detrusor smooth muscle of the guinea-pig bladder. Br J Pharmacol 141: 183–193.

20. Petkov GV (2012) Role of potassium ion channels in detrusor smooth muscle function and dysfunction. Nat Rev Urol 9: 30–40.

21. Hristov KL, Parajuli SP, Soder RP, Cheng Q, Rovner ES, et al. (2012) Suppression of human detrusor smooth muscle excitability and contractility via pharmacological activation of large conductance Ca^{2+}-activated K^+ channels. Am J Physiol Cell Physiol: C1632–1641.

22. Hayase M, Hashitani H, Kohri K, Suzuki H (2009) Role of K$^+$ channels in regulating spontaneous activity in detrusor smooth muscle in situ in the mouse bladder. J Urol 181: 2355–2365.

23. Heppner TJ, Bonev AD, Nelson MT (1997) Ca^{2+}-activated K$^+$ channels regulate action potential repolarization in urinary bladder smooth muscle. Am J Physiol 273: C110–117.

24. Brown SM, Bentcheva-Petkova LM, Liu L, Hristov KL, Chen M, et al. (2008) Beta-adrenergic relaxation of mouse urinary bladder smooth muscle in the absence of large-conductance Ca^{2+}-activated K$^+$ channel. Am J Physiol Renal Physiol 295: F1149–1157.

25. Herrera GM, Nelson MT (2002) Differential regulation of SK and BK channels by Ca^{2+} signals from Ca^{2+} channels and ryanodine receptors in guinea-pig urinary bladder myocytes. J Physiol 541: 483–492.

26. Petkov GV, Bonev AD, Heppner TJ, Brenner R, Aldrich RW, et al. (2001) Beta1-subunit of the Ca^{2+}-activated K$^+$ channel regulates contractile activity of mouse urinary bladder smooth muscle. J Physiol 537: 443–452.

27. Petkov GV, Nelson MT (2005) Differential regulation of Ca^{2+}-activated K$^+$ channels by beta-adrenoceptors in guinea pig urinary bladder smooth muscle. Am J Physiol Cell Physiol 288: C1255–1263.

28. Sprossmann F, Pankert P, Sausbier U, Wirth A, Zhou XB, et al. (2009) Inducible knockout mutagenesis reveals compensatory mechanisms elicited by constitutive BK channel deficiency in overactive murine bladder. FEBS J 276: 1680–1697.

29. Hristov KL, Chen M, Kellett WF, Rovner ES, Petkov GV (2011) Large-conductance voltage- and Ca^{2+}-activated K$^+$ channels regulate human detrusor smooth muscle function. Am J Physiol Cell Physiol 301: C903–912.

30. Meredith AL, Thorneloe KS, Werner ME, Nelson MT, Aldrich RW (2004) Overactive bladder and incontinence in the absence of the BK large conductance Ca^{2+}-activated K$^+$ channel. J Biol Chem 279: 36746–36752.

31. Soder RP, Petkov GV (2011) Large conductance Ca^{2+}-activated K$^+$ channel activation with NS1619 decreases myogenic and neurogenic contractions of rat detrusor smooth muscle. Eur J Pharmacol 670: 252–259.

32. Xin W, Cheng Q, Soder RP, Petkov GV (2012) Inhibition of phosphodiesterases relaxes detrusor smooth muscle via activation of the large-conductance voltage-and Ca^{2+}-activated K$^+$ channel. Am J Physiol Cell Physiol 302: C1361–1370.

33. Chang S, Gomes CM, Hypolite JA, Marx J, Alanzi J, et al. (2010) Detrusor overactivity is associated with downregulation of large-conductance calcium- and voltage-activated potassium channel protein. Am J Physiol Renal Physiol 298: F1416–1423.

34. Layne JJ, Nausch B, Olesen SP, Nelson MT (2010) BK channel activation by NS11021 decreases excitability and contractility of urinary bladder smooth muscle. Am J Physiol Regul Integr Comp Physiol 298: R378–384.

35. Christ GJ, Day NS, Day M, Santizo C, Zhao W, et al. (2001) Bladder injection of "naked" hSlo/pcDNA3 ameliorates detrusor hyperactivity in obstructed rats in vivo. Am J Physiol Regul Integr Comp Physiol 281: R1699–1709.

36. Melman A, Bar-Chama N, McCullough A, Davies K, Christ G (2007) Plasmid-based gene transfer for treatment of erectile dysfunction and overactive bladder: results of a phase I trial. Isr Med Assoc J 9: 143–146.

37. Melman A, Biggs G, Davies K, Zhao W, Tar MT, et al. (2008) Gene transfer with a vector expressing Maxi-K from a smooth muscle-specific promoter restores erectile function in the aging rat. Gene Ther 15: 364–370.

38. Thorneloe KS, Meredith AL, Knorn AM, Aldrich RW, Nelson MT (2005) Urodynamic properties and neurotransmitter dependence of urinary bladder contractility in the BK channel deletion model of overactive bladder. Am J Physiol Renal Physiol 289: F604–610.

39. Aydin M, Wang HZ, Zhang X, Chua R, Downing K, et al. (2012) Large-conductance calcium-activated potassium channel activity, as determined by whole-cell patch clamp recording, is decreased in urinary bladder smooth muscle cells from male rats with partial urethral obstruction. BJU Int 110: E402–408.

40. Afeli SA, Rovner ES, Petkov GV (2012) SK but not IK channels regulate human detrusor smooth muscle spontaneous and nerve-evoked contractions. Am J Physiol Renal Physiol 303: F559–568.

41. Hamill OP, Marty A, Neher E, Sakmann B, Sigworth FJ (1981) Improved patch-clamp techniques for high-resolution current recording from cells and cell-free membrane patches. Pflugers Arch 391: 85–100.

42. Horn R, Marty A (1988) Muscarinic activation of ionic currents measured by a new whole-cell recording method. J Gen Physiol 92: 145–159.

43. Livak KJ, Schmittgen TD (2001) Analysis of relative gene expression data using real-time quantitative PCR and the 2(−Delta Delta C(T)) Method. Methods 25: 402–408.

44. Li L, Jiang C, Song B, Yan J, Pan J (2008) Altered expression of calcium-activated K and Cl channels in detrusor overactivity of rats with partial bladder outlet obstruction. BJU Int 101: 1588–1594.

45. Nardi A, Olesen SP (2008) BK channel modulators: a comprehensive overview. Curr Med Chem 15: 1126–1146.

16

Cortical Implication in Lower Voluntary Muscle Force Production in Non-Hypoxemic COPD Patients

Francois Alexandre[1,2]*, **Nelly Heraud[2]**, **Nicolas Oliver[2]**, **Alain Varray[1]**

1 Movement To Health Laboratory, Euromov, University of Montpellier 1, Montpellier, France, **2** Clinique du Souffle La Vallonie, Fontalvie, Lodève, France

Abstract

Recent studies have shown that muscle alterations cannot totally explain peripheral muscle weakness in COPD. Cerebral abnormalities in COPD are well documented but have never been implicated in muscle torque production. The purpose of this study was to assess the neural correlates of quadriceps torque control in COPD patients. Fifteen patients (FEV_1 $54.1 \pm 3.6\%$ predicted) and 15 age- and sex-matched healthy controls performed maximal (MVCs) and submaximal (SVCs) voluntary contractions at 10, 30 and 50% of the maximal voluntary torque of the knee extensors. Neural activity was quantified with changes in functional near-infrared spectroscopy oxyhemoglobin (fNIRS-HbO) over the contralateral primary motor (M1), primary somatosensory (S1), premotor (PMC) and prefrontal (PFC) cortical areas. In parallel to the lower muscle torque, the COPD patients showed lower increase in HbO than healthy controls over the M1 ($p<0.05$), PMC ($p<0.05$) and PFC areas ($p<0.01$) during MVCs. In addition, they exhibited lower HbO changes over the M1 ($p<0.01$), S1 ($p<0.05$) and PMC ($p<0.01$) areas during SVCs at 50% of maximal torque and altered motor control characterized by higher torque fluctuations around the target. The results show that low muscle force production is found in a context of reduced motor cortex activity, which is consistent with central nervous system involvement in COPD muscle weakness.

Editor: Andrea Macaluso, University of Rome Foro Italico, Italy

Funding: FA was partially supported by a grant in aid from the French Ministry through the Association Nationale de la Recherche et de la Technology (National Agency for Research and Technology). The authors did not receive other specific funding for this work. The funders had no role in study design, data collection and analysis, decision to publish, or preparation of the manuscript.

Competing Interests: The authors have declared that no competing interests exist.

* Email: francois.alexandre@fontalvie.fr

Introduction

Peripheral muscle dysfunction is very frequent in COPD and has major consequences. The loss of muscle force in COPD patients has become a matter of heightened concern because it implies exercise limitation [1], increased use of health care resources [2], and higher mortality [3]. The involvement of muscle atrophy in this loss was established several years ago [4]. However, several elements point to the existence of other explanatory mechanisms. For instance, a recent study reported that COPD patients exhibit a decline in muscle force even when their muscle mass is comparable to that of healthy controls [5]. In addition, the lower muscle force across GOLD stages (between GOLD I and IV) is not explained by smaller muscle cross-sectional areas [6]. Therefore, other mechanisms should be explored to enhance understanding of the pathophysiology of muscle weakness in COPD.

A decline in muscle force can be caused by alterations in the muscle and/or the nervous system [7]. Interestingly, several studies have assessed the cerebral properties in COPD patients and reported small cerebral vessel disease [8], gray matter deficits [9], white matter lesions [9,10] and neuronal dysfunction [11]. At a more functional level, COPD patients exhibit lengthening peripheral [12] and central [13] nervous conduction times, alterations in motor cortex excitability [14], and cognitive

disorders [9,10]. In contrast, the potential repercussions over the central motor drive and muscle performance are unknown.

A few studies have evaluated muscle activation in COPD using the twitch interpolation technique [15–17], an indirect assessment of the central motor drive. However, the results were discrepant [15–17] and no definitive conclusions could be drawn. The discrepancies may be explained by the poor sensitivity of this technique at near maximal force, which makes it difficult to discriminate two populations during maximal voluntary contractions (MVCs) [18]. Thus, the question of nervous system involvement in COPD muscle weakness remains unanswered.

An alternative to circumvent the limitations of twitch interpolation could be the use of neuroimaging techniques. Force output is directly related to cortical activity as measured by functional magnetic resonance imaging (fMRI) [19] and functional near infrared spectroscopy (fNIRS) [20]. The fNIRS oxy- (HbO) and deoxy-hemoglobin (HbR) signals are strongly correlated with the blood-oxygen-level-dependent (BOLD) fMRI signal, and they are widely acknowledged to be reliable for functional cortical activity assessment in various conditions [21–23]. In addition, fNIRS has been validated for the study of neural activity in a wide range of populations, such as the elderly [23] and COPD [24], stroke [25], and obese patients [26] during various motor tasks, including MVCs [26]. Whereas fMRI restricts body movement within the enclosed chamber, fNIRS presents a high signal-to-noise ratio and relatively poor sensitivity to motion artifacts, making it the more suitable for cortical activity assessment during exercise [27,28].

Given the numerous cerebral alterations in COPD that have never been linked with poor muscle force production, the purpose of this study was to assess the fNIRS-neural correlates of quadriceps contraction at maximal and submaximal intensity in COPD patients. We hypothesized lower activity over motor cortical areas in COPD patients than healthy controls during quadriceps contractions.

Materials and Methods

Subjects

Fifteen COPD patients and 15 age- and sex-matched sedentary healthy subjects were recruited for the study. The participation criteria for the COPD patients were forced expiratory volume in the 1st second (FEV_1) between 30 and 80% of the predicted values, with no exacerbation or weight loss in the month preceding the study. No patient had taken part in a rehabilitation program in the previous 12 months. The non-inclusion criteria for the participants were an inability to give written consent, inability to perform the experimental maneuvers, impaired visual function, use of drugs known to impair brain function, current or past alcohol abuse, and neurologic or neuromuscular disease. All participants gave written consent. Procedures were approved by the local Ethics Committee (Comité de protection des personnes Sud Est VI, number AU980) and complied with the principles of the Declaration of Helsinki for human experimentation. The study was registered at www. clinicaltrials.gov as NCT01679782.

Design

All participants underwent a medical examination, including evaluation of resting pulmonary function, body composition and clinical parameters, before taking part in the study. The protocol consisted of maximal and submaximal voluntary contractions of the knee extensors, during which cortical activity was assessed non-invasively from changes in fNIRS signals [22,25]. The exercise protocol is presented in Figure 1. After determination of the dominant leg, the participants performed a standardized warm-up of the knee extensors by repeating 20 submaximal voluntary contractions for 2 s every 5 s. They next performed three maximal voluntary contractions (MVCs) and three submaximal voluntary contractions (SVCs) at 10, 30 and 50% of the maximal voluntary torque twice in random order. Each MVC lasted for 5 s and two successive MVCs were separated by a 2-min resting period. Each SVC lasted for 20 s and two successive SVCs were separated by a 1.5 min resting period. The random draw to determine the order of the SVCs took place immediately after the three MVCs had been performed and the target torques calculated. A last MVC was performed to ensure the absence of neuromuscular fatigue at the end of the exercise testing.

Mechanical recordings

Subjects were comfortably seated on a dedicated ergometer for knee extensor testing (Quadriergoforme, Aleo Industrie, Salome, France) with a 30° back inclination. Chair adjustments were made to ensure that the foot, patella and coxofemoral articulation of the dominant leg were in the same axis. The knee angle was set to 110°. The pelvis and the proximal extremity of the patella were securely attached to the chair in order to minimize movements of adjacent muscles. In addition, the head was supported by a neck brace to avoid potential head motion. Torque of the knee extensors during the contractions was recorded with a strain gauge torque sensor (Captels, Saint Mathieu de Treviers, France). The acquired analog signal was converted into digital data (DA conversion) through an acquisition system (Biopac MP100, Biopac Systems, Santa Barbara, CA, USA) and instantaneously relayed to a screen to give visual feedback. During each MVC and each SVC, subjects were verbally encouraged to ensure maximal muscle torque and to maintain the force requirement, respectively. Before the SVCs, the target torque was clearly indicated to the subjects via the computer monitor and they received visual feedback of their performance during the contractions.

Cortical activity assessment

A continuous wave multichannel functional near-infrared spectroscopy (fNIRS) system (Oxymon Mark III, Artinis, the Netherlands) was used at two wavelengths in the near-infrared range (nominal wavelengths of 760 and 850 nm) to detect regional concentration changes in oxyhemoglobin (HbO) and deoxyhemoglobin (HbR) during cortical activation over cortical motor areas. fNIRS is based on neurovascular coupling: when neural activity increases, the increase in regional cerebral blood flow is ten times higher than the increase in regional oxygen consumption. Thus, as the increase in regional cerebral blood flow greatly exceeds the increase in oxygen consumption, neuronal hemodynamic concentration is closely coupled with the increase in regional cerebral blood flow, which turns into local hyperoxygenation [29] and subsequent increase in HbO with a decrease in HbR [30]. The fNIRS-measured hemoglobin is comparable to the BOLD-fMRI signal and mainly reflects changes in cortical gray matter hemodynamic [22]. The fNIRS optodes were held by a cap fixated by several bands surrounding the subject's head. A total of nine channels were positioned over the contralateral primary motor (M1), primary somatosensory (S1), premotor (PMC) and prefrontal (PFC) cortical areas in accordance with the modified EEG 10-10 system [31] (Figure 2a). The source-detector spacing was set to 3.5 cm. During probe placement, Oxysoft software (V6.0, Artinis, the Netherlands) allowed real time assessment of the quality of the fNIRS signal for each channel based on the light source power level and the receiver gain. Hemoglobin concentrations were corrected by implementing a specific differential pathlength factor ($4.99 + 0.067 \times age^{0.814}$), in order to convert the

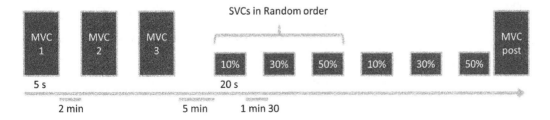

Figure 1. Experimental Design. MVC: Maximal Voluntary Contraction, SVC: Submaximal Voluntary Contraction.

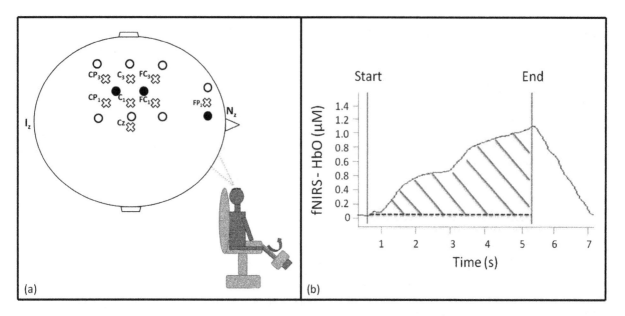

Figure 2. Measurement of cortical activity by functional near-infrared spectroscopy (fNIRS). a) fNIRS optode placement. Three receivers (black circles) and seven emitters (white circles) were set over the scalp, resulting in 9 measured channels. The crosses represent the reference points used to target primary sensory (CP_3 - CP_1), primary motor (C_3 - C_1), premotor (FC_1 - FC_3) and prefrontal cortical areas (FP_1) according to the modified international EEG 10-10 system. I_z: Inion, N_z: Nasion.b) Example of a functional near-infrared spectrospcopy oxyhemoglobin signal (fNIRS-HbO) during a maximal voluntary contraction in one subject. Hatched area represents the area under the curve of HbO (as index of neural activity).

concentration changes in HbO and HbR to M units [32]. The fNIRS signal was low-pass filtered (finite impulse response) using a cut-off frequency of 0.7 Hz. The sampling rate was set at 10 Hz. To avoid systemic bias, we also monitored the pulsed arterial oxygen saturation (SpO_2) in a restricted group of patients (n = 12). The oximetry probe (Weinman, Hamburg, Deutshland) was placed on the index finger and the participants were asked to keep their hand motionless throughout the experiment.

Data analysis

During MVCs, maximal quadriceps torque (Q_{MVC}) was calculated over the highest 500-ms plateau of torque during the best trial of the three MVCs.

During SVCs, task matching was evaluated by averaging and comparing the mean performed torque versus the target torque. In addition, during each SVC, the motor control was assessed from the fluctuations around the target. An inaccuracy index (Inaccuracy$_{index}$) was calculated and represents the RMS (root mean square) of the difference between produced and target torques during the 20 s of submaximal voluntary contractions expressed as a percentage of the target torque [33]. The normalization by the target torque is necessary because the torque variability is known to be proportional to the torque level [34].

Changes in cortical activity were determined from HbO variations as previously described [25]. HbO signals with artifacts or a too-low signal-to-noise ratio were marked and excluded from the analyses under a visual pre-processing analysis [35]. During the best trial of the three MVCs and of the more accurate SVCs at 10, 30 and 50% of Q_{MVC}, the area under the curve of HbO normalized over time was used as an index of neural activity (Figure 2b).

The data, taken from the four channels over the M1 area, the two channels over the S1 area, and the two channels over the PMC area were averaged, resulting in the overall response of, respectively, the M1, S1 and PMC areas.

Before the beginning of exercise testing, resting HbO was calculated for each cortical area over a 2-min resting period, respecting the same analysis process as aforementioned.

Statistical analysis

All statistical analyses were performed using Statistica software (StatSoft, Inc., version 6.0, Tulsa, OK, USA). All data were examined for normality using a Shapiro-Wilk test. Differences in subject characteristics and variables recorded during MVCs were tested between controls and patients using an unpaired Student's t-test. Absence of neuromuscular fatigue was tested using a two-way analysis of variance (ANOVA) with group as between-subject factor (COPD and controls) and condition (before and after exercise testing) as within-subject factor. The Inaccuracy$_{index}$ and HbO recorded during SVCs were tested using a two-way ANOVA with group as between-subject factor and torque level (10, 30 and 50% of Q_{MVC}) as within-subject factor. Analysis of covariance (ANCOVA) with adjustment for Q_{MVC} was used to ensure that the difference in HbO between patients and controls was not due to a difference in muscle torque between the groups. Task compliance during SVCs was tested with a three-way ANOVA with group as between-subject factor and condition (target versus performed) and torque level (10, 30 and 50% of Q_{MVC}) as two within-subject factors. The underlying assumptions of ANOVA were checked using a Levene test (homogeneity of the variance) and a Mauchly test (sphericity of the variance). When the ANOVA F ratio was significant ($p < 0.05$), the means were compared by a LSD post-hoc test. Data are reported as means and standard error of the mean (SE).

Results

Subject characteristics

The subject characteristics are given in Table 1. Consistent with the matching, no difference in the gender ratio or age was observed between patients and controls. Weight, body mass index

Table 1. Characteristics of the subjects included in the study.

	Control(n = 15)	COPD(n = 15)	p-value
Gender M/F	10/5	10/5	
Age yrs	61 (2.9)	62.8 (2.5)	NS (0.64)
Weight kg	75.8 (3.3)	72.8 (4.2)	NS (0.57)
BMI kg.m^{-2}	25.8 (1)	25.3 (1.3)	NS (0.76)
FEV$_1$ L	3.1 (0.2)	1.5 (0.2)	<0.001
FEV$_1$ % pred	104.5 (3)	54.1 (3.6)	<0.001
FEV$_1$/FVC	73.1 (1.1)	49.7 (2.4)	<0.001
FFM kg	55.3 (3)	53.9 (3)	NS (0.73)
FFMI kg.m^{-2}	18.6 (0.5)	18.8 (0.7)	NS (0.92)
Voorrips AU	7.4 (1.25)	6.5 (1.35)	NS (0.64)
PaO$_2$ mmHg		72.9 (2.8)	
PaCO$_2$ mmHg		37.4 (1.4)	

BMI: Body Mass Index, FEV$_1$: Force Expiratory Volume in 1 s, FVC: Force Vital Capacity, FFM: Fat-Free Mass, FFMI: Fat-Free Mass Index. NS: no significant difference between controls and COPD patients. Values are mean (SE).

and fat-free mass index exhibited no significant differences (p> 0.05). According to the Voorrips questionnaire [36], the level of physical activity was comparable for patients and controls (p = 0.64).

Control of absence of desaturation and fatigue during exercise testing

SpO$_2$ remained stable for all patients during both MVCs and SVCs. The mean ΔSpO2 was $0.01\pm0.12\%$ during MVCs (p = 0.98) and $0.017\pm0.19\%$ during SVCs (p = 0.98).

Absence of neuromuscular fatigue was checked by changes in Q$_{MVC}$ after the protocol. Both patients and controls exhibited no

significant differences in Q$_{MVC}$ (condition and interaction F ratio ranged from 0.17 to 1.10, p ranged from 0.31 to 0.68).

Maximal voluntary contractions

Q$_{MVC}$ was significantly lower by 24.8% in COPD patients compared with controls (131.9 ± 16.6 and 175.4 ± 24.9 Nm, respectively, for patients and controls, t = 2.5, p<0.05).

The regional HbO during MVCs is shown in Figure 3. Compared with controls, patients showed significantly lower HbO changes over M1 (t = 2.1, p<0.05), PMC (t = 2.3, p<0.05) and PFC (t = 3.1, p<0.01). In contrast, HbO changes during MVCs were comparable between patients and controls over S1 (t = 0.3, p = 0.74).

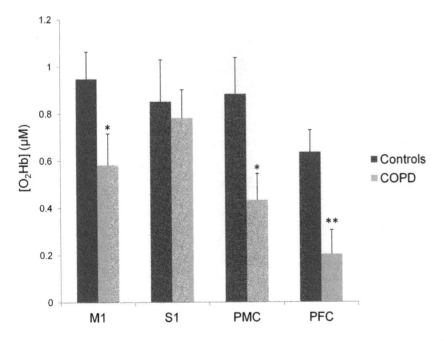

Figure 3. HbO changes during maximal voluntary contractions over primary motor (M1), primary sensory (S1), premotor (PMC) and prefrontal (PFC) cortex areas. * p<0.05 and ** p<0.01 significantly different from controls.

Submaximal voluntary contractions (SVCs)

Task matching during SVCs was checked by comparing the performed torque with the target torque (Figure 4). No significant differences were found between performed and target torques for patients or controls at the three submaximal torque levels (F ranged from 0.31 to 2.22, p ranged from 0.15 to 0.74). In contrast, the Inaccuracy$_{index}$ was significantly higher in patients compared with controls for all submaximal torque levels (F = 7.99, p<0.001). At 10, 30 and 50% of Q_{MVC}, the Inaccuracy$_{index}$ was 7.04±0.59 vs 5.15±0.62, 4.6±0.44 vs 3.46±0.58, and 4.83±0.47 vs 3.69±0.78 in patients and controls, respectively.

The regional HbO as a function of torque level is shown in Figure 5.

Over the M1 area, HbO was significantly increased compared with resting values, from 30% of Q_{MVC} in controls (p<0.001) and from 50% of Q_{MVC} in patients (p<0.01). Compared with controls, patients showed significantly lower HbO changes at 30% and 50% of Q_{MVC} (respectively, p<0.05 and p<0.01).

Over the S1 area, HbO was significantly increased compared with resting values, from 50% of Q_{MVC} in controls (p<0.001). In patients, HbO did not change significantly whatever the submaximal torque (p ranged from 0.34 to 0.49). In addition, at 50% of Q_{MVC}, HbO changes were significantly lower in COPD patients than in controls (0.26±0.09 vs 0.59±0.18 μM, p<0.05).

Over the PMC area, HbO was significantly increased compared with resting values, from 30% of Q_{MVC} in patients and controls (systematically p<0.01). Compared with controls, patients showed lower HbO changes at 50% of Q_{MVC} (0.25±0.13 vs 0.72±0.12 μM, p<0.01).

Over the PFC area, HbO was significantly increased compared with resting values, at 50% of Q_{MVC} in patients and controls (systematically p<0.05). There was no difference in HbO changes

between patients and controls for any submaximal torque level (F ranged from 0.75 to 0.9, p ranged from 0.35 to 0.53).

The impact of the patients' lower absolute torque values compared with controls on HbO changes was checked using an ANCOVA. Consistently with respect to Figure 6 and adjusting for Q_{MVC}, HbO remained significantly lower over M1 at 30% and 50% of Q_{MVC} in patients compared with controls (all p<0.05). Similarly, the observed effects in HbO changes over the S1, PMC and PFC areas were unaffected when Q_{MVC} was added as a covariable: HbO changes remained significantly lower over the S1 and PMC areas in patients at 50% of Q_{MVC} (all p<0.05), but comparable between the patients and controls over the PFC area (F ranged from 0.01 to 2, p ranged from 0.17 to 0.99).

Discussion

The present study is the first to assess the neural correlates of quadriceps contractions in COPD patients. The main findings were lower HbO changes over the M1, PMC and PFC areas during maximal voluntary contractions in the COPD patients compared with controls. In addition, the COPD patients showed lower HbO changes than controls over the M1 area at 30% and 50% of Q_{MVC} and over the S1 and PMC areas at 50% of Q_{MVC}. Last, the COPD patients exhibited greater torque fluctuations around the target than controls.

The COPD patients exhibited 24.8% lower muscle force than healthy controls. This is consistent with the usual torque deficit reported in the literature in moderate COPD patients, which ranges from 20% to 30% [37]. The neural correlates of quadriceps torque were simultaneously recorded with the non-invasive neuroimaging fNIRS technique [22,25] over major cortical areas for movement generation. Our results show smaller HbO

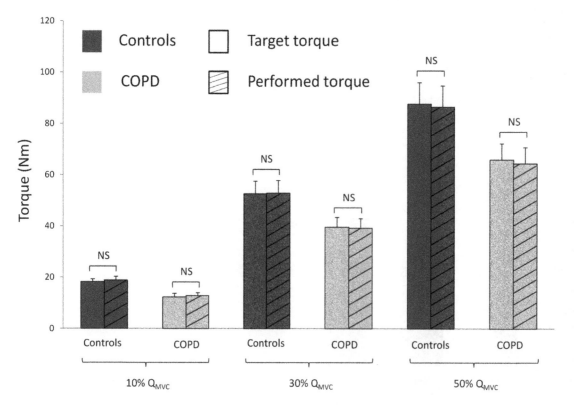

Figure 4. Performed torque versus target torque during submaximal voluntary contractions at 10, 30 and 50% of maximal quadriceps torque (Q_{MVC}). NS: Non-significant difference between target and performed torque.

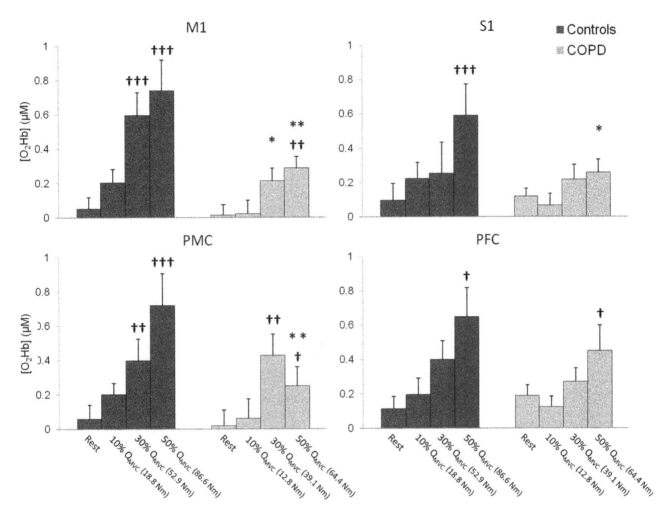

Figure 5. HbO changes during submaximal quadriceps contractions as a function of % of maximal quadriceps torque (Q_{MVC}) over primary motor (M1), primary sensory (S1), premotor (PMC) and prefrontal (PFC) cortex areas. Values in parenthesis on the x axis indicate the mean torque performed at the given % of maximal quadriceps torque. Significant differences from rest: [†] $p < 0.05$ [††] $p < 0.01$ and [†††] $p < 0.001$. Significant differences between controls and patients: * $p < 0.05$, ** $p < 0.01$ and *** $p < 0.001$.

increases over the M1, PMC and PFC areas in the COPD patients during MVCs. These results cannot be due to oxygen desaturation because the exercise did not induce SpO_2 changes. Similarly, it may not be explained by lower resting cerebral blood flow due to resting blood gases abnormalities because cerebrovascular reactivity to hypoxemia (increase in cerebral blood flow when PaO_2 decreases) is preserved in COPD [38,39]. According to the neurovascular coupling principle (as previously explained in the methods section), the data thus obtained with the fNIRS technique suggest a smaller local hyperoxygenation at the cortex in COPD patients compared with healthy controls. These results support lower neural activity in these patients, which would explain the decreased voluntary torque via reduced cortical motor output, and is coherent with the cerebrovascular damage and gray matter deficit described in the literature [8,9].

During the submaximal voluntary contractions, we found a smaller HbO increase in the patients over the three main cortical areas of the frontal lobe involved in the execution and control of visual-motor tasks [40], at 30 and 50% of Q_{MVC} over the M1 area, and at 50% over the PMC and S1 areas. These results complete and support the findings of Vivodtzev et al. [17], who indirectly showed lower activation in COPD for comparable submaximal

force levels with the twitch interpolation technique. In parallel to the altered neural activity, we found an increase in the inaccuracy index for submaximal torque levels in the COPD patients compared with controls, indicating greater torque fluctuations around the target in patients. Such torque fluctuations, known as dysmetria, are classic signs of lesions in the cerebellum [41], a subcortical area whose main function is the control and coordination of movement and whose output travels to motor and premotor cortex [42]. Interestingly, the dysmetria reported in the patients did not impact the task matching, as they were able to reach the required target (mean values). Hence, to summarize, the COPD patients were able to reach the desired target at submaximal intensities but with lower motor drive and high fluctuations, indicating less efficient motor control.

Given the difference in absolute torque value between the COPD patients and controls, we sought to ensure that the lower neural activity did not result from the lower muscle torque developed by the patients. As shown in Figure 6, for any given absolute torque value, increases in HbO were always about twice lower in the patients over M1. This agrees with the analysis of covariance, which indicated that adjusting for maximal voluntary torque had no impact on the difference in HbO changes between

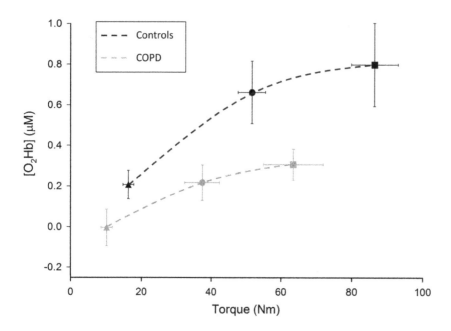

Figure 6. HbO changes over M1 as a function of absolute torque value at 10 (triangular shape), 30 (circular shape) and 50% (square shape) of the maximal voluntary torque.

the COPD patients and controls. Taken together, these results provide new insight into the functional limitations in COPD patients, as the lower neural activity (lower increase in HbO) cannot be explained by either lower muscle torques or a lack of patient motivation or cooperation.

"In a previous study, Higashimoto et al. [24] recorded neural activity over the PFC area during a whole-body exercise that induced an increase in dyspnea score in both COPD patients and controls during testing, with the increase being higher in COPD. The authors reported a clear tendency toward smaller HbO changes in the COPD patients compared with healthy controls, although it did not reach the significance threshold. In addition, they reported correlations between the increase in dyspnea score and the increase in PFC activity during the exercise testing. These results raised the possibility of lower neural activity during whole-body exercise in COPD that might have been hidden by the greater increase in dyspnea-induced PFC activation [24]. Our findings are consistent with and complete the results of Higashimoto et al. [24], because a local exercise carried out without any dyspnea confirmed that the COPD patients had lower cortical activity."Several factors have been suggested to explain the cerebral alterations in COPD but the exact mechanisms remain unclear. These factors notably include inflammation, oxidative stress, hypoxemia and vascular disease [43]. In accordance with other studies [10], we report cerebral alterations in stable non-hypoxemic COPD patients, ruling out a determining role for hypoxemia. Understanding the mechanisms of the brain impairment in COPD patients has become a major issue. Our results provide new insight into the extrapulmonary effects of COPD on the brain and suggest new directions for research in order to

optimize treatment for muscle force recovery in COPD. Further, they suggest the interest of early physical activity for COPD patients, given the potential effects of exercise on cerebral plasticity and neuroprotection [44], although this has yet to be specifically investigated in COPD.

In summary, COPD patients showed lower HbO changes over cortical motor areas during maximal and submaximal voluntary contractions of the knee extensors. This impairment was associated with a decrease in the maximal voluntary torque and altered motor control. The results provide the first evidence that the knee extensors of patients with stable moderate COPD cannot be optimally driven by the brain. Our findings highlight a lower motor cortex activity during quadriceps contraction in COPD and are consistent with an involvement of the central nervous system in the COPD quadriceps torque impairment. To optimize muscle force recovery in COPD patients, interventions targeting neuroprotection and neuroplasticity must be strongly considered.

Acknowledgments

The authors would like to thank Prof. Stephane Perrey for the use of the NIRS equipment funded by a grant in aid from the Languedoc-Roussillon Region Council (AVENIR). Further, the authors wish to thanks Jean-Paul Micallef for his assistance in the development of experimental materials.

Author Contributions

Conceived and designed the experiments: FA NH AV. Performed the experiments: FA NO. Analyzed the data: FA AV. Contributed reagents/materials/analysis tools: FA NH AV. Wrote the paper: FA NH NO AV.

References

1. Gosselink R, Troosters T, Decramer M (1996) Peripheral muscle weakness contributes to exercise limitation in COPD. Am J Respir Crit Care Med 153: 976–980.

2. Decramer M, Gosselink R, Troosters T, Verschueren M, Evers G (1997) Muscle weakness is related to utilization of health care resources in COPD patients. Eur Respir J 10: 417–423.

3. Swallow EB, Reyes D, Hopkinson NS, Man WD, Porcher R, et al. (2007) Quadriceps strength predicts mortality in patients with moderate to severe chronic obstructive pulmonary disease. Thorax 62: 115–120.

4. Bernard S, LeBlanc P, Whittom F, Carrier G, Jobin J, et al. (1998) Peripheral muscle weakness in patients with chronic obstructive pulmonary disease. Am J Respir Crit Care Med 158: 629–634.

5. Menon MK, Houchen L, Harrison S, Singh SJ, Morgan MD, et al. (2012) Ultrasound assessment of lower limb muscle mass in response to resistance training in COPD. Respir Res 13: 119.

6. Shrikrishna D, Patel M, Tanner RJ, Seymour JM, Connolly BA, et al. (2012) Quadriceps wasting and physical inactivity in patients with COPD. Eur Respir J 40: 1115–1122.

7. Clark BC, Manini TM (2008) Sarcopenia = / = dynapenia. J Gerontol A Biol Sci Med Sci 63: 829–834.

8. Lahousse L, Vernooij MW, Darweesh SK, Akoudad S, Loth DW, et al. (2013) Chronic obstructive pulmonary disease and cerebral microbleeds. The Rotterdam Study. Am J Respir Crit Care Med 188: 783–788.

9. Zhang H, Wang X, Lin J, Sun Y, Huang Y, et al. (2013) Reduced regional gray matter volume in patients with chronic obstructive pulmonary disease: a voxel-based morphometry study. AJNR Am J Neuroradiol 34: 334–339.

10. Dodd JW, Chung AW, van den Broek MD, Barrick TR, Charlton RA, et al. (2012) Brain structure and function in chronic obstructive pulmonary disease: a multimodal cranial magnetic resonance imaging study. Am J Respir Crit Care Med 186: 240–245.

11. Shim TS, Lee JH, Kim SY, Lim TH, Kim SJ, et al. (2001) Cerebral metabolic abnormalities in COPD patients detected by localized proton magnetic resonance spectroscopy. Chest 120: 1506–1513.

12. Oncel C, Baser S, Cam M, Akdag B, Taspinar B, et al. (2010) Peripheral neuropathy in chronic obstructive pulmonary disease. COPD 7: 11–16.

13. Kirkil G, Tug T, Ozel E, Bulut S, Tekatas A, et al. (2007) The evaluation of cognitive functions with P300 test for chronic obstructive pulmonary disease patients in attack and stable period. Clin Neurol Neurosurg 109: 553–560.

14. Hopkinson NS, Sharshar T, Ross ET, Nickol AH, Dayer MJ, et al. (2004) Corticospinal control of respiratory muscles in chronic obstructive pulmonary disease. Respir Physiol Neurobiol 141: 1–12.

15. Mador MJ, Deniz O, Aggarwal A, Kufel TJ (2003) Quadriceps fatigability after single muscle exercise in patients with chronic obstructive pulmonary disease. Am J Respir Crit Care Med 168: 102–108.

16. Seymour JM, Ward K, Raffique A, Steier JS, Sidhu PS, et al. (2012) Quadriceps and ankle dorsiflexor strength in chronic obstructive pulmonary disease. Muscle Nerve 46: 548–554.

17. Vivodtzev I, Flore P, Levy P, Wuyam B (2008) Voluntary activation during knee extensions in severely deconditioned patients with chronic obstructive pulmonary disease: benefit of endurance training. Muscle Nerve 37: 27–35.

18. Herbert RD, Gandevia SC (1999) Twitch interpolation in human muscles: mechanisms and implications for measurement of voluntary activation. J Neurophysiol 82: 2271–2283.

19. van Duinen H, Renken R, Maurits NM, Zijdewind I (2008) Relation between muscle and brain activity during isometric contractions of the first dorsal interosseus muscle. Hum Brain Mapp 29: 281–299.

20. Derosiere G, Perrey S (2012) Relationship between submaximal handgrip muscle force and NIRS-measured motor cortical activation. Adv Exp Med Biol 737: 269–274.

21. Strangman G, Culver JP, Thompson JH, Boas DA (2002) A quantitative comparison of simultaneous BOLD fMRI and NIRS recordings during functional brain activation. Neuroimage 17: 719–731.

22. Sato H, Yahata N, Funane T, Takizawa R, Katura T, et al. (2013) A NIRS-fMRI investigation of prefrontal cortex activity during a working memory task. Neuroimage 83: 158–173.

23. Mehagnoul-Schipper DJ, van der Kallen BF, Colier WN, van der Sluijs MC, van Erning IJ, et al. (2002) Simultaneous measurements of cerebral oxygenation changes during brain activation by near-infrared spectroscopy and functional magnetic resonance imaging in healthy young and elderly subjects. Hum Brain Mapp 16: 14–23.

24. Higashimoto Y, Honda N, Yamagata T, Matsuoka T, Maeda K, et al. (2011) Activation of the prefrontal cortex is associated with exertional dyspnea in chronic obstructive pulmonary disease. Respiration 82: 492–500.

25. Lin PY, Chen JJ, Lin SI (2013) The cortical control of cycling exercise in stroke patients: an fNIRS study. Hum Brain Mapp 34: 2381–2390.

26. Mehta RK, Shortz AE (2013) Obesity-related differences in neural correlates of force control. Eur J Appl Physiol.

27. Perrey S (2008) Non-invasive NIR spectroscopy of human brain function during exercise. Methods 45: 289–299.

28. Ekkekakis P (2009) Illuminating the black box: investigating prefrontal cortical hemodynamics during exercise with near-infrared spectroscopy. J Sport Exerc Psychol 31: 505–553.

29. Fox PT, Raichle ME, Mintun MA, Dence C (1988) Nonoxidative glucose consumption during focal physiologic neural activity. Science 241: 462–464.

30. Colier WN, Quaresima V, Oeseburg B, Ferrari M (1999) Human motor-cortex oxygenation changes induced by cyclic coupled movements of hand and foot. Exp Brain Res 129: 457–461.

31. (1994) Guideline thirteen: guidelines for standard electrode position nomenclature. American Electroencephalographic Society. J Clin Neurophysiol 11: 111–113.

32. Duncan A, Meek JH, Clemence M, Elwell CE, Fallon P, et al. (1996) Measurement of cranial optical path length as a function of age using phase resolved near infrared spectroscopy. Pediatr Res 39: 889–894.

33. Chow JW, Stokic DS (2011) Force control of quadriceps muscle is bilaterally impaired in subacute stroke. J Appl Physiol (1985) 111: 1290–1295.

34. Missenard O, Mottet D, Perrey S (2008) Muscular fatigue increases signal-dependent noise during isometric force production. Neurosci Lett 437: 154–157.

35. Minagawa-Kawai Y, van der Lely H, Ramus F, Sato Y, Mazuka R, et al. (2011) Optical brain imaging reveals general auditory and language-specific processing in early infant development. Cereb Cortex 21: 254–261.

36. Voorrips LE, Ravelli AC, Dongelmans PC, Deurenberg P, Van Staveren WA (1991) A physical activity questionnaire for the elderly. Med Sci Sports Exerc 23: 974–979.

37. Mador MJ, Bozkanat E (2001) Skeletal muscle dysfunction in chronic obstructive pulmonary disease. Respir Res 2: 216–224.

38. Yildiz S, Kaya I, Cece H, Gencer M, Ziylan Z, et al. (2012) Impact of COPD exacerbation on cerebral blood flow. Clin Imaging 36: 185–190.

39. Albayrak R, Fidan F, Unlu M, Sezer M, Degirmenci B, et al. (2006) Extracranial carotid Doppler ultrasound evaluation of cerebral blood flow volume in COPD patients. Respir Med 100: 1826–1833.

40. Nishimura Y, Onoe H, Morichika Y, Tsukada H, Isa T (2007) Activation of parieto-frontal stream during reaching and grasping studied by positron emission tomography in monkeys. Neurosci Res 59: 243–250.

41. Manto M, Bower JM, Conforto AB, Delgado-Garcia JM, da Guarda SN, et al. (2012) Consensus paper: roles of the cerebellum in motor control–the diversity of ideas on cerebellar involvement in movement. Cerebellum 11: 457–487.

42. Paulin MG (1993) The role of the cerebellum in motor control and perception. Brain Behav Evol 41: 39–50.

43. Dodd JW, Getov SV, Jones PW (2010) Cognitive function in COPD. Eur Respir J 35: 913–922.

44. Kramer AF, Erickson KI (2007) Capitalizing on cortical plasticity: influence of physical activity on cognition and brain function. Trends Cogn Sci 11: 342–348.

17

Sustained Maximal Voluntary Contraction Produces Independent Changes in Human Motor Axons and the Muscle They Innervate

David A. Milder, Emily J. Sutherland, Simon C. Gandevia, Penelope A. McNulty*

Neuroscience Research Australia, Sydney and University of New South Wales, Sydney, Australia

Abstract

The repetitive discharges required to produce a sustained muscle contraction results in activity-dependent hyperpolarization of the motor axons and a reduction in the force-generating capacity of the muscle. We investigated the relationship between these changes in the adductor pollicis muscle and the motor axons of its ulnar nerve supply, and the reproducibility of these changes. Ten subjects performed a 1-min maximal voluntary contraction. Activity-dependent changes in axonal excitability were measured using threshold tracking with electrical stimulation at the wrist; changes in the muscle were assessed as evoked and voluntary electromyography (EMG) and isometric force. Separate components of axonal excitability and muscle properties were tested at 5 min intervals after the sustained contraction in 5 separate sessions. The current threshold required to produce the target muscle action potential increased immediately after the contraction by 14.8% ($p<0.05$), reflecting decreased axonal excitability secondary to hyperpolarization. This was not correlated with the decline in amplitude of muscle force or evoked EMG. A late reversal in threshold current after the initial recovery from hyperpolarization peaked at -5.9% at ~35 min ($p<0.05$). This pattern was mirrored by other indices of axonal excitability revealing a previously unreported depolarization of motor axons in the late recovery period. Measures of axonal excitability were relatively stable at rest but less so after sustained activity. The coefficient of variation (CoV) for threshold current increase was higher after activity (CoV 0.54, $p<0.05$) whereas changes in voluntary (CoV 0.12) and evoked twitch (CoV 0.15) force were relatively stable. These results demonstrate that activity-dependent changes in motor axon excitability are unlikely to contribute to concomitant changes in the muscle after sustained activity in healthy people. The variability in axonal excitability after sustained activity suggests that care is needed when using these measures if the integrity of either the muscle or nerve may be compromised.

Editor: William Phillips, University of Sydney, Australia

Funding: This work was supported by the National Health and Medical Research Council of Australia and the New South Wales Office of Science and Medical Research. The funders had no role in study design, data collection and analysis, decision to publish, or preparation of the manuscript.

Competing Interests: The authors have declared that no competing interests exist.

* E-mail: p.mcnulty@neura.edu.au

Introduction

The repetitive activity required to generate a sustained voluntary contraction produces changes in both the muscle and its motor nerve supply. In the nerve there is an activity-dependent decrease in the excitability of motor axons secondary to hyperpolarization caused by overactivity of the electrogenic Na^+-K^+ pump [1–3]. In the muscle there is a progressive decrease in its force-generating capacity [4]. There is a long-held view that the contractile and biochemical properties of a muscle are determined, at least in part, by their innervating motor axons [5] and that the properties of the motoneurones, motor units and muscles in the healthy system are tightly coupled [6–9]. Although sustained activity produces equivalent discharges in both the motor axons and the muscle, Ishihara and colleagues [10] concluded that chronic activity-dependent changes were more pronounced in the muscle than its nerve supply. The association between acute activity-dependent changes in nerve and muscle, their magnitude and the time course of their recovery is uncertain.

Threshold tracking has been used to examine the biophysical properties of human peripheral motor axons in vivo at rest (see [11,12]) and in response to acute, sustained voluntary activity in healthy subjects [13–15]. More recently, it has been used to understand the pathophysiology of chronic disease states by examining activity-dependent changes in axonal excitability of diabetic neuropathy [16], amyotrophic lateral sclerosis [17] and chemotherapy-induced neuropathy [18]. In this technique changes in motor axon excitability are inferred from changes in the current required to generate a muscle action potential of predetermined amplitude [12] on the assumption that the measured changes in axonal excitability are reproducible and do not reflect a change in muscle properties. Similarly, activity-dependent decreases in muscle force with sustained activity are assumed to be independent of any change in excitability of the innervating motor axons [4]. These assumptions have never been directly tested.

The relationship between the properties of motoneurones, their axons and innervated muscle fibres is maintained in response to exercise [19]. The diameter of a motor axon is correlated to the electromechanical properties of the muscle fibres including contractile speed and maximal tetanic tension [20,21]. For instance, compared with large motor axons, smaller motor axons

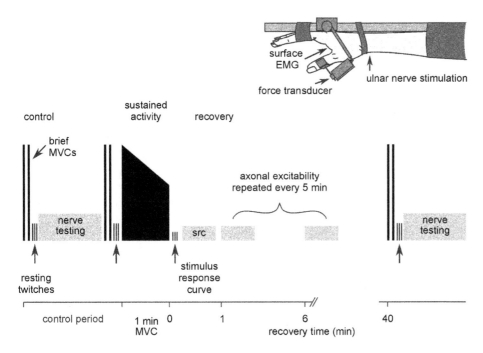

Figure 1. Schematic representation of the experimental setup and protocol. The experimental setup is viewed from above. The experimental protocol (not shown to scale) consisted of a control period, a sustained 1-min adductor pollicis MVC, and the recovery period. The "nerve testing" rectangle represents the TRONDNF protocol. After the stimulus-response curve (src) one component of axonal excitability was measured every 5 min for 40 min through the recovery period in 4 experimental sessions with measures of muscle force in the 5th session.

innervate muscle fibres that produce less force, are less susceptible to fatigue, and have a greater reliance on oxidative phosphorylation [22]. This matching of properties also occurs during maximal contractions, so that declining motor axon discharge rates 'match' the slowing contractile speed of muscle fibres (see [4]). The transmission of impulses from the nerve to the muscle is reliable and robust because the safety margin at the neuromuscular junction ensures synaptic efficacy even during vigorous and sustained muscle activation [23]. Although action potential propagation is less secure at branch points and in terminal axons, complete block is rare except in the case of focal demyelination (e.g. [2]) and is unlikely to explain any disocciation in activity-dependent changes between the muscle and its motor innervation.

In this study we investigated whether activity-dependent reductions in the force-generating capacity of the muscle were directly associated with activity-dependent changes in motor axon excitability in healthy subjects who performed a standardised sustained voluntary task. The TROND protocol introduced in 2000 was the first semi-automated threshold tracking program (see [12]), and since then "multi-tracking" protocols have been implemented (e.g. [13]). We used the TROND protocol of threshold tracking to examine the excitability of the ulnar motor axons innervating the adductor pollicis muscle. Five parameters that could be rapidly measured were examined in detail, each of which reflected different biophysical properties of the motor axons [11,12]. Despite its speed, multi-tracking was not used because it does not allow a detailed analysis of each parameter. In addition to measuring ulnar nerve excitability, activity-dependent changes in the adductor pollicis muscle were examined during brief maximal evoked and voluntary contractions before and after a sustained 1-min contraction sufficient to induce significant reductions in force (ie fatigue). Our aim was to investigate systematically the relationship between the changes, and the reproducibility of these

changes, in both the muscle and its nerve under physiological conditions.

Methods

Activity-dependent changes in adductor pollicis and its ulnar nerve supply were studied in the right arm of ten healthy subjects (5 men, 5 women; mean age 26 years; age range 21–42 years). All were right-handed. The study tested five specific aspects of nerve and muscle function at 5 min intervals after 1 min of sustained voluntary muscle activity. Thus each subject was tested on five separate occasions separated by at least 48 hours. Informed written consent was obtained prior to the experimental procedures which were approved by the Human Research Ethics Committee, University of New South Wales. All experiments were conducted in accordance with the Declaration of Helsinki.

Experimental setup

Subjects sat with the test forearm supported, semi-pronated and immobilised by strapping. The wrist and digits II–V were also restrained (Fig. 1). The thumb was positioned in 75% of each subject's maximal abduction, the optimal position on the length-tension curve for adductor pollicis (McNulty PA unpublished data). Isometric adduction force was measured using a 350 N load cell (XTRAN, Applied Measurement Australia) strapped to the interphalangeal joint of the thumb. The force signal was amplified 1170 times, filtered from DC to 20 Hz (AMA2044B, Applied Measurement Australia), digitised at 2 kHz with a 1401 data acquisition card and analysed using Spike2 software (Cambridge Electronic Design, UK). Temperature was monitored at the site of nerve stimulation and maintained above 32°C using radiant heat and blankets as required.

Surface electrodes (10 mm Ag/AgCl) were used for nerve stimulation and electromyographic (EMG) recording. For nerve stimulation the cathode was positioned at the site producing an optimal muscle action potential in adductor pollicis, typically just proximal to the wrist crease and medial to the tendon of flexor carpi ulnaris. The anode was placed ~10 cm more proximal. A switch was used to alternate between two current sources, one for testing axonal excitability and the other for testing muscle properties. For testing axonal excitability, a computer-controlled bipolar constant-current stimulator (DS5, Digitimer, UK) delivered rectangular stimuli of different pulse width, amplitude and polarity. For testing resting muscle force, rectangular pulses (0.1 ms duration) were delivered from a constant-current stimulator (DS7AH, Digitimer, UK).

EMG activity was recorded in a belly-tendon configuration with the cathode on the belly of adductor pollicis and the anode 30 mm distal. EMG signals were amplified 200 times and filtered from 10 Hz to 1 kHz (IP511, Grass, USA) with 50 Hz mains noise removed (Humbug, Quest Scientific, Canada). The EMG signal was sampled at 10 kHz (PCI-6221, National Instruments, USA) for axonal excitability testing, and at 5 kHz with a 1401 data acquisition card and Spike2 software (Cambridge Electronic Design, UK) for testing muscle properties.

Axonal excitability testing

Activity-dependent changes in the excitability of motor axons innervating adductor pollicis were studied using a computerised threshold tracking program and the TRONDNF protocol (QTRACS, Institute of Neurology, UK). Unless otherwise stated, 1 ms test pulses were delivered at 2 Hz. Threshold tracking began with a stimulus-response curve to determine the maximum compound muscle action potential (M_{max}), the amplitude of which was measured from baseline to negative peak. The target potential was set to 40% M_{max}, which corresponds to the steepest point on the stimulus-response curve and is the level most commonly used in clinical studies (e.g. [18,24]). Changes in the current required to elicit this target potential (the threshold current) were tracked throughout the protocol. A decrease in threshold current represented an increase in axonal excitability and vice versa. To confirm that changes in axonal excitability following sustained activity were due to hyperpolarization, multiple components were measured at 5 min intervals, including the strength-duration relationship, threshold electrotonus, current-threshold relationship and the recovery cycle in separate experiments. Threshold tracking was based on M_{max} rather than force output to allow for accurate measurement of all components of axonal excitability [25].

To derive the strength-duration time constant (τ_{SD}) and rheobase, stimuli with durations of 0.2, 0.4, 0.6, 0.8 and 1.0 ms were given. For threshold electrotonus, changes in threshold current were determined at intervals from −10 to 200 ms relative to the onset of a 100 ms subthreshold conditioning pulse that was either depolarizing (+20% and +40% of threshold current) or hyperpolarizing (−20% and −40% of threshold current). The current-threshold relationship was measured by delivering a test pulse at the end of a 200 ms depolarizing or hyperpolarizing subthreshold conditioning pulse, graded in 10% steps from +50% to −100% of threshold current. for this relationship the decreases in threshold current are conventionally plotted on the x-axis while the strength of the conditioning pulses are plotted on the y-axis, despite the dependent variable being the decrease in threshold current (see [12]). The recovery cycle was used to measure changes in threshold current at 18 intervals from 2 to 200 ms after a 1 ms supramaximal stimulus. For further details of threshold tracking procedures, see Kiernan and colleagues [12] and Krishnan and colleagues [26].

Muscle testing

To assess maximal voluntary force, subjects were instructed to contract adductor pollicis by pulling the interphalangeal joint of the thumb towards the web space between digits II–III. To ensure voluntary contractions were maximal, standardised verbal encouragement and visual force feedback were provided. Subjects were allowed to reject any contraction they considered not to be maximal. MVC force was established as the peak response during 3 brief, 2–3 s maximal efforts prior to the experimental protocol. Three supramaximal stimuli were delivered at 1 Hz immediately after the MVC to assess the twitch force of a fully potentiated muscle during relaxation. To ensure all motor axons were stimulated, the stimulus intensity was 150% of that required to produce M_{max}. Pilot studies that tracked the amplitude of M_{max} throughout the protocol demonstrated that this stimulus intensity was sufficient to produce M_{max} even after 1 min of maximal voluntary activity of adductor pollicis and that the stimulus did not become submaximal in the following 40 min (see below).

Protocol

This protocol is a modification of that used in previous studies and was designed so that changes in each measured parameter could be quantified systematically at the same constant interval following standardised voluntary activity. All subjects participated in 5 sessions so that each of four components of axonal excitability began at the same interval after the end of the sustained voluntary contraction regardless of their order in a full TRONDNF protocol. Muscle properties were tested in the same manner in the 5th session. The protocol consisted of a control period in which baseline values were established, a sustained contraction, and the recovery period (Fig. 1). In the control period subjects performed 2 brief, 2–3 s MVCs immediately before 3 resting twitches were evoked. This was followed by the TRONDNF protocol, 2 brief MVCs and 3 resting twitches. In the sustained contraction subjects performed a 1-min MVC, followed immediately by 3 resting twitches. The recovery period began with a repeat of the stimulus-response curve to update the amplitude of the target potential used for threshold tracking. One parameter of axonal excitability was then measured every 5 min for 8 cycles in the first four experimental sessions. The first cycle began 1 min after the end of the MVC. In these sessions the strength-duration relationship, threshold electrotonus, current-threshold relationship and the recovery cycle were measured. Voluntary and resting twitch forces were measured in the fifth session at the same intervals. Testing continued for 40 min and finished with 2 brief MVCs, 3 resting twitches and a final TRONDNF protocol.

The amplitude of M_{max} (and consequently the target potential) was updated immediately after the 1-min MVC but not updated for another 40 min. If the size of the target potential changed markedly during this 40 min period, it may have resulted in an incorrect estimation of changes in axonal excitability. Consequently, two control experiments were performed on 5 subjects during which the amplitude of M_{max} and the target potential was updated with a stimulus-response curve every 5 min prior to the measurement of either the strength-duration relationship or the recovery cycle. Updating the amplitude and threshold current of the target potential in this way did not alter the pattern of recovery for axonal excitability.

Data analysis

Measures of axonal excitability. Changes in the current required to generate the target potential (40% M_{max}) were normalised to the threshold current value in the first stimulus-response curve. Using Weiss's law, the linear regression of threshold charge on stimulus duration was used to derive τ_{SD} and rheobase (see Fig. 2B). For threshold electrotonus, three time periods of interest were identified a priori. The first of these, S1, reflects the slow spread of subthreshold conditioning pulses to the internode (Burke et al., 2001). With depolarizing currents, S1 was measured 10–20 ms after the start of the 40% depolarizing conditioning pulse (TEd^{40}_{10-20}). For hyperpolarizing currents, S1 was measured 10–20 ms (TEh^{40}_{10-20}), 20–40 ms (TEh^{40}_{20-40}) and 90–100 ms (TEh^{40}_{90-100}) after the start of the 40% hyperpolarizing conditioning pulse. S2, the second period of interest, reflects axonal accommodation to depolarizing currents (Burke et al., 2001). It was measured 40–60 ms (TEd^{40}_{40-60}) and 90–100 ms (TEd^{40}_{90-100}) after the start of the 40% depolarizing conditioning pulse. Finally, the under- ($TEd^{40}_{undershoot}$) and overshoot ($TEh^{40}_{overshoot}$) in axonal excitability were measured ~40 and ~90 ms and after the offset of the conditioning pulses, respectively. For the current-threshold relationship, the resting IV slope was measured as the gradient between the data points for −10%, 0% and +10% conditioning pulses. Minimum IV slope was derived from the smallest gradient between any 3 adjacent data points. Hyperpolarizing IV slope was the gradient between −80%, −90% and −100% conditioning pulse data, while depolarizing IV slope was the gradient between +30%, +40% and +50% conditioning pulse data. For the recovery cycle, the durations of the refractory and superexcitable periods were extrapolated from the intercept of the curve and the x-axis of the curve (see Fig. 2D). The amplitude of superexcitability was calculated from the mean of three responses at adjacent interstimulus intervals at which the reduction in threshold current was maximal while its extent was calculated as area under the curve. The amplitude of subexcitability was calculated from the mean of three responses at adjacent interstimulus intervals beyond 10 ms at which the increase in threshold current was maximal.

Measures of EMG and force. The EMG signal of the sustained contraction was root mean square (RMS) processed using a 125 ms sliding window. The amplitude of EMG and force was measured as an average over 50 ms both at the start of the 1-min MVC around the absolute peak force, and immediately before the subject was instructed to relax. The resting M_{max} was measured as amplitude (baseline to negative peak and peak-to-peak) and as total area of the potential.

Statistical analysis. Activity-induced changes in indices of axonal excitability were assessed using one-way repeated measures ANOVA with post-hoc Holm-Sidak pairwise comparisons for normally distributed data, and one-way repeated measures ANOVA on ranks with post-hoc Tukey tests for data that were not normally distributed. Sustained activity-induced changes in muscle force, M_{max} amplitude and voluntary EMG were assessed using paired t-tests. Pearson and Spearman correlations were used for data that were normally and not normally distributed, respectively. To evaluate reproducibility, a coefficient of variation (CoV) for within-subject data was calculated. The data were normally distributed unless otherwise stated and are presented as mean and 95% confidence interval. Data that were not normally distributed are presented as median and interquartile range [IQR]. Statistical analysis was performed using SigmaStat (Systat, USA). Results were considered significant when $p < 0.05$.

Results

Changes in axonal excitability parameters immediately after the 1-min MVC were consistent with axonal hyperpolarisation. After the initial recovery there was a late reversal in axonal-excitability. Following maximal voluntary activity there were changes in

muscle properties including resting twitch and peak voluntary force, the amplitude of M_{max}, and voluntary EMG. However, none of these changes was correlated with reductions in axonal excitability. Finally, measures of axonal excitability were relatively stable at rest but less so after sustained activity.

Changes in axonal excitability immediately after sustained activity

Stimulus-response curve. After the sustained maximal contraction the stimulus-response curve shifted to the right, indicating more current was required to produce the target compound muscle action potential (Fig. 2A). The mean increase in threshold current was 14.8% [9.7–20.0%] ($p < 0.05$). This reflected a decrease in the excitability of motor axons. When the stimulus intensity was normalised to the current required to produce 50% of M_{max}, the slope of the curve did not change significantly after the sustained contraction.

Strength-duration relationship (τ_{SD} and rheobase). τ_{SD} decreased from 0.51 ms [0.47–0.55 ms] in the control period to 0.47 ms [0.44–0.49 ms] 1 min after the sustained contraction ($p < 0.05$) (Fig. 2B). Rheobase increased from 4.1 mA [3.3–4.9 mA] to 4.7 mA [3.7–5.6 mA] ($p < 0.05$).

Threshold electrotonus. Changes in threshold electrotonus after sustained activity are presented in Figure 2C. For depolarizing currents, S1 measured at TEd^{40}_{10-20} (see Methods), increased from control values of 67.7% [64.2–71.2%] to 70.1% [65.8–74.4%] after the sustained contraction ($p < 0.05$). S2, measured at TEd^{40}_{40-60} and TEd^{40}_{90-100}, increased from 51.2% [46.4–56.0%] and 44.2% [40.0–48.4%] to 53.41% [49.1–57.8%] and 47.8% [43.2–52.4%], respectively ($p < 0.05$). $TEd^{40}_{undershoot}$ decreased from −19.2% [−21.7−−16.7%] to −15.5% [−17.6−−13.3%] ($p < 0.05$).

For hyperpolarizing currents, there was no significant change in TEh^{40}_{10-20} after sustained activity. However, TEh^{40}_{20-40} and TEh^{40}_{90-100} increased from median values of −88.5% [−101.2−−85.9%] and −115.2% [−140.0−−112.8%] to −94.1% [−102.3−−89.1%] and −130.2% [−151.8−−119.7%], respectively ($p < 0.05$). $TEh^{40}_{overshoot}$ decreased from 13.9% [12.1–15.6%] to 9.1% [5.7–12.4%] ($p < 0.05$).

Current-threshold relationship. The sustained contraction produced changes in the current-threshold relationship (Fig. 2D). Changes in the slope of the IV curve are illustrated in Figure 2E. After the sustained contraction resting IV slope decreased from a control value of 0.56 [0.50–0.62] to 0.49 [0.42–0.56] ($p < 0.05$). There was no significant change in the depolarizing, hyperpolarizing or minimum IV slopes.

Recovery cycle. The duration of the refractory period decreased from 2.9 ms [2.6–3.1 ms] to 2.6 ms [2.4–2.8 ms] after the sustained contraction ($p < 0.05$) (Fig. 2F). The amplitude of the relative refractory period measured at 2.5 ms decreased from 12.9% [4.0–21.9%] in the control period to 2.1% [−5.7–9.9%] ($p < 0.05$). There was no significant change in the amplitude of superexcitability after the 1-min MVC, but its duration and area increased. The duration increased from 15.8 ms [14.1–17.6 ms] to 20.3 ms [16.4–24.2 ms] while the area increased by 32.7% [18.4–47.0%] ($p < 0.05$). The amplitude of subexcitability did not change significantly.

Time course of recovery in axonal excitability

Threshold current returned to control values by 6 min (Fig. 3A). Other indices that had recovered by 6 min were τ_{SD}, rheobase, TEd^{40}_{10-20}, TEd^{40}_{40-60}, TEd^{40}_{90-100}, TEh^{40}_{20-40}, TEh^{40}_{90-100}, resting IV slope, and the duration and area of superexcitability. Indices with slower time courses of recovery were (i) the magnitude

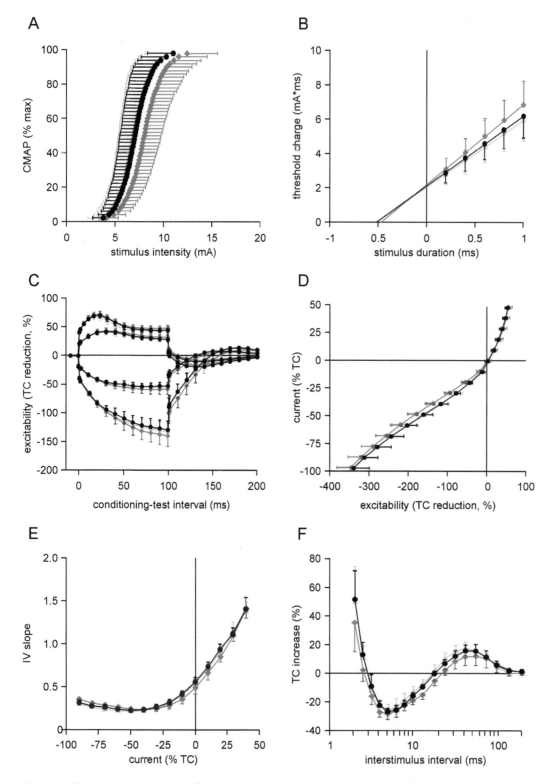

Figure 2. Changes in components of axonal excitability after sustained activity. Black symbols: control data; red symbols: data recorded after the 1 min sustained contraction; blue symbols: data recorded after the 40 min recovery period. A: stimulus-response curves with the CMAP normalised to M_{max}. B: charge-duration curves. τ_{SD} and rheobase were derived from the x-intercepts and gradients of the linear regressions, respectively. C: threshold electrotonus. D: current-threshold relationship. E: slope of the current-threshold relationship. F: recovery cycle. Four subjects were excluded from the data at an interstimulus interval of 2 ms only because the output of the stimulator was insufficient to produce the target potential. Data presented as mean ± 95% confidence intervals. TC: threshold current.

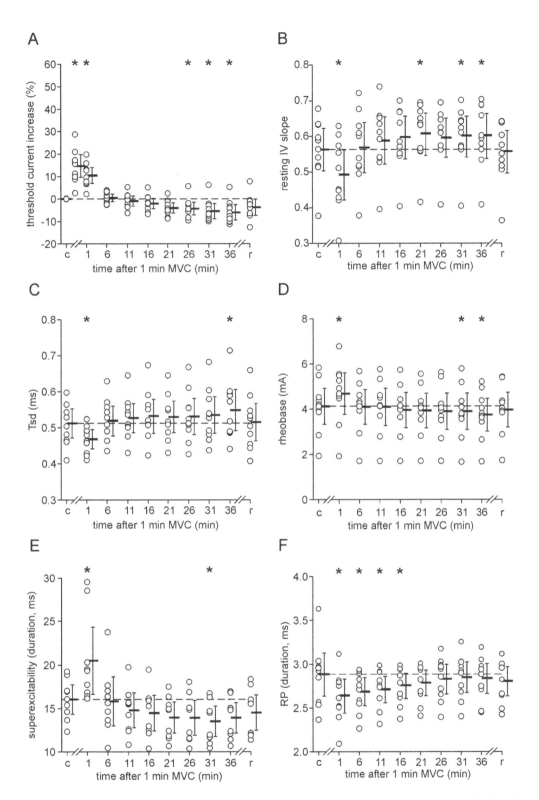

Figure 3. Recovery of axonal excitability after sustained activity. Open symbols represent the data for each subject; pooled data are presented as mean (solid bars) and 95% confidence intervals. A: threshold current. B: resting IV slope. C: τ_{SD}. D: rheobase. D: the duration of the superexcitable period. F: the duration of the refractory period (RP). *: $p < 0.05$.

and duration of the relative refractory period, which returned to control values by 21 min (Fig. 3F) and (ii) $TEd^{40}_{undershoot}$, which had not returned to control values by 40 min.

After the initial recovery period threshold current showed a late reversal which was significant at 26 min [−4.2%; −7.2−−1.3%], 31 min [−5.2%; −8.7−−1.8%] and 36 min [−5.9%; −9.4−−2.3%] ($p < 0.05$) (Fig. 3A). This late reversal also occurred for resting IV slope at 21, 31 and 36 min (Fig. 3B); τ_{SD} at 31 min (Fig. 3C); rheobase at 31 and 36 min (Fig. 3D); the duration of superexcitability at 31 min (Fig. 3E); and the area of super-excitability at 26, 31 and 36 min (p<0.05).

Changes in M_{max}, voluntary EMG, twitch force and maximal voluntary force

There was a significant decrease in the (updated) peak amplitude of M_{max} after the sustained contraction. The baseline to negative-peak amplitude decreased from 11.1 mV [9.6–12.6 mV] to 9.7 mV [8.4–11.0 mV] and the peak-to-peak amplitude decreased from 19.1 mV [16.3–22.0 mV] to 17.2 mV [14.7–19.7 mV] (p<0.001). However, the area of M_{max} did not change significantly (Fig. 4A). At the start of the 1-min MVC the amplitude of voluntary EMG was 0.9 mV (RMS) [0.8–.0 mV]. This decreased to 0.6 mV [0.5–0.7 mV] at the end of the contraction (p<0.001; Fig. 4B).

Resting twitch force decreased by 42% after the sustained contraction, from 9.5 N [6.3–12.6 N] before the 1-min MVC to 5.1 N [3.7–6.5 N] (p<0.001) after the 1-min MVC (Fig. 4C). Peak voluntary force was 68.3 N [52.9–83.7 N] at the start of the 1-min MVC and this decreased to 30.9 N [23.5–38.3 N] at the end of the contraction (p<0.001), a decline of 55% (Fig. 4D).

Relationship between changes in axonal and muscle properties

There were no significant correlations between the decrease in motor axonal excitability measured as the increase in the threshold current required to produce 40% of M_{max} in the updated stimulus-response curve, and the decline in the area or amplitude of the twitch force in the relaxed muscle (Fig 5A). Importantly, there was no significant correlation between decreased motor axon excitability and the decline in maximal voluntary muscle output, whether measured as EMG or force (Fig. 5B).

Intersession variability

The repeated testing protocol allowed for the assessment of inter-session variability. Some measures were relatively stable between sessions including the majority of axonal excitability indices at rest, such as threshold current measured before the 1 min-MVC [CoV (median and IQR) 0.12; 0.06–0.18]; and the extent of voluntary force production, measured as the force decline during the 1-min MVC [CoV 0.12; 0.06–0.18]. The decline in resting twitch force after the 1-min MVC was of was slightly more variable [CoV 0.15; 0.23–0.44]. The increase in threshold current following sustained activity was most variable [CoV 0.54; 0.33–0.65], and its coefficient of variation was significantly higher than that for threshold current at rest or the reduction in force during the 1-min MVC (p<0.05).

Discussion

In this study we systematically investigated the relationship between activity-dependent changes in the adductor pollicis muscle and the motor axons of its ulnar nerve supply. Our key finding was that the changes in the adductor pollicis muscle were independent of the activity-dependent changes in the motor axons despite the same high demand on both the muscle and its nerve supply. This suggests that decreased axonal excitability makes no contribution to the reduction in the force-generating capacity of the muscle that occurs as a consequence of sustained voluntary activity, ie fatigue. This is the first study to examine the reproducibility of activity-dependent changes in motor axons and muscles. We found that the observed increase in threshold

current was the least reproducible parameter studied, and that measures of axonal excitability are significantly more variable after voluntary muscle activity than at rest or for any measure of muscle output. A novel observation was a reversal in the excitability of the motor axons, most noticeably of threshold current, that occurred late in recovery period and presumably reflects the delayed deactivation of currents opposing hyperpolarization. These results provide a note of caution when using axonal excitability threshold tracking in diseases that may affect the muscle and nerve differently. In such cases a change in the properties of the muscle cannot necessarily be used as the basis for inferring a change in the properties of the motor axon membrane.

Decreased motor axonal excitability reflected hyperpolarization

The pattern of changes in multiple indices of axon function suggests that decreased axonal excitability with sustained activity was caused by hyperpolarization. Specifically, τ_{SD} declined and rheobase increased, consistent with a hyperpolarization-induced reduction in the persistent Na^+ current (I_{NaP}) at the node [27,28]. The increased absolute magnitude of the threshold electrotonus, S1 and S2 produced a 'fanned out' appearance [29], reflecting increased resistance of the internodal membrane due to a hyperpolarization-mediated reduction in K^+ channel activation [11]. In contrast, both $TEd^{40}_{undershoot}$ and $TEh^{40}_{overshoot}$ decreased in absolute magnitude, resulting in a 'fanned in' appearance. Resting IV slope decreased, suggesting a decreased input conductance of the axon secondary to hyperpolarization [30]. The decrease in relative refractory period suggests a reduction in Na^+ channel inactivation [11]. The duration and area of superexcitability increased, presumably due to an augmented depolarizing afterpotential secondary to a hyperpolarization-mediated inactivation of K^+ channels with fast kinetics (K_f) [31]. Overall, these changes reflected nodal and intermodal hyperpolarization.

There is a discrepancy between the findings on axonal changes of the present study and the results of Kuwabara and colleagues [13]. In the latter study the authors reported an increase in the threshold current of the relative refractory period (measured at 2 ms) following a sustained contraction lasting ~3 min despite having expected a decline because of hyperpolarization. The amplitude of M_{max} was decreased when evoked by closely spaced (2–4 ms) paired pulses, which was proposed to reflect activity-dependent conduction block at distal axon branch points and nerve terminals [13], shown to be sites of lowered safety margin [32–34]. In the present study there was no evidence of a transient increase in the refractory period. Kuwabara and colleagues [13] measured activity-dependent changes in the recovery cycle at only two interstimulus intervals within the refractory (2 ms) and superexcitable (7 ms) periods. In contrast, the recovery cycle test used here as part of the TRONDNF protocol, worked backwards from 200 to 2 ms, taking ~2 min to "reach" the relative refractory period. This delay may contribute to the difference in findings between the present study and that of Kuwabara and colleagues [13]. However, the physiological relevance of any conduction block with 2–4 ms interstimulus intervals is uncertain because they correspond to motoneurone firing rates of ~250–500 Hz, which are rarely encountered in human motor tasks [35], except briefly in ballistic efforts [36] or with doublet discharges [37].

Late reversal in axonal excitability

A late reversal in threshold current followed the initial recovery from hyperpolarization. This pattern was mirrored by other

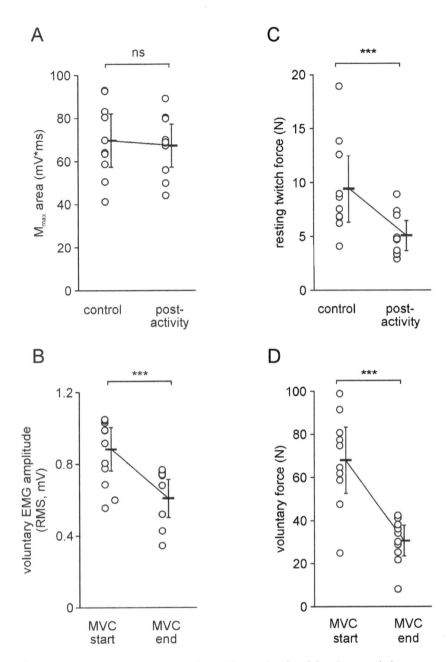

Figure 4. Changes in muscle properties with sustained activity. Open symbols represent the mean for each subject across 5 experimental sessions; pooled data for 10 subjects are shown beside the individual data as mean (solid bars) and 95% confidence intervals. A: there was no change in the area of M_{max} after the sustained contraction; B: there was a significant change in the resting twitch force immediately after the 1-min MVC compared to control values; C: the peak amplitude of the voluntary EMG was significantly larger at the start than at the end of the 1-min MVC; D: peak voluntary force was significantly smaller at the end of the 1-min MVC than at the start demonstrating an activity-dependent reduction in the force-generating capacity of the muscle (ie fatigue). ns: not significant; ***: p<0.001.

indices of axonal excitability including τ_{SD} and superexcitability, suggesting the reversal in threshold current reflected a subsequent depolarization. This late period of axonal depolarization has not previously been reported following voluntary activity, perhaps because recovery has not been followed for >20 min. Kiernan and colleagues [38] measured the recovery of median motor axons for ~35 min after 10 min of 8 Hz electrical stimulation. Although not noted by the authors, a late reversal in threshold current as observed here is evident in their Figure 1A. Similar phenomena have been reported in animal studies. Specifically, depolarizing reversals in membrane potential occurred in motoneurones of the

cat [39] and sensory ganglion neurones of the mouse [40] following hyperpolarizing pulses, albeit over much shorter time courses (~200 ms). Presumably these reversals were mediated by the delayed deactivation of a hyperpolarization-activated cation current known as I_h [40], an internodal rectifying channel that counters hyperpolarization by permitting a net inward cationic current [26,41].

We know of no animal studies that applied hyperpolarizing pulses of very long duration (minutes) to motor axons; nor has this been done in human studies due to the discomfort involved. Nevertheless, we propose that the late reversal in threshold current

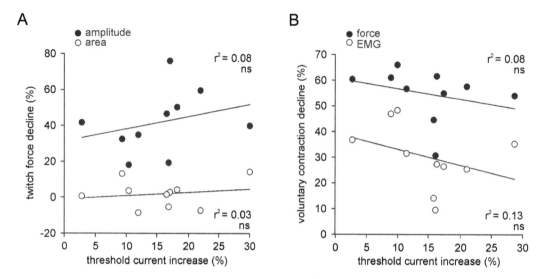

Figure 5. Relationship between the activity-dependent changes in muscle output and axonal excitability. Symbols represent the mean for each subject across 5 experimental sessions. A: There was no relationship between the activity-dependent increases in threshold current and the decline in the amplitude (black symbols) or area (white symbols) of resting twitch force. B: Similarly, there was no relationship between increases in threshold current and the decline in voluntary force (black symbols) and voluntary EMG (white s). ns: not significant.

in this study reflected delayed I_h deactivation as changes in axonal excitability after voluntary activity represent a balance between the opposing actions on membrane potential of the Na^+-K^+ pump [1] and I_h [40–42]. Immediately after sustained activity, the electrogenic effects of the Na^+-K^+ pump predominate, resulting in hyperpolarization. Later in the recovery period when the Na^+-K^+ pump is less active, the effects of I_h may predominate, particularly given its slow kinetics of deactivation [43], resulting in a net depolarization of the motor axon [44].

Repeated axonal excitability testing is unlikely to have contributed to this delayed depolarisation. A study by Howells and colleagues [45] demonstrated that measures of axonal excitability are highly reproducible within a subject during the same experimental session, despite the session involving repeated stimuli and multiple excitability protocols. The stability of threshold tracking over a prolonged time period (6 hours) in the absence of activity has also been demonstrated [46].

Magnitude of activity-dependent changes

The decline in muscle force after the sustained contraction in the present study was similar to previous reports of ~50% (e.g. [47]). The reported decrease in axonal excitability in median motor axons has been more variable, ranging from ~38% [14,15] to~15% [48]. The decline of 14.8% in the present study is similar to the decline of 18.3% in a previous study of 20 subjects after a 1-min MVC of adductor pollicis [49]. This smaller decline in excitability may reflect different experimental protocols. Measurement of the stimulus-response curve in the present study was completed after the sustained contraction and took ~30 s. This unavoidable delay may have produced an underestimation of excitability changes. However, the updated stimulus-response curve was critical to adjust for sustained activity-induced changes in the amplitude of the target muscle action potential (see above).

The magnitude of axonal excitability changes may also reflect the nerve and muscle tested. Previous studies examined median motor axons innervating abductor pollicis brevis [13,15]. Changes in the present study are consistent with the only other study to have examined sustained activity of ulnar motor axons innervating adductor pollicis [49]. Differences in biophysical properties have

been reported at rest for ulnar and median motor axons [50], and perhaps these differences affect the magnitude of hyperpolarization following sustained activity. Specifically, the change in threshold electrotonus in the hyperpolarizing direction was smaller in ulnar motor axons than in median motor axons [50]. This was interpreted to reflect a difference in the activity of I_h, with respect to either the specific isoform of the HCN channel or threshold for activation [50]. It is possible that this limits the extent of hyperpolarisation in ulnar motor axons, and produces a more prominent late reversal in axonal excitability.

It is difficult to compare the magnitude of these excitability changes to those in disease states because of the choice of nerve and muscle. Previous studies of neuropathic nerves were conducted using the median nerve and abductor pollicis brevis muscle (e.g. [16,17]) rather than the ulnar nerve and adductor pollicis of this study. Not all neuropathies are associated with a change in the extent of activity-dependent hyperpolarisation. For example, for patients with end-stage kidney disease there was an 18.4% decrease in axonal excitability after a 1-min MVC [48], but this was not significantly different to healthy controls (15.0%) or this study. For neuropathies associated with a substantial change in the extent of hyperpolarisation there is significant variation according to disease state. Patients with diabetic neuropathy had a small decrease in axonal excitability (13.1%), thought to reflect dysfunction of the Na^+-K^+ pump [16], while patients with amyotrophic lateral sclerosis had a larger increase (36.5%), thought to be due to higher discharge rates of the surviving motor axons [17].

Reproducibility

Variability of axonal excitability indices at rest have been studied in motor axons of the median [46] and ulnar nerves [50]. However, this is the first study to report the reproducibility of decreases in axonal excitability after sustained activity. After sustained activity the increase in threshold current (reflecting decreased axonal excitability) was the most variable within-subjects measure. This was despite the reproducibility of reductions in voluntary force during the 1-min MVC, which was facilitated by the standardisation of the MVC in this study, unlike previous reports. This suggests the extent of axonal hyperpolarization with sustained voluntary contractions is intrinsically variable. This variability may be related to day-to-day fluctuations in factors affecting Na^+-K^+ pump activity, including resting membrane potential [51], and electrolyte status [52].

Relationship between changes in motor axonal excitability and properties of the muscle

This is the first study to assess the correlation between decreases in motor axonal excitability and muscle output, such as correlated reductions in axonal excitability and resting twitch force. No correlation was observed, so that activity-dependent changes in axonal excitability were not correlated with activity-dependent changes in adductor pollicis despite the widespread assumption that the properties of motoneurones, their axons and the innervated muscle fibres are closely matched [6–9].This finding also suggests that muscle force production is not compromised by activity-induced axonal hyperpolarization in healthy subjects, presumably due to the large safety margin for saltatory conduction [53,54] and at the neuromuscular junction [23]. Conduction block predominantly occurs in disease states with localised demyelinating neuropathies [55,56].

In conclusion, we have shown that the activity-dependent changes that occur in the muscle after sustained activity follow different time courses to, and are not correlated with, changes that occur in its motor nerve supply. In the healthy population such changes do not impede impulse conduction, even after intense but brief maximal voluntary activity. These results provide confidence that the safety margin of both the motor axons and the neuromuscular junction is more than sufficient to accommodate sudden increases in sustained activity. Our data suggest that although these methods are robust in healthy adults, care is required when interpreting activity-dependent neuromuscular excitability changes with pathologies.

Acknowledgments

We are grateful to Professor D Burke for helpful discussion and comments on the manuscript.

Author Contributions

Conceived and designed the experiments: PMcN Performed the experiments: DM, ES Analyzed the data: DM, ES, PMcN Wrote the manuscript: DM, ES, SG, PMcN

References

1. Ritchie JM, Straub RW (1957) The hyperpolarization which follows activity in mammalian non-medullated fibres. J Physiol 136: 80–97.
2. Bostock H, Grafe P (1985) Activity-dependent excitability changes in normal and demyelinated rat spinal root axons. J Physiol 365: 239–257.
3. Kaji R, Sumner AJ (1989) Ouabain reverses conduction disturbances in single demyelinated nerve fibers. Neurology 39: 1364–1368.
4. Gandevia S (2001) Spinal and supraspinal factors in human muscle fatigue. Physiol Rev 81: 1725–1789.
5. Buller AJ, Eccles JC, Eccles RM (1960) Interactions between motoneurones and muscles in respect of the characteristic speeds of their responses. J Physiol 150: 417–439.
6. Henneman E, Somjen G, Carpenter DO (1965) Functional Significance of Cell Size in Spinal Motoneurons. J Neurophysiol 28: 560–580.
7. Burke R (1981) Motor units: anatomy, physiology, and functional organization. In: J . Brookhart and V . Mountcastle, editors. Handbook of Physiology, Section 1: The Nervous System. Bethesda: American Physiological Society. pp. 345–422.
8. Kernell D (1992) Organized variability in the neuromuscular system: a survey of task-related adaptations. Arch Ital Biol 130: 19–66.
9. Enoka RM (1995) Morphological features and activation patterns of motor units. J Clin Neurophysiol 12: 538–559.
10. Ishihara A, Roy RR, Ohira Y, Edgerton VR (2003) Motoneuron and sensory neuron plasticity to varying neuromuscular activity levels. Exerc Sport Sci Rev 31: 51–57.
11. Burke D, Kiernan MC, Bostock H (2001) Excitability of human axons. Clin Neurophysiol 112: 1575–1585.
12. Kiernan MC, Burke D, Andersen KV, Bostock H (2000) Multiple measures of axonal excitability: a new approach in clinical testing. Muscle Nerve 23: 399–409.
13. Kuwabara S, Lin CSY, Mogyoros I, Cappelen-Smith C, Burke D (2001) Voluntary contraction impairs the refractory period of transmission in healthy human axons. J Physiol 531: 265–275.
14. Kuwabara S, Cappelen Smith C, Lin CSY, Mogyoros I, Burke D (2002) Effects of voluntary activity on the excitability of motor axons in the peroneal nerve. Muscle Nerve 25: 176–184.
15. Vagg R, Mogyoros I, Kiernan MC, Burke D (1998) Activity-dependent hyperpolarization of human motor axons produced by natural activity. J Physiol 507: 919–925.
16. Krishnan AV, Lin CSY, Kiernan MC (2008) Activity-dependent excitability changes suggest Na+/K+ pump dysfunction in diabetic neuropathy. Brain 131: 1209–1216.
17. Vucic S, Krishnan AV, Kiernan MC (2007) Fatigue and activity dependent changes in axonal excitability in amyotrophic lateral sclerosis. J Neurol Neurosurg Psychiatry 78: 1202–1208.
18. Park SB, Lin CSY, Krishnan AV, Goldstein D, Friedlander ML, et al. (2011) Utilizing natural activity to dissect the pathophysiology of acute oxaliplatin-induced neuropathy. Exp Neurol 227: 120–127.
19. Edstrom L, Grimby L (1986) Effect of exercise on the motor unit. Muscle Nerve 9: 104–126.
20. McPhedran AM, Wuerker RB, Henneman E (1965) Properties of motor units in a heterogeneous pale muscle (m. gastrocnemius) of the cat. J Neurophysiol 28: 85–99.
21. McPhedran AM, Wuerker RB, Henneman E (1965) Properties of motor units in a homogeneous red muscle (soleus) of the cat. J Neurophysiol 28: 71–84.
22. Henneman E, Olson CB (1965) Relations between structure and function in the design of skeletal muscles. J Neurophysiol 28: 581–598.
23. Wood SJ, Slater CR (2001) Safety factor at the neuromuscular junction. Prog Neurobiol 64: 393–429.
24. Z'Graggen WJ, Lin CS, Howard RS, Beale RJ, Bostock H (2006) Nerve excitability changes in critical illness polyneuropathy. Brain 129: 2461–2470.
25. Trevillion L, Howells J, Jankelowitz S, Burke D (2004) Axonal excitability measured by tracking twitch contraction force. Muscle Nerve 30: 437–443.
26. Krishnan AV, Lin CSY, Park SB, Kiernan MC (2009) Axonal ion channels from bench to bedside: a translational neuroscience perspective. Prog Neurobiol 89: 288–313.
27. Bostock H, Rothwell J (1997) Latent addition in motor and sensory fibres of human peripheral nerve. J Physiol 498: 277–294.
28. Bostock H, Cikurel K, Burke D (1998) Threshold tracking techniques in the study of human peripheral nerve. Muscle Nerve 21: 137–158.
29. Nodera H, Kaji R (2006) Nerve excitability testing and its clinical application to neuromuscular diseases. Clin Neurophysiol 117: 1902–1916.
30. Kiernan MC, Bostock H (2000) Effects of membrane polarization and ischaemia on the excitability properties of human motor axons. Brain 123: 2542–2551.
31. David G, Modney B, Scappaticci KA, Barrett JN, Barrett EF (1995) Electrical and morphological factors influencing the depolarizing after-potential in rat and lizard myelinated axons. J Physiol 489: 141–157.
32. Deschenes M, Landry P (1980) Axonal branch diameter and spacing of nodes in the terminal arborization of identified thalamic and cortical neurons. Brain Res 191: 538–544.
33. Brigant JL, Mallart A (1982) Presynaptic currents in mouse motor endings J Physiol 333: 619–636.
34. Debanne D, Guerineau NC, Gahwiler BH, Thompson SM (1997) Action-potential propagation gated by an axonal I(A)-like K+ conductance in hippocampus. Nature 389: 286–289.
35. Bellemare F, Woods JJ, Johansson R, Biglandritchie B (1983) Motor-unit discharge rates in maximal voluntary contractions of 3 human muscles. J Neurophysiol 50: 1380–1392.
36. Van Cutsem M, Duchateau J, Hainaut K (1998) Changes in single motor unit behaviour contribute to the increase in contraction speed after dynamic training in humans. J Physiol 513: 295–305.
37. Simpson JA (1969) Terminology of electromyography. Electroencephalogr Clin Neurophysiol 26: 224–226.
38. Kiernan MC, Lin CSY, Burke D (2004) Differences in activity-dependent hyperpolarization in human sensory and motor axons. J Physiol 558: 341–349.
39. Ito M, Oshima T (1965) Electrical behaviour of the motoneurone membrane during intracellularly applied current steps. J Physiol 180: 607–635.
40. Mayer ML, Westbrook GL (1983) A voltage-clamp analysis of inward (anomalous) rectification in mouse spinal sensory ganglion neurones. J Physiol 340: 19–45.
41. Baker M, Bostock H, Grafe P, Martius P (1987) Function and distribution of three types of rectifying channel in rat spinal root myelinated axons. J Physiol 383: 45–67.

42. Soleng AF, Chiu K, Raastad M (2003) Unmyelinated axons in the rat hippocampus hyperpolarize and activate an H current when spike frequency exceeds 1 Hz. J Physiol 552: 459–470.

43. Pape HC (1996) Queer current and pacemaker: the hyperpolarization-activated cation current in neurons. Annual Review of Physiology 58: 299–327.

44. Howells J, Trevillion L, Bostock H, Burke D (2012) The voltage dependence of Ih in human myelinated axons. J Physiol 590: 1625–1640.

45. Howells J, Czesnik D, Trevillion L, Burke D (2013) Excitability and the safety margin in human axons during hyperthermia. J Physiol 591: 3063–3080.

46. Tomlinson S, Burke D, Hanna M, Koltzenburg M, Bostock H (2010) In vivo assessment of HCN channel current (I(h)) in human motor axons. Muscle Nerve 41: 247–256.

47. Bigland-Ritchie B, Johansson R, Lippold O, Woods J (1983) Contractile speed and EMG changes during fatigue of sustained maximal voluntary contractions. J Neurophysiol 50: 313–324.

48. Krishnan AV, Phoon RKS, Pussell BA, Charlesworth JA, Bostock H, et al. (2006) Neuropathy, axonal Na+/K+ pump function and activity-dependent excitability changes in end-stage kidney disease. Clin Neurophysiol 117: 992–999.

49. Sutherland E (2010) The different time course of recovery of human muscle and nerve properties after a sustained maximal voluntary contraction. Sydney: University of New South Wales.

50. Murray JE, Jankelowitz SK (2011) A comparison of the excitability of motor axons innervating the APB and ADM muscles. Clin Neurophysiol 122: 2290–2293.

51. Rakowski RF, Gadsby DC, De Weer P (1989) Stoichiometry and voltage dependence of the sodium pump in voltage-clamped, internally dialyzed squid giant axon. J Gen Physiol 93: 903–941.

52. Morita K, David G, Barrett JN, Barrett EF (1993) Posttetanic hyperpolarization produced by electrogenic Na(+)-K+ pump in lizard axons impaled near their motor terminals. J Neurophysiol 70: 1874–1884.

53. Tasaki I (1939) The electro-saltatory transmission of the nerve impulse and the effect of narcosis upon the nerve fiber. Am J Physiol 127: 211–227.

54. Stämpfli R (1954) Saltatory conduction in nerve. Physiol Rev 34: 101–112.

55. Cappelen Smith C, Kuwabara S, Lin CSY, Mogyoros I, Burke D (2000) Activity dependent hyperpolarization and conduction block in chronic inflammatory demyelinating polyneuropathy. Ann Neurol 48: 826–832.

56. Kaji R, Bostock H, Kohara N, Murase N, Kimura J, et al. (2000) Activity-dependent conduction block in multifocal motor neuropathy. Brain 123: 1602–1611.

18

Fatigue Effect on Low-Frequency Force Fluctuations and Muscular Oscillations during Rhythmic Isometric Contraction

Yen-Ting Lin[1,2], Chia-Hua Kuo[2], Ing-Shiou Hwang[3,4]*

1 Physical Education Office, Asia University, Taichung, Taiwan, 2 Department of Sports Sciences, University of Taipei, Taipei, Taiwan, 3 Department of Physical Therapy, College of Medicine, National Cheng Kung University, Tainan, Taiwan, 4 Institute of Allied Health Sciences, National Cheng Kung University, Tainan, Taiwan

Abstract

Continuous force output containing numerous intermittent force pulses is not completely smooth. By characterizing force fluctuation properties and force pulse metrics, this study investigated adaptive changes in trajectory control, both force-generating capacity and force fluctuations, as fatigue progresses. Sixteen healthy subjects (20–24 years old) completed rhythmic isometric gripping with the non-dominant hand to volitional failure. Before and immediately following the fatigue intervention, we measured the gripping force to couple a 0.5 Hz sinusoidal target in the range of 50–100% maximal voluntary contraction. Dynamic force output was off-line decomposed into 1) an ideal force trajectory spectrally identical to the target rate; and 2) a force pulse trace pertaining to force fluctuations and error-correction attempts. The amplitude of ideal force trajectory regarding to force-generating capacity was more suppressed than that of the force pulse trace with increasing fatigue, which also shifted the force pulse trace to lower frequency bands. Multi-scale entropy analysis revealed that the complexity of the force pulse trace at high time scales increased with fatigue, contrary to the decrease in complexity of the force pulse trace at low time scales. Statistical properties of individual force pulses in the spatial and temporal domains varied with muscular fatigue, concurrent with marked suppression of gamma muscular oscillations (40–60 Hz) in the post-fatigue test. In conclusion, this study first reveals that muscular fatigue impairs the amplitude modulation of force pattern generation more than it affects the amplitude responsiveness of fine-tuning a force trajectory. Besides, motor fatigue results disadvantageously in enhancement of motor noises, simplification of short-term force-tuning strategy, and slow responsiveness to force errors, pertaining to dimensional changes in force fluctuations, scaling properties of force pulse, and muscular oscillation.

Editor: Ramesh Balasubramaniam, University of California, Merced, United States of America

Funding: The authors have no support or funding to report.

Competing Interests: The authors have declared that no competing interests exist.

* E-mail: ishwang@mail.ncku.edu.tw

Introduction

When muscles are exhausted, they cannot generate enough force to achieve a target level because of a reduction in force-generating capacity. Muscular fatigue typically manifests as variations in the amplitude and spectrum of surface electromyograms (EMG); however, myoelectrical manifestations of a fatigued muscle vary with the load characteristics of a fatigue protocol [1,2], such as static versus dynamic contractions [3] and maximal versus submaximal contractions [4,5]. An invariant measure of change in an exhausted contraction appears to be increases in the size of force fluctuations [6,7], traditionally viewed as enhancement of background noises in motor drive [8,9]. Although a larger size of force fluctuations with fatigue progress may impair task quality, how time-dependent structure of force fluctuations varies with fatigue is little understood. The structure of force fluctuations can be indexed with different nonlinear analyses (such as entropy measures, detrended fluctuation analysis, recurrence quantification analysis, and so on), which describe the complexity of force fluctuations by assessing the degree of predictability of fluctuations over a force data stream [10,11,12]. For an un-fatigued muscle, the size and the complexity of force fluctuations are influenced by

separate control processes [10,11]. Increases in the complexity of force fluctuations do not necessarily undermine task quality, but they do reflect the engagement of error corrections. Force tracking with visual feedback results in better tracking congruency, smaller force fluctuations, and greater complexity of force fluctuations than force tracking without visual feedback [13,14]. Also, in aged adults, force fluctuations are greater in size but less complex for constant-force level tasks [15].

Force fluctuations are ascribed to numerous discrete blocks of pulse elements in a force profile [11,16]. The genesis of force pulse elements in a continuous force profile is related to the sampled processes, with which the central nervous system could intermittently approximate the ideal movement against feedback delays in the visuomotor system [17,18]. Several studies have also emphasized the roles of the pulse elements in an additive accuracy control mechanism to remedy trajectory deviations with the feedback or feedforward process [16,19,20]. Force pulse elements are scaled and superimposed onto ideal force trajectory to tune force deviations from a priori standard [21]. A smoother force output with less fluctuation indicates a lower number of error corrections and successful blending of pulse elements [22]. We argue that the

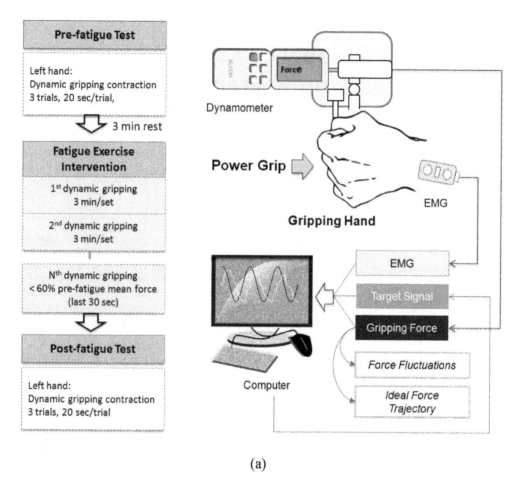

(a)

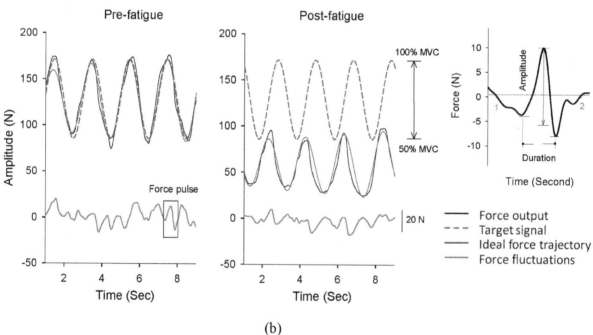

(b)

Figure 1. Experiment procedure, system setup, and data recording. (a) Schematic diagrams of the apparatus and fatigue protocol, (b) Typical recordings of force and target signals in the pre-fatigue and post-fatigue tests. The force signal was decomposed into a ideal force trajectory and a force pulse trace, visibly smaller after fatiguing contraction. Measures of amplitude and duration of a force pulse in the force pulse trace are displayed.

scaling of force pulses co-varies with adaptive changes in force fluctuations with fatigue development, underlying variations in peripherally derived afferent information [23,24,25], lowering of the recruitment threshold of motor units [26,27], and variable firing rates of motoneurons [28], and so on.

The present study investigated fatigue effect on force-generating capacity and force-tuning strategy during rhythmic force-tracking, by characterizing organizational properties of the rhythmic force component of the target rate (ideal force trajectory) and force fluctuations (corrective actions). On account of target constraints to produce the criterion force, rhythmic force-tracking has higher task demand on force-tuning properties than a constant-load contraction [15,29]. Rhythmic force-tracking with specific rate coding for the patterned muscle contraction [30,31] exhibits more frequent and evident force adjustments than static contraction [29]. To our knowledge, research has not been conducted to investigate force-tuning strategies of a muscle following rhythmic fatiguing contraction with the size and the complexity of force fluctuations. Moreover, if responsiveness of force tuning is not fully a corollary of force-generating capacity, motor fatigue could differently impact accuracy and efficiency of force production. Another goal of this study was to link feature changes in force fluctuations with EMG oscillations in a fatigued muscle, as previous studies have shown that beta (13–20 Hz) and gamma (40–60 Hz) cortico-muscular rhythms are crucial for force stabilization during static and rhythmic isometric contraction [32,33,34]. Our main hypotheses were that 1) the fatigue effect would result in differential adaptations in rhythmic force component of the target rate (ideal force trajectory) and force fluctuations (corrective actions); 2) the size, the complexity, and spectral components of the force fluctuations would reduce after fatiguing contraction, and 3) fatigue-related modulation of force fluctuations would concur with suppression of muscular oscillations. The present findings could lend novel insight into the internal coding of motor commands for an exhausted muscle to tune force trajectory during rhythmic isometric contraction.

Methods

Subjects. Sixteen subjects (20–24 years, all males) were convenience samples recruited from the department of the university. The subjects had completed a previous study in our laboratory, so that they were skilled at the rhythmic isometric gripping prior to the experiment. All subjects were self-reported as being right-handed, and none had symptoms or signs of neuromuscular diseases. The research project was approved by an authorized institutional human research review board of the Chung-Shan University Hospital, Taiwan. All subjects signed informed consents before the experiment in accordance with the Declaration of Helsinki.

Experimental procedures. The subjects sat on a chair with their non-dominant (left) hands placed on the touch plate of a force gauge fixed firmly on the test table. The standard position for all subjects was shoulder flexion of 0 degrees, elbow flexion of 90 degrees, and the wrist in the neutral position. The subjects were informed that they would be using the non-dominant hand to complete three 20-second trials of isometric power gripping in a rhythmic manner in the pre-fatigue and post-fatigue tests, conducted prior to and following the fatigue intervention (Fig. 1(a)). The fatigue intervention was intended to cause a remarkable difference in mean force level of rhythmic force output between the pre-fatigue and post-fatigue tests. In the beginning of the experiment, the maximal voluntary contraction of power gripping was predetermined for the non-dominant hand with

visual feedback, by selecting the peak force from three sets of 3-s maximal gripping contractions separated by 3 minutes each.

Following 3 minutes of rest, three trials of the pre-fatigue test were measured with inter-trial intervals of at least 1 minute. After that, the subjects performed the fatiguing protocol, which contained several contraction trials of 3-minute rhythmic isometric power gripping similar to that used in the pre-fatigue test. There was no resting period between the trials in the fatiguing protocol. The fatiguing protocol continued until the mean force output in the last 30 seconds of the last trial was lower than 60% of the mean force level of the pre-fatigue test. Three successive trials of the post-fatigue test, without resting periods, were completed similarly to the pre-fatigue test.

The force-tracking paradigm used in the pre-fatigue test, fatigue exercise intervention, and the post-fatigue test was rhythmic isometric power gripping. The subjects manipulated the position of a manual cursor on a computer monitor, which was linearly proportional to the force exerted by the gripping hand. The subjects performed rhythmic isometric contraction in the range of 50%–100% of maximal gripping force in order to couple the manual cursor with a 0.5 Hz sinusoidal target wave. The target signal moved vertically in a range of 7.2° of visual angle (i.e., 3.6° above and 3.6° below the eye level on the screen). The manual cursor and the target curve were displayed on the computer monitor as on-line visual guidance for force tracking. Prior to the experiment, the subjects were allowed for a few practice trials to get familiar with rhythmic gripping following by a rest period without causing fatigue. In case of motor fatigue, the subjects could not exert sufficient force output to keep with the target trace, especially when the mean force level and range of force modulation were smaller than those of the pre-fatigue condition.

A digital force gauge (sensitivity: 0.01 N, bandwidth = DC-1 kHz, Model: 9820P, AIKOH, Japan) connected to an analog amplifier (Model: PS-30A-1, Entran, UK) was used to measure the gripping force that the subjects exerted on the touch plate. The bipolar surface electrode units (1.1 cm in diameter, gain = 365, CMRR = 102 dB, Imoed Inc., USA) were used to measure the left flexor digitorum superficialis (FDS). The muscle activity of the FDS was recorded by placing the electrode at an oblique angle approximately 4 cm above the wrist on the palpable muscle mass. The target signal, force output, and EMG were sampled at 1 kHz using a custom program on a Labview platform (National Instruments, Austin, TX, USA).

Data processing. Gripping force was down-sampled to 100 Hz in off-line analysis and then conditioned with a low-pass filter (cut-off frequency: 6 Hz) [20], such that physiological tremor in 8–12 Hz was excluded. The exclusion of physiological tremor in 8–12 Hz was because it is an involuntary movement irrelevant to corrective actions. Only force components of lower frequency below 4 Hz could be considered as sensorimotor process for voluntary movement control [15,20,21]. The mean gripping force in an experimental trial was thus obtained by averaging the conditioned gripping force profile in the pre-fatigue and post-fatigue tests. The tracking congruency was assessed with the correlation coefficient between the target trajectory and gripping force profile. Then the force profile was further decomposed into two time series, the ideal force trajectory and the force pulse trace (Fig. 1(b)) [20,35]. The ideal force trajectory was a smooth 0.5 Hz sinusoidal wave that approximated the force profile of rhythmic isometric gripping in amplitude. Therefore, the ideal force trajectory represented an ideal force trajectory with the identical spectral component to target rate. In contrast, the force pulse trace was an irregular component of gripping force and a major source of force fluctuations. Force pulse trace could be obtained by conditioning the force output with a zero-phasing notch filter that passes all frequencies except for a target rate at 0.5 Hz. The transfer function of the notch filter ($H(z)$) in this study was

$$H(Z) = b_0 \frac{(1 - e^{j\omega_0}z^{-1})(1 - e^{-j\omega_0}z^{-1})}{(1 - re^{j\omega_0}z^{-1})(1 - re^{-j\omega_0}z^{-1})}, \quad r = .9975, \quad \omega_0 = \pi/360.$$

We obtained the ideal force trajectory by subtracting the gripping force from the force pulse trace (RMS_{FP}). The amplitudes of the ideal force trajectory profile (RMS_{IF}) and force pulse trace were calculated by root mean square. The amplitude ratio ($R_{IF/FP}$) of the ideal force trajectory to force pulse trace was the RMS value of the ideal force trajectory divided by the RMS of the force pulse trace. $R_{IF/FP}$ estimated the ratio of the regular component of gripping force relative to the irregular component of gripping force.

The spectral distribution of the force pulse trace was calculated with the Welch method. A Hanning window was applied to each artifact-free 2.048-second epoch of the force pulse trace with an overlap of 0.512 seconds. The spectral density was calculated using a fast Fourier transform, and the spectral resolution was 0.02 Hz. Mean frequency and mode frequency were determined from the spectral profile of the force pulse trace. Spectral dispersion of the force pulse trace was defined as the spectral ranges between the 10th and 90th percentiles of the power spectra. We also quantified the complexity variations in a force pulse trace with multi-scale entropy (MSE), or sample entropy (SampEn) across different time scales [36,37]. The calculation of the MSE consisted of three steps. First, obtain the coarse-grained sequences

of down-sampled force pulse trace $\{x(\tau)\} X^{(j)} = 1/n \sum_{i=(j-1)n}^{jn} z_i,$

where $\{z_1, z_2, ..., z_N\}$ is the time series of force pulse trace and τ is the time scale. Next, sample entropy $\{SampEn(m,r,N)^{(\tau)}, \tau = 1,2,...40\}$ for each coarse-grained sequence $\{X(\tau)\}$ were calculated. Sample entropy measures the negative natural logarithm of an estimate of the conditional probability that epochs of length m that match point-wise within a tolerance level (r) also match at the next point. The mathematical formula of sample entropy was

$$SampEn(m,r,N) = \ln\left(\frac{\sum_{i=1}^{N-m} n_i^m}{\sum_{i=1}^{N-m-1} n_i^{m+1}}\right) = \ln\left(\frac{n_n}{n_d}\right), \text{ where } r = 20\% \text{ of}$$

where the standard deviations of $X(\tau)$ and $m = 2$. Finally, the MSE areas in low and high time scales were defined as summation of the SampEn in the time scales 1–5 and 25–40, respectively.

That is, MSE area of low time scale $= \sum_{\tau=1}^{5} SampEn^{(\tau)}$ and

MSE area of high time scale $= \sum_{\tau=25}^{40} SampEn^{(\tau)}$. MSE area has been shown to be robust in measuring the complexity of biological time-series [36,37], with a higher MSE area indicating a noisier structure. The time scale for MSE was 10 ms after down-sampling (100 Hz).

The spatial and temporal parameters of individual force pulses were characterized. Pulse amplitude was defined as the difference between a local maximum and the average value of the two nearest minima (Fig. 1(b)) [20,35]. To exclude insignificant force pulses contributed by random noise, this study defined the threshold pulse amplitude as the upper limit of a 95% confidence interval of the pulse amplitude in the relaxed condition before the fatiguing contraction. Only force pulses exceeding the threshold amplitude were considered meaningful. The pulse duration of these meaningful force pulses was the time between two successive local minima in the force pulse trace. Mean kurtosis and mean

skewness of the pulse amplitude and pulse duration of the tracking trials in the pre-fatigue and post-fatigue tests were averaged.

Band-pass filters were used to condition the EMG of the left FDS muscles (pass band: 1~400 Hz). The RMS values and mean frequencies of the EMG for the FDS muscles were determined in the pre-fatigue and post-fatigue tests. In addition, we estimated the power spectrum of the rectified EMG, as rectification of surface EMG is thought to highlight the spectral peaks that symbolize common oscillatory inputs or the mean firing rate of an active muscle [38–40]. The spectral profiles of rectified EMG of the three trials in the pre-fatigue and post-fatigue tests were averaged and normalized with the mean spectral amplitude to reduce population variability. Spectral peaks in the alpha (8–12 Hz) and gamma (40–60 Hz) bands were obtained from the mean standardized spectral profile of rectified EMG. The power spectra of the un-rectified and rectified EMG were estimated with the Welch method and a fast Fourier transform (Hanning window: 2.048-second epoch with an overlap of 0.512 seconds). The spectral resolution for FDS EMG was 0.244 Hz. Signal processing was completed using a MATLAB script (The Mathworks Inc., Natick, MA, USA).

Statistical analyses. The force variables (ideal force trajectory and force pulse trace) as well as EMG variables of the three trials in the pre-fatigue and post-fatigue tests were averaged for each subject. Hotelling's T^2 statistics and post-hoc analysis with Bonferoni corrections were used to examine the significance of parametric changes due to the fatigue effect, by contrasting tracking outcomes (mean gripping force and tracking congruency), force amplitude variables (RMS_{IF}, RMS_{FP}, and $R_{IF/FP}$), EMG variables (RMS, mean frequency, alpha spectral peak, and gamma spectral peak), spectral features of force pulse trace (mean frequency, mode frequency, and spectral dispersion), complexity of force pulse trace (MSE areas in high and low time scales), temporal force pulse characteristics (pulse duration, duration kurtosis, and duration skewness), and spatial force pulse characteristics (pulse amplitude, amplitude kurtosis, and amplitude skewness) between the pre-fatigue and post-fatigue tests. Pearson's correlation was used to examine the significance of correlation between force pulse metrics and the size (RMS of force pulse trace)/the complexity (MSE areas) of force variability in the pre-fatigue and post-fatigue conditions. Statistical analysis was completed with the SPSS 15.0 statistical package (SPSS Inc., Armonk, NY, USA). The significance level was set at 0.05. Data reported in the texts, figures, and tables are presented as mean ± standard error (SE).

Results

Hotelling's T^2 statistics suggested a fatigue effect on force variables (Wilks's $\Lambda = .075$, $P<.001$). The mean force level was smaller in the post-fatigue test (71.15 ± 3.68 N) than in the pre-fatigue test (119.65 ± 5.04 N)($P<.001$). Namely, mean force level in the post-fatigue test was $59.79 \pm 2.16\%$ of that in the pre-fatigue test. Tracking congruency in the post-fatigue test ($.266 \pm .054$) was markedly smaller than that in the pre-fatigue test ($.757 \pm .028$)($P<.001$). Force measures confirmed failure of the gripping task in the post-fatigue test.

Figure 1(b) contrasts the force profile, ideal force trajectory, and force pulse trace between the pre-fatigue and post-fatigue tests from a typical subject. This plot clearly reveals that the capacity of rhythmic force regulation and mean force level in the post-fatigue test were lower than those in the pre-fatigue test. Table 1 presents the means and standard errors for the amplitudes of ideal force trajectory and force pulse trace, as well as the amplitude ratio of ideal force trajectory to force pulse trace ($R_{IF/FP}$) before and after the fatiguing exercise. Hotelling's T^2 statistic suggested a significant fatigue effect on those force pulse variables (Wilks'$\Lambda = .29$, $P = .001$). RMS values of the ideal force trajectory and force pulse trace were significantly smaller in the post-fatigue test ($P<.001$). It is worth noting that $R_{IF/FP}$ was smaller in the post-fatigue test (pre-fatigue: 5.36 ± 0.18 vs. post-fatigue: 4.35 ± 0.22)($P<.01$), specifying a non-parallel amplitude reduction for the ideal force trajectory and force pulse trace due to fatigue, with greater suppression on the ideal force trajectory than on the force pulse trace.

The left plots in Figure 2 show spectral variations in the force pulse trace from two typical subjects after the fatigue exercise intervention. Hotelling's T^2 statistic showed that spectral features of the force pulse trace were subject to the fatigue effect (Wilks' $\Lambda = 0.280$, $P<.001$). The mean frequency and mode frequency of the force pulse trace in the post-fatigue test were much lower than those in the pre-fatigue test (mean frequency: pre-fatigue: 1.48 ± 0.13 Hz, post-fatigue: 1.21 ± 0.17 Hz)(mode frequency: pre-fatigue: 1.28 ± 0.22 Hz; post-fatigue: 0.78 ± 0.32 Hz)($P<.001$) (Fig. 2, upper right). In addition, the force pulse trace in the post-fatigue test had a wider spectral dispersion than did that in the pre-fatigue test ($P = .024$)(Fig. 2, lower right). Figure 3 shows the results of multi-scale entropy (MSE) analysis to contrast the complexity of the force pulse traces before and after the fatigue intervention. The SampEn curves of the force pulse traces were visibly different for the pre-fatigue and post-fatigue tests (Fig. 3, left). The complexity of the force pulse traces in different time scales were estimated in terms of the area under the SampEn curves. The results of Hotelling T^2 statistics suggested a significant fatigue effect on MSE areas of the low time scale (1–5) and the high time scale (25–40)(Wilks' $\Lambda = 0.370$, $P = .001$), though they were modulated in an opposite manner. The MSE area of the low time scale in the post-fatigue test was smaller (had greater regularity) than that of the pre-fatigue test ($P<.01$), whereas the MSE area of the high time scale in the post-fatigue test was larger (had greater complexity) than that in the pre-fatigue test ($P<.001$)(Fig. 3, right).

Scaling properties of individual force pulses before and after the fatigue intervention exercise are contrasted in Table 2. Spatial scaling of force pulses was subject to the fatigue intervention (Wilks' $\Lambda = .183$, $P<.001$), with a smaller pulse amplitude in the post-fatigue test ($P<.001$). Fatigue intervention did not significantly alter the amplitude kurtosis ($P = .714$) or amplitude skewness of force pulses ($P = .208$). Temporal scaling of force pulses was also subject to the fatigue intervention (Wilks' $\Lambda = .279$,

$P = .001$). The pulse duration was smaller in the post-fatigue test than in the pre-fatigue test ($P<.001$). Moreover, fatigue intervention also led to significant enhancements of duration kurtosis ($P = .001$) and duration skewness ($P = .003$) in the post-fatigue test. Table 3 shows the results of Pearson's correlation between the size of a force pulse and force pulse metrics in the pre-fatigue and post-fatigue tests. In the pre-fatigue test, force pulse RMS was related to pulse amplitude ($r = .935$, $P<.001$). In addition to pulse amplitude ($r = .958$, $P<.001$), force pulse RMS was a function of pulse duration ($r = .576$, $P = .019$) in the post-fatigue test. Table 4 shows Pearson's correlation between the force pulse complexity and statistical properties of the force pulse variables. In the pre-fatigue condition, the MSE area of the force pulse was not related to the statistical properties of the force pulse variables, except for a significant correlation between duration skewness and MSE area in high time scales ($r = .537$, $P = .032$). In the post-fatigue test, however, MSE areas of force pulses in low and high time scales were negatively related to skewness and kurtosis of pulse amplitude ($r = -.499\sim-.699$, $P<.05$).

After the fatigue exercise intervention, the results of Hotelling T^2 statistics suggested a significant fatigue effect on EMG variables (Wilks's $\Lambda = .274$, $P = .002$). Post-hoc analysis suggested that the root mean square of EMG (pre-fatigue: 44.79 ± 5.23 μV; post-fatigue: 14.93 ± 2.4 μV) and mean frequency of un-rectified EMG (pre-fatigue: 56.51 ± 1.91 Hz; post-fatigue: 48.61 ± 2.15 Hz) decreased after the fatigue intervention ($P<.001$). Reductions in the mean frequency and amplitude of FDS EMG suggested a fatigued state of the muscle in the post-fatigue test. Figure 4 contrasts the pooled power spectrum of the rectified EMG and mean spectral peaks of the FDS muscle between the pre-fatigue and post-fatigue tests. Two prominent spectral peaks in the alpha (8–12 Hz) and gamma bands (40–60 Hz) were enhanced with the rectification process (Fig. 4, left). Post-hoc analysis revealed that the standardized amplitude of gamma muscular oscillation in the post-fatigue test (1.29 ± 0.07) was significantly smaller than that in the pre-fatigue test (1.81 ± 0.16)($P = 0.01$)(Fig. 4, right). However, the alpha muscular oscillation was not significantly affected by the fatigue intervention ($P = 0.555$).

Discussion

The designated fatiguing protocol led to task failure, as evidenced with the EMG (reductions in amplitude and mean frequency) and force behavior (declines in mean force level and tracking congruency) variables. We presented several novel findings on fatigue-related modulations of force fluctuations and muscular oscillation. Muscular fatigue impaired the balance between regular and irregular force components ($R_{IF/FP}$), as a result of more pronounced amplitude suppression on the ideal force trajectory than on the force pulse trace. Muscular fatigue altered force-tuning strategies during rhythmic isometric contraction, underlying subsidence in higher spectral components and changes in complexity in force fluctuations. Fatigue also modified statistical properties of force pulse metrics, such that the size and the complexity of force fluctuations were differently represented by scaling of force pulses in the pre-fatigue and post-fatigue tests. The changes in force fluctuation properties co-varied with suppression of gamma muscular oscillation by the fatigue effect.

Fatigue-related variations in ideal force trajectory and force pulse trace

In this study, the force outputs during rhythmic isometric gripping were dichotomized into the ideal force trajectory and force pulse trace. One of the methodological merits of the

Table 1. The contrast of amplitude variables of the ideal force trajectory and force pulse between pre-fatigue and post-fatigue.

Amplitude variable[1]	Pre-fatigue	Post-fatigue
RMS$_{IF}$ (N)[3]	29.57 ± 2.04	15.30 ± 1.89***
RMS$_{FP}$ (N)[4]	5.59 ± 0.40	3.34 ± 0.30***
R$_{IF/FP}$[5]	5.36 ± 0.18	4.35 ± 0.22++
Statistics	$\Lambda = 0.290$, $P = .001$[2]	

[1]Values were presented as mean $\pm$ se.
[2]Post-hoc for pre-fatigue vs. post-fatigue (***: post-fatigue<pre-fatigue, $P<.001$; ++: post-fatigue<pre-fatigue, $P<.01$).
[3]RMS$_{IF}$: root mean square of ideal force trajectory.
[4]RMS$_{FP}$: root mean square of force pulse trace.
[5]R$_{IF/FP}$ denotes amplitude ratio of the ideal force trajectory to force pulse trace.

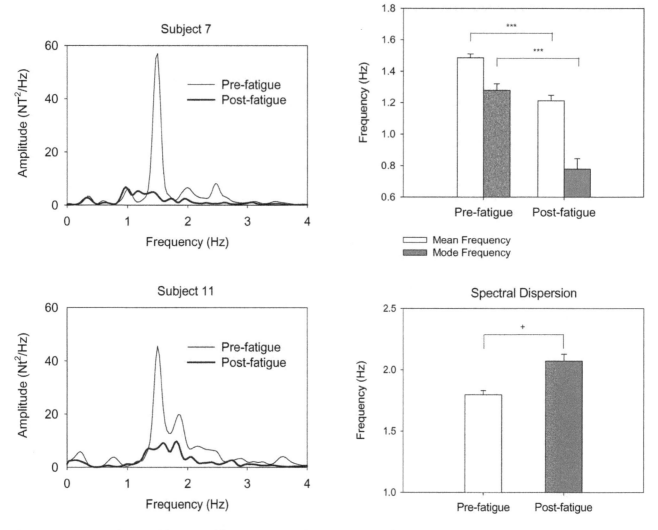

Figure 2. Contrasts of spectral features of force pulse trace between the pre-fatigue and post-fatigue tests. Spectral profiles of force pulse trace for two typical subjects are shown in the left plots. Fatigue effect on mean frequency, mode frequency and spectral dispersion of force pulse trace is summarized in the right plots. (***: Post-fatigue<Pre-fatigue, $P<.001$; †: Post-fatigue>Pre-fatigue, $P<.05$).

dichotomy is to firstly specify imbalance between ideal and irregular force components due to motor fatigue. Akin to kinematic submovements [17,20,35], force pulse trace of irregular nature represents many corrective attempts to remedy tracking mismatches, whereas ideal force trajectory symbolizes a priori force drive to couple rhythmic target movement. Also, ideal force trajectory is reminiscent of force command stabilizing the referent configuration trajectory, and force pulse trace is the emergent pattern complementary to the target goal, according to the lambda-hypothesis [41,42]. Central to the interpretations, we noted reduction in the capacities to produce force in a rhythmic manner and to tune force trajectory for suppression of the ideal force trajectory and force pulse trace in the post-fatigue test (Table 1). A smaller $R_{IF/FP}$ in the post-fatigue test further validated a more pronounced amplitude suppression on the ideal force trajectory due to motor fatigue (pre-fatigue: 5.36±0.18 vs. post-fatigue: 4.35±0.22). The non-parallel inhibition provides novel evidence that force fine-tuning is not a completely corollary of rhythmic force-generating capacity. Ideal pattern generation and error correction of force production were likely to be separated control processes, such that ideal force trajectory and force

fluctuations were differentially affected by motor fatigue. According to the optimal feedback control framework [43], ideal force trajectory resembles to an efference copy of the force command (or open-loop control) used to state estimates of the force-tracking maneuver and force fluctuations reflect the solution to reproduce target kinematic pattern in an optimization process [43,44]. In view of amplitude suppression, the ability to fine-tune force trajectory was less damaged by the fatiguing protocol than the capacity to generate rhythmic force was. Previous studies using static fatigue protocol have shown that fatigue increases in relative force variability [45,46]. Our finding generalized the concept to rhythmic isometric contraction in terms of reduced $R_{IF/FP}$ in the post-fatigue condition, implying the probability to miss the target increases if the same force pattern is planned during fatigue.

Changes in force pulse trace in the complexity and spectral features also lend novel insight into force trajectory control in a fatigued muscle. In the pre-fatigue test, a force pulse trace was composed of stereotypical force pulses with the major power spectrum spanning below 2 Hz (Fig. 2, left) [15,16]. In case of motor fatigue, the force pulse trace was downward modulated to a lower spectral band below 1 Hz (Fig. 2, right). It is known that

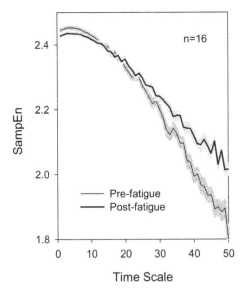

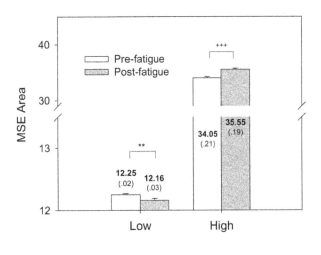

Figure 3. Contrasts of SampEn versus time scales and MSE area between pre-fatigue and post-fatigue tests. Time scale for MSE plot in temporal domain is 10 ms. (**: Post-fatigue<Pre-fatigue, $P<.01$; +++: Post-fatigue>Pre-fatigue, $P<.001$)(SampEn: sample entropy; MSE: multi-scale entropy).

central- or muscular-based perception could be impaired by motor fatigue [47,48].The slower oscillations in the force pulse trace, a biomarker of inability to produce sufficiently frequent corrective responses, was partly attributable to lacking timely feedback of real motor status. Besides, motor fatigue brought about marked complexity changes in force fluctuations (Fig. 3). In a fatigued state, the MSE area at low time scales of 1–5 became smaller, reminiscent of an increase in short-range correlation commonly observed in changed physiological complexity with aging and diseases [49]. An inherent part of transient loss of complexity in the force pulse trace is speculated to be an increase in the number of motoneurons d more than once in a short interval (doublets or triplets) during fatiguing contractions [50], a compensatory mechanism to escalate the central excitatory outflow to offset fatigue-induced increases in peripheral conduction impedance [51,52]. According to the MSE algorithm, brief force events caused by short-term repetitive discharges of motoneurons could be counted as matching each other, when force pulse data were

less coarse-grained at small time scales. The reduction in force fluctuation irregularity at low time scales functionally indicates a short-term simplification of trajectory control. Running counter to that at the low time scales, the enhancement of the MSE area at high time scales (25–40) in the post-fatigue test suggested that the long-range correlation of the force pulse trace were reduced. In terms of MSE area, the complexity increment of long-range force fluctuations seems to overpower the decrease in short-range force fluctuation (Fig. 3, left), comparable with an increase in force irregularity (increase in ApEn) for older adults during a sinusoidal force task [15]. Fatigue-related increase in long-range complexity could result from motor noises following fatigue [11], and additive randomness in force pulse data was mathematically invariant to more coarse-grained averaging using large time scales [36,37]. MSE analysis reveals an opposite trend of force fluctuation complexity in low and high time scales. The fact speaks for interaction of at least two regulatory systems, which operate over a wide range of temporal scales underlying force tuning of a fatigued muscle.

Temporal and spatial scaling of force pulse during fatigued rhythmic isometric gripping

The scaling properties of individual force pulses were also subject to the fatigue effect. In addition to an apparent inhibitory modulation on force pulse (fundamental elements of force output),

Table 2. Hotelling's T^2 statistics for force pulse variables in the pre-fatigue and post-fatigue tests.

Force pulse variable[1]	Pre-fatigue	Post-fatigue
Amplitude (N)	9.48±0.56	4.60±0.45***
Amplitude Kurtosis	2.99±0.09	3.09±0.14
Amplitude Skewness	0.56±0.05	0.63±0.05
Duration (Sec)	0.41±0.01	0.36±0.01***
Duration Kurtosis	0.46±0.07	3.13±0.10++
Duration Skewness	0.46±0.04	0.73±0.04++
Statistics	$\Lambda_{amplitude} = 0.183, P = .000^2$	
	$\Lambda_{duration} = 0.279, P = .001^2$	

[1]Values were presented as mean ± se.
[2]Post-hoc for pre-fatigue vs. post-fatigue (***: post-fatigue<pre-fatigue, $P<.001$; ++: post-fatigue>pre-fatigue, $P<.01$).

Table 3. Pearson's correlation coefficients between the size of force fluctuations and force pulse metrics.

(n = 16)	Pre-fatigue RMS_FP[1]	Post-fatigue RMS_FP[1]
Amplitude	r = .935, P = .000***	r = .958, P = .000***
Duration	r = .211, P = .432	r = .576, P = .019*

[1]RMS_FP represents root mean square of force pulse trace.
*: $P<.05$;
***: $P<.001$.

Rectified EMG Power Spectrum

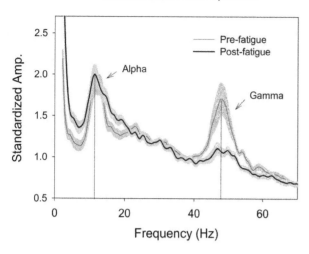 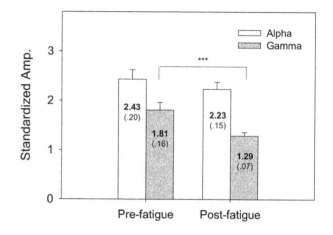

Figure 4. Fatigue effect on pooled spectral profiles and spectral features of the rectified EMG. Two spectral peaks in the 8–12 Hz and 40–60 Hz bands were noted, and the 40–60 Hz spectral peak was visibly suppressed after fatiguing exercise. (***: Post-fatigue<Pre-fatigue, P<.001).

we also note different representations of force fluctuations with force pulse metrics due to fatigue effect. In particular, the size of force fluctuations in the post-fatigue test became a function of pulse duration that was originally independent of force fluctuations for an un-fatigued muscle (Table 3). On account of the use of intermittent visual feedback for a visuomotor task [16,18,19], the fact that temporal scaling became a function of the size of force fluctuations seemingly related to increasing visual mismatches between the force output and target signal following fatigue-induced strength decrease (Fig. 1(b)). The feedback blur could add to extra computational load to remedy tracking deviations [44], such that the size of force fluctuations depended in part on temporal scaling of force pulses during the exhausted force-tracking. Fatigue also altered representation of the complexity of force fluctuations with force pulses (Table 4). The complexity of force pulse traces at high time scales was positively related to the temporal scaling property of force pulses (duration skewness) in the pre-fatigue test; however, the complexity of force pulse traces was negatively related to spatial scaling properties of force pulses (amplitude kurtosis and amplitude skewness) in the post-fatigue test. Despite that no known physiological mechanisms can directly explain such a variation in scaling properties due to fatigue, our findings clearly revealed that the size and complexity of force

fluctuations were more constrained by known statistical properties of force pulse metrics after fatigue.

Fatigue effect on oscillatory muscular activities during rhythmic isometric gripping

In addition to force fluctuation properties, waning of gamma EEG oscillation (40–60 Hz) was noted as a new EMG manifestation of motor fatigue during rhythmic isometric contraction (Fig. 4). Research has shown that corticomuscular coherence in the gamma band manifested with phasic movement [32,54] and repetitive isotonic contraction [34]. For an un-fatigued muscle, gamma synchrony is believed to involve in global alertness to integrate sensory-motor information when a motor task entails temporal control of phasic patterns [32,33,54]. Although we did not directly measure the corticomuscular coherence (rectified EMG-EEG coherence), it was likely that spectral peaks of the rectified EMG could be muscular oscillations in the peripheral part of corticomuscular coherence [32,53]. Consequently, it was not surprising to observe a prominent gamma muscular oscillation in the pre-fatigue test for successful execution of rhythmic isometric gripping. In post-fatigue test, the waning of gamma muscular oscillation indicates a failure of rapid recalibration of the neuromuscular plant demanded by the rhythmic force output,

Table 4. Pearson's correlation coefficients between the complexity of force fluctuations and statistical properties of force pulse.

(n = 16)	Pre-fatigue		Post-fatigue	
	MSE$_{LTS}$[1]	MSE$_{HTS}$[2]	MSE$_{LTS}$[1]	MSE$_{HTS}$[2]
Amplitude Kurtosis	r = −.192, P = .477	r = .011, P = .969	r = −.634, P = .008**	r = −.499, P = .049*
Amplitude Skewness	r = −.462, P = .072	r = .355, P = .177	r = −.699, P = .003**	r = −.518, P = .040*
Duration Kurtosis	r = −.225, P = .402	r = .078, P = .774	r = .099, P = .716	r = .106, P = .695
Duration Skewness	r = −.066, P = .808	r = .537, P = .032	r = −.034, P = .901	r = .010, P = .970

[1]MSE$_{LTS}$ represents multi-scale entropy area of low time scale 1–5.
[2]MSE$_{HTS}$ represents multi-scale entropy area of low time scale 25–40.
*: P<.05;
**: P<.01.

including reduced capacities in force pattern generation and tracking mismatches for rhythmic contraction. Another prominent muscular oscillation during rhythmic isometric gripping was in the alpha band (8–12 Hz), which could be physiological/force tremor [1,2] or coherent modulation of motor unit discharge during quasi-sinusoidal isometric contraction [55]. However, alpha muscular oscillation is not susceptible to the fatigue effect, when EMG amplitude was normalized.

Some methodological considerations

First, contrary to a focused definition of muscle fatigue by quantifying the decline in maximal force capacity [56,57], the present study used a non-classical fatigue measurement to characterize and force generation pattern and force fluctuations at the moment of task failure. Hence, more exactly, changes in force behavior identified in this study reflect physiological mechanisms associated with inability of continuing force-tracking maneuver [57]. Next, because the subjects failed to keep in line with the target signal in the post-fatigue trials, fatigue-related changes in force behavior might be affected by feedback blur that added to extra computational load on the control of force accuracy during exhausted tracking [44]. Ideally, to specify strength decrement, the target signal should be timely adjusted to force performance for feedback accuracy. In practice, it was technically difficult to display optimal target trace based on prediction of varying fatigue states across individuals. Finally, this study required to produce force oscillations up to 100% MVC, which might exhaust the subjects and biased force measures in the pre-

fatigue trials. However, we noted that almost all the subjects could successfully achieve the target goal, because tentative maximal effort during rhythmic force-tracking was less arduous than MVC that was determined by averaging 3-second sustained maximal isometric contraction.

Conclusions

The present study adds to the increasing body of literature on force control in a fatigued muscle by characterizing force fluctuation properties and muscular oscillation. We firstly revealed that motor fatigue led to more amplitude suppression on ideal force pattern than on force fluctuations. Motor fatigue also results in structural changes in force fluctuations due to rescaling of force pulses in the temporal and spatial domains. A spectral shift of the force fluctuations to lower frequency bands and complexity changes in force fluctuations suggest that a fatigued neuromuscular plant with enhanced motor noises inclines to use a simplified force-tuning strategy, so that the plant is not responsive to rapid trajectory deviations for rhythmic force outputs. Suppression of 40–60 Hz muscular oscillation is likely the source of the characteristic changes in force behaviors, underlying lack of a sensible motor drive to produce rhythmic force output.

Author Contributions

Conceived and designed the experiments: YTL CHK ISH. Performed the experiments: YTL. Analyzed the data: YTL ISH. Contributed reagents/materials/analysis tools: YTL ISH. Wrote the paper: YTL ISH.

References

1. Huang CT, Hwang IS, Huang CC, Young MS (2006) Exertion dependent alternations in force fluctuations and limb acceleration during sustained fatiguing contraction. Eur J Appl Physiol 97: 362–371.
2. Huang CT, Huang CC, Young MS, Hwang IS (2007) Age effect on fatigue-induced limb acceleration as a consequence of high-level sustained submaximal contraction. Eur J Appl Physiol 100: 675–683.
3. Masuda K, Masuda T, Sadoyama T, Inaki M, Katsuta S (1999) Changes in surface EMG parameters during static and dynamic fatiguing contractions. J Electromyogr Kinesiol 9: 39–46.
4. Mottram CJ, Jakobi JM, Semmler JG, Enoka RM (2005) Motor-unit activity differs with load type during a fatiguing contraction. J Neurophysiol 93: 1381–1392.
5. Taylor JL, Gandevia SC (2008) A comparison of central aspects of fatigue in submaximal and maximal voluntary contractions. J Appl Physiol 104: 542–550.
6. Contessa P, Adam A, De Luca CJ (2009) Motor unit control and force fluctuation during fatigue. J Appl Physiol 107: 235–243.
7. Missenard O, Mottet D, Perrey S (2009) Factors responsible for force steadiness impairment with fatigue. Muscle Nerve 40: 1019–1032.
8. Meyer DE, Abrams RA, Kornblum S, Wright CE, Smith JE (1988) Optimality in human motor performance: ideal control of rapid aimed movements. Psychol Rev 95: 340–370.
9. Schmidt RA, Zelaznik H, Hawkins B, Frank JS, Quinn JT Jr (1979) Motor-output variability: a theory for the accuracy of rapid motor acts. Psychol Rev 47: 415–451.
10. Slifkin AB, Newell KM (1999) Noise, information transmission, and force variability. J Exp Psychol Hum Percept Perform 25: 837–851.
11. Slifkin AB, Newell KM (2000) Variability and noise in continuous force production. J Mot Behav 32: 141–150.
12. Li K, Marquardt TL, Li ZM (2013) Removal of visual feedback lowers structural variability of inter-digit force coordination during sustained precision pinch. Neurosci Lett 545: 1–5.
13. Jordan K, Newell KM (2004) Task goal and grip force dynamics. Exp Brain Res 156: 451–457.
14. Kuznetsov NA, Riley MA (2010) Spatial resolution of visual feedback affects variability and structure of isometric force. Neurosci Lett 470: 121–125.
15. Vaillancourt DE, Newell KM (2003) Aging and the time and frequency structure of force output variability. J Appl Physiol 94: 903–912.
16. Sosnoff JJ, Newell KM (2005) Intermittency of visual information and the frequency of rhythmical force production. J Mot Behav 37: 325–334.
17. Miall RC, Weir DJ, Stein JF (1993) Intermittency in human manual tracking tasks. J Mot Behav 25: 53–63.
18. Navas F, Stark L (1968) Sampling or intermittency in hand control system dynamics. Biophys J 8: 252–302.
19. Slifkin AB, Vaillancourt DE, Newell KM (2000) Intermittency in the control of continuous force production. J Neurophysiol 84: 1708–1718.
20. Pasalar S, Roitman AV, Ebner TJ (2005) Effects of speeds and force fields on submovements during circular manual tracking in humans. Exp Brain Res 163: 214–25.
21. Selen LP, van Dieën JH, Beek PJ (2006) Impedance modulation and feedback corrections in tracking targets of variable size and frequency. J Neurophysiol 96: 2750–2759.
22. Dipietro L, Krebs HI, Fasoli SE, Volpe BT, Hogan N (2009) Submovement changes characterize generalization of motor recovery after stroke. Cortex 45: 318–324.
23. Taylor JL, Butler JE, Gandevia SC (2000) Changes in muscle afferents, motoneurons and motor drive during muscular fatigue. Eur J Appl Physiol 83: 106–115.
24. Gandevia SC (2001) Spinal and supraspinal factors in human muscular fatigue. Physiol Rev 81: 1725–1789.
25. Allen TJ, Leung M, Proske U (2010) The effect of fatigue from exercise on human limb position sense. J Physiol 588: 1369–1377.
26. Carpentier A, Duchateau J, Hainaut K (2001) Motor unit behaviour and contractile changes during fatigue in the human first dorsal interosseus. J Physiol (London) 534: 903–912.
27. Vila-Chã C, Falla D, Correia MV, Farina D (2012) Adjustments in motor unit properties during fatiguing contractions after training. Med Sci Sports Exerc 44: 616–624.
28. Westad C, Westgaard RH, De Luca CJ (2003) Motor unit recruitment and derecruitment induced by brief increase in contraction amplitude of the human trapezius muscle. J Physiol (London) 552: 645–656.
29. Chen YC, Lin YT, Huang CT, Shih GL, Yang ZR, et al. (2013) Trajectory adjustments underlying task-specific intermittent force behaviors and muscular rhythms. PloS One 8(9): e74273.
30. Iyer MB, Christakos CN, Ghez C (1994) Coherent modulations of human motor unit discharges during quasi-sinusoidal isometric muscle contractions. Neurosci Lett 170(1): 94–8.
31. Sosnoff JJ, Vaillancourt DE, Larsson L, Newell KM (2005) Coherence of EMG activity and single motor unit discharge patterns in human rhythmical force production. Behav Brain Res 158: 301–310.
32. Andrykiewicz A, Patino L, Naranjo JR, Witte M, Hepp-Reymond MC, et al. (2007) Corticomuscular synchronization with small and large dynamic force output. BMC Neurosci 8: 101.
33. Gwin JT, Ferris DP (2012) Beta- and gamma-range human lower limb corticomuscular coherence. Front Hum Neurosci 6: 258.
34. Muthukumaraswamy SD (2010) Functional properties of human primary motor cortex gamma oscillations. J Neurophysiol 104: 2873–2885.

35. Roitman AV, Massaquoi SG, Takahashi K, Ebner TJ (2004) Kinematic analysis of manual tracking in monkeys: characterization of movement intermittencies during a circular tracking task. J Neurophysiol 91: 901–911.

36. Costa M, Goldberger AL, Peng CK (2002) Multiscale entropy analysis of complex physiologic time series. Phys Rev Lett 89: 068102.

37. Costa M, Priplata AA, Lipsitz LA, Wu Z, Huang NE, et al. (2007) Noise and poise: Enhancement of postural complexity in the elderly with a stochastic-resonance-based therapy. Europhys Lett 77: 68008.

38. Boonstra TW, Breakspear M (2012) Neural mechanisms of intermuscular coherence: implications for the rectification of surface electromyography. J Neurophysiol 107: 796–807.

39. Myers LJ, Lowery M, O'Malley M, Vaughan CL, Heneghan C, et al. (2003) Rectification and non-linear pre-processing of EMG signals for cortico-muscular analysis. J Neurosci Methods 124: 157–165.

40. Stegeman DF, van de Ven WJ, van Elswijk GA, Oostenveld R, Kleine BU (2010) The alpha-motoneuron pool as transmitter of rhythmicities in cortical motor drive. Clin Neurophysiol 121: 1633–1642.

41. Feldman AG, Ostry DJ, Levin MF, Gribble PL, Mitnitski AB (1998) Recent tests of the equilibrium-point hypothesis (lambda model). Motor Control 2: 189–205

42. Singh T, Vardahan SK, Zatsiorsky VM, Latash ML (2010) Adaptive increase in force variance during fatigue in tasks with low redundancy. Neurosci Lett 485: 204–207.

43. Diedrichsen J, Shadmehr R, Ivry RB (2010) The coordination of movement: optimal feedback control and beyond. Trends Cogn Sci 14(1): 31–39.

44. Bays PM, Wolpert DM (2007) Computational principles of sensorimotor control that minimize uncertainty and variability. J Physiol 578(Pt 2): 387–96.

45. Bedrov YA, Dick OE, Romanov SP (2007) Role of signal-dependent noise during maintenance of isometric force. Biosystems 89: 50–57

46. Missenard O, Mottet D, Perrey S (2008) Muscular fatigue increases signal-dependent noise during isometric force production. Neurosci Lett 437: 154–157.

47. Jones LA (1995) The senses of effort and force during fatiguing contractions. Adv Exp Med Biol 384: 305–313.

48. Park WH, Leonard CT, Li S (2007) Perception of finger forces within the hand after index finger fatiguing exercise. Exp Brain Res 182: 169–177.

49. Goldberger AL, Peng CK, Lipsitz LA (2002) What is physiologic complexity and how does it change with aging and disease? Neurobiol Aging 23(1): 23–6.

50. Desmedt JE, Godaux E (1978) Ballistic contractions in fast or slow human muscles: discharge patterns of single motor units. J Physiol (London) 285: 185–196.

51. Andersen B, Felding UA, Krarup C (2012) Increased probability of repetitive spinal motoneuron activation by transcranial magnetic stimulation after muscular fatigue in healthy subjects. J Appl Physiol 112: 832–840.

52. Z'Graggen WJ, Humm AM, Durisch N, Magistris MR, Rösler KM (2005) Repetitive spinal motor neuron discharges following single transcranial magnetic stimuli: a quantitative study. Clin Neurophysiol 116: 1628–1637.

53. Schoffelen JM, Poort J, Oostenveld R, Fries P (2011) Selective movement preparation is subserved by selective increases in corticomuscular gamma-band coherence. J Neurosci 31: 6750–6758.

54. Omlor W, Patino L, Hepp-Reymond MC, Kristeva R (2007) Gamma-range corticomuscular coherence during dynamic force output. Neuroimage 34: 1191–1198.

55. Iyer MB, Christakos CN, Ghez C (1994) Coherent modulations of human motor unit discharges during quasi-sinusoidal isometric muscle contractions. Neurosci Lett 170: 94–98.

56. Househam E, McAuley J, Charles T, Lightfoot T, Swash M (2004) Analysis of force profile during a maximum voluntary isometric contraction task. Muscle Nerve 29: 401–408.

57. Enoka RM, Duchateau J (2008) Muscle fatigue: what, why and how it influences muscle function. J Physiol 586: 11–23.

19

The Single-Bout Forearm Critical Force Test: A New Method to Establish Forearm Aerobic Metabolic Exercise Intensity and Capacity

J. Mikhail Kellawan, Michael E. Tschakovsky*

School of Kinesiology and Health Studies, Queen's University, Kingston, Ontario, Canada

Abstract

No non-invasive test exists for forearm exercise that allows identification of power-time relationship parameters (W', critical power) and thereby identification of the heavy-severe exercise intensity boundary and scaling of aerobic metabolic exercise intensity. The aim of this study was to develop a maximal effort handgrip exercise test to estimate forearm critical force (fCF; force analog of power) and establish its repeatability and validity. Ten healthy males (20–43 years) completed two maximal effort rhythmic handgrip exercise tests (repeated maximal voluntary contractions (MVC); 1 s contraction-2 s relaxation for 600 s) on separate days. Exercise intensity was quantified via peak contraction force and contraction impulse. There was no systematic difference between test 1 and 2 for $fCF_{peak\ force}$ (p = 0.11) or $fCF_{impulse}$ (p = 0.76). Typical error was small for both $fCF_{peak\ force}$ (15.3 N, 5.5%) and $fCF_{impulse}$ (15.7 N·s, 6.8%), and test re-test correlations were strong ($fCF_{peak\ force}$, r = 0.91, ICC = 0.94, p<0.01; $fCF_{impulse}$, r = 0.92, ICC = 0.95, p<0.01). Seven of ten subjects also completed time-to-exhaustion tests (TTE) at target contraction force equal to $10\% < fCF_{peak\ force}$ and $10\% > fCF_{peak\ force}$. TTE predicted by W' showed good agreement with actual TTE during the TTE tests (r = 0.97, ICC = 0.97, P<0.01; typical error 0.98 min, 12%; regression fit slope = 0.99 and y intercept not different from 0, p = 0.31). MVC did not predict $fCF_{peak\ force}$ (p = 0.37), $fCF_{impulse}$ (p = 0.49) or W' (p = 0.15). In conclusion, the poor relationship between MVC and fCF or W' illustrates the serious limitation of MVC in identifying metabolism-based exercise intensity zones. The maximal effort handgrip exercise test provides repeatable and valid estimates of fCF and should be used to normalize forearm aerobic metabolic exercise intensity instead of MVC.

Editor: Stephen E. Alway, West Virginia University School of Medicine, United States of America

Funding: M.E. Tschakovsky was funded by Natural Sciences and Engineering Council of Canada (NSERC) Discovery Grant 250367- 06, Canada Foundation for Innovation and Ontario Innovation Trust Infrastructure Grants, Queen's University Chancellor's Research Award. J. Mikhail Kellawan was funded by the Ontario Graduate Scholarship, the Ontario Graduate Scholarship in Science and Technology, and the R.S. McLaughlin Fellowship. The funders had no role in study design, data collection and analysis, decision to publish, or preparation of the manuscript.

Competing Interests: The authors have declared that no competing interests exist.

* E-mail: mt29@queensu.ca

Introduction

The forearm handgrip exercise model is an important model for investigation of factors affecting, and mechanisms determining, O_2 supply matching of exercising muscle O_2 demand [1–3]. This is because such experiments are at best difficult, or at worst impossible, to perform in other exercise modalities. Furthermore, the forearm musculature has specific relevance for occupational settings and activities of daily living. In large muscle mass exercise models, non-invasive gas exchange can be used to identify ventilatory threshold and maximal oxygen uptake which can readily identify aerobic metabolic capacity, aerobic metabolic exercise intensity domains and the impact of interventions on these. Unfortunately there is currently no non-invasive exercise test that can provide this for the forearm handgrip exercise model.

Forearm exercise intensity is typically identified based on % of an individual's maximum voluntary contraction (MVC) [2–4]. This is somewhat surprising since it has been well-established that %MVC is not related to metabolic exercise intensity domains [5,6]. For example, Kent-Braun et al. [6] demonstrated that during progressive %MVC increases in dorsiflexion exercise the % MVC at which transitions across metabolic domains occur varied

considerably between individuals. Saugen et al. [5] found marked between-subject differences in both time course and magnitude of PCr and pH changes during 40% MVC exercise in otherwise similar subjects.

A potential alternative approach would be to identify what has been traditionally referred to as the critical power (CP) which is the maximal power output that still results in a metabolic steady state characterized by a plateau in $\dot{V}O_2$ and in inorganic phosphate [7–9]. In exercise above CP, exhaustion is precipitated by progressive fatigue and failure to stabilize metabolic state which may in part reflect depletion of a fixed anaerobic energy reserve, and likely also reflects the net effect of factors determining muscle force production for a given motor drive (i.e. factors determining muscle fatigue). The resulting fixed amount of work that can be performed above CP is termed W'. In exercise just below CP, exhaustion is precipitated by progressive fatigue despite a stable metabolic state. The stabilizing of PCr below but not above CP and the sensitivity of CP to manipulations of O_2 delivery (increased with hyperoxia and decreased with hypoxia) indicate that CP is the maximal exercise intensity at which aerobic ATP production can completely match ATP demand [10–12]. These characteristics speak to the potential for CP as a means of

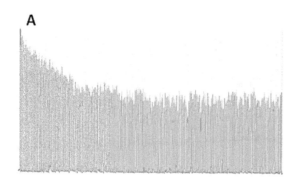

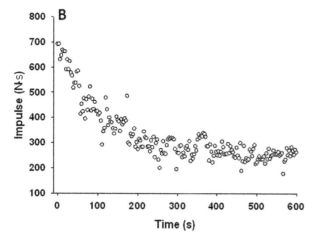

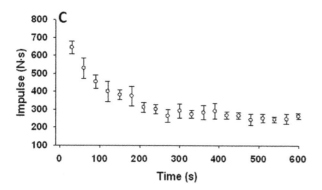

Figure 1. Force output during a 10 min maximal effort handgrip exercise test in a representative subject. Panel A: Raw force trace output **Panel B:** Impulse force of contraction plotted for all contractions during the test. **Panel C:** Impulse force averaged into 30 s time bins. Error bars indicate the contraction-to-contraction variability within each 30 s time bin.

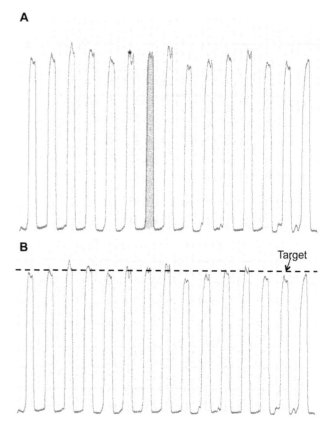

Figure 2. Force tracings from a representative subject. Panel A: Raw force trace depicting the data points used for calculation of the peak force (single *) and force impulse (shaded grey area) **Panel B:** Raw force trace during constant intensity handgrip exercise at target force of 10%>$fCF_{peak\ force}$. Arrow indicates first of three consecutive contractions where target force was not achieved, and represents the time at which exhaustion occurred.

quantifying muscle aerobic metabolic function, identifying aerobic exercise intensity domains, and assessing the impact of interventions on these in the forearm exercise model.

Recently, Burnley [13] validated a single bout, all-out intermittent isometric quadriceps contraction test to estimate CP quantified as knee extensor torque analog of CP. However, findings in this model cannot be assumed to apply to other small muscle mass exercise models. Accordingly, we have developed a maximal effort rhythmic isometric handgrip exercise test to estimate forearm critical intensity (fCF; force analog of CP). Such a test would allow both the identification of exercise intensity in terms of a measure of aerobic metabolic capacity, and the

quantification of cross-sectional and both acute and chronic longitudinal intervention effects on said aerobic capacity. The aim of our study was to determine the repeatability and validity of the fCP estimated from this test. A secondary aim was to determine to what extent MVC was related to fCF and W'.

We hypothesized that fCF as quantified by the plateau in exercise intensity in the last 30 s of a 10 min maximal effort rhythmic isometric handgrip exercise test would demonstrate good between-day test-retest repeatability. Furthermore, we hypothesized that this exercise fCF plateau would be a valid representation of CP as reflected by a good agreement between time to exhaustion (TTE) during constant intensity exercise above fCF and TTE predicted for that exercise intensity based on the W' estimated from the maximal effort test. Finally, we hypothesized that MVC would not be related to either fCF or W'.

Materials and Methods

Subjects

Ten healthy recreationally active males (20–43 years) volunteered to participate in the study.

Ethics Statement

After receiving a complete verbal and written description of the experimental protocol and potential risks, each subject provided

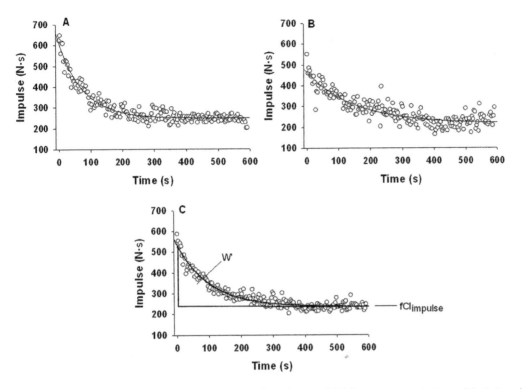

Figure 3. Curve fitting approach to determining fCF$_{impulse}$ and W′ for a representative subject. Panel A: Test 1 plot of contraction impulses with line of best fit. **Panel B:** Test 2 plot of contraction impulses with line of best fit. **Panel C:** Average of Test 1 and Test 2, showing line of best fit, the fCF$_{impulse}$, and the area between fCF$_{impulse}$ and the line of best fit of the average contraction impulse which is W′.

signed consent to the experimental procedures that were approved by the Queen's University Health Sciences Research Ethics Board (HSREB) in accordance with the terms of the Declaration of Helsinki on research ethics.

Experimental Design

All subjects experienced an initial familiarization visit. This was followed by two experimental visits separated by a minimum of 48 hours in which the subjects performed maximal effort rhythmic isometric handgrip exercise (i.e. fCF) tests. The first of these visits was within 24 hrs of the familiarization visit (visit details below). Seven subjects completed two additional visits separated by at least 24 hrs involving rhythmic handgrip exercise tests to exhaustion at a target intensity equal to 10% above fCF quantified as peak force (fCF$_{peak\ force}$) or to a maximum of 20 min at 10% below fCF$_{peak\ force}$ based on the higher of the two fCF$_{peak\ force}$ estimates. All experimental sessions were conducted in a temperature-controlled laboratory (20–22°C) after a minimum of 2 hrs post-prandial and 12 hrs of abstaining from exercise and caffeine.

Familiarization Trials

Familiarization trials were ~30 min long. They involved having the participant perform maximal contractions at 1 s contraction to 2 s relaxation work cycle for three minutes at a time in order to become familiar with maintaining contraction intensity for 1 s based on visual feedback of continuously displayed force output (Powerlab, ADInstruments, Sydney, Australia) and audio and visual cues from a metronome.

Maximal Effort Rhythmic Isometric Forearm Handgrip Critical Intensity Test (fCF)

Upon arrival at the laboratory, subjects lay supine with the experimental arm (left) extended 90° at heart level as previously described [14]. After a period of acclimatization (~5–10 min) subjects performed 3 maximal voluntary contraction (MVC) efforts separated by 1 minute. The highest of these was identified as the target contraction force for the maximal effort test. Data collection began with an initial 2 min period of quiet rest, followed by 10 min of rhythmic handgrip maximal voluntary contractions (1 s contraction to 2 s relaxation duty cycle). The 10 min duration of the maximal effort test was established during prior pilot work using a 10 min duration test in which it was observed that, while tests consistently resulted in subjects reaching a plateau by the last of the 10 min, some subjects did not reach a plateau prior to this time. Therefore 10 min was used for this duty cycle. It should be noted that the duration of the test would be expected to decrease with a higher contraction/relaxation duty cycle as the total work performed per unit time would be increased. Likewise it would be expected to increase with a lower contraction/relaxation duty cycle. Subjects observed their force output continuously displayed on a computer screen (Powerlab, ADInstruments, Sydney, Australia) (Fig. 1A) and attempted to reach their maximum force on every contraction. Subjects received constant verbal encouragement and coaching by a research assistant to achieve a "square wave" during each maximal voluntary contraction and to engage only the muscles of the forearm.

Time-to-exhaustion Above and Below fCF$_{impulse}$ Estimate

The constant intensity rhythmic handgrip exercise trials were performed at the same duty cycle as the maximal effort fCF test. The target force equal to 10% above or 10% below fCF$_{peak\ force}$

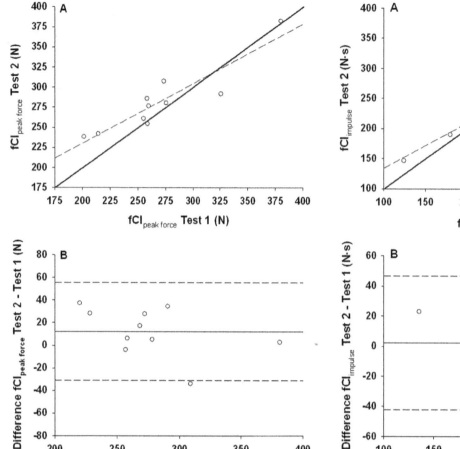

Figure 4. Test-retest correlations of fCF_{peak force}. **Panel A:** fCF as peak force. Line of identity is shown as a solid line and the fitted regression as a dashed line. **Panel B:** Bland-Altman plot of fCF_{peak force}. Mean difference between test 1 and test 2 (bias; solid line) ±43.2 N 95% limits of agreement (dashed lines).

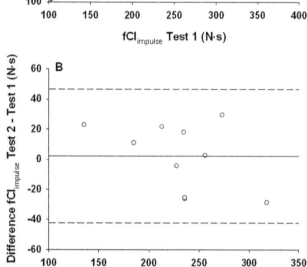

Figure 5. Test-retest correlations of fCF_{impulse}. **Panel A:** fCF as force impulse. Line of identity is shown as a solid line and the fitted regression as a dashed line. **Panel B:** Bland-Altman plot of fCF_{impulse}. Mean difference between test 1 and test 2 (bias; solid line). ±44.5 N·s 95% limits of agreement (dashed lines).

was identified on the computer display screen with a target line. Time-to-exhaustion (TTE) was identified as the time of the first of three consecutive contraction efforts where the subject was unable to achieve the target force despite strong encouragement (Fig. 2B). All participants were stopped if they reached 20 min of exercise.

Data Acquisition and Analysis

Handgrip force was obtained using an electronic handgrip dynamometer (ADInstruments, Sydney, Australia) connected to a data acquisition system sampling at 200 Hz (Powerlab, ADInstruments, Sydney, Australia) and recorded on a personal computer. For each contraction during a maximal effort test, we quantified both the peak contraction force and the integral of the force tracing (Impulse; see Fig. 2A).

To determine the fCF_{peak force} and the fCF_{impulse} estimate for each test we obtained a line of best fit (LBF) for a 3 parameter exponential decay function ($f = y0 + a \cdot \exp^{(-bx)}$) fit to the plot of contraction impulse vs. time and contraction peak force vs. time (Sigmaplot 12.0 curve fit software; see Fig. 3 A). The last 30 s of the curve fit was used to quantify the fCF_{impulse} and the fCF_{peak force}. To quantify the W' for each subject we averaged the two maximal effort tests to obtain a single plot of contraction impulse

vs. time. We then fit this with the same 3 parameter decay function and quantified fCF_{impulse} from the last 30 s of the curve fit. W' was then determined by calculating the contraction impulse in excess of the fCF_{impulse} (EI_{fCF Test}) for each contraction

$$EI_{fCF\ Test} = LBF\ contraction\ impulse f - CF_{impulse} \quad (1)$$

and then calculating the sum of these (see Fig. 3C). To obtain a subject's predicted TTE based on this W', we first quantified the excess impulse for each contraction occurring during the constant supra-fCF_{impulse} intensity exercise test (EI_{Constant Intensity Test})

$$EI_{Constant\ Intensity\ Test} = contraction\ impulse f - CF_{impulse} \quad (2)$$

and then calculated the average of these (AEI_{Constant Intensity Test}). Since a contraction occurred every 3 seconds, a given contraction's EI_{Constant Intensity Test} would contribute to depletion of W' every 3 seconds. Therefore we could calculate the predicted TTE (min)

$$TTE\ (min) = W'/AEI_{Constant\ Intensity\ Test} \cdot 3\ s \cdot 1\ min/60\ s. \quad (3)$$

Table 1. Forearm critical intensity peak force (fCF$_{peak\ force}$) and its test-retest repeatability.

Subject	fCF$_{peak\ force}$ Test 1 (N)	fCF$_{peak\ force}$ Test 2 (N)	fCF$_{peak\ force}$ Mean (N)	SD (N)	Difference Score Test 2–Test 1 (N)	CV (%)
1	259.4	276.7	268.1	12.2	17.3	4.6
2	258.4	254.7	256.6	2.6	−3.7	1.0
3	201.1	238.5	219.8	26.5	37.5	12.0
4	213.9	242.2	228.1	20.0	28.2	8.7
5	379.8	382.8	381.3	2.1	2.9	0.5
6	275.3	280.6	277.9	3.7	5.3	1.3
7	254.8	261.1	258.0	4.5	6.3	1.7
8	273.2	307.7	290.4	24.4	34.5	8.4
9	258.0	285.9	271.9	19.7	27.9	7.2
10	325.6	291.9	308.7	23.8	−33.7	7.7
Mean	270.0	282.2	276.1	14.0	12.2	5.5
(SD)	(51.3)	(41.7)	(45.5)	(10)	(21.6)	–

CV – coefficient of variation. The "mean" CV is the typical error as a % of the grand mean.

Statistical Analysis

Repeatability of the fCF test was quantified as follows. First, a paired-t test was conducted to detect if there was a systematic difference between test 1 and test 2 for each of fCF$_{peak\ force}$ and fCF$_{impulse}$. Second, the standard error of measurement or typical error (the standard deviation (SD) of difference in scores/$\sqrt{2}$) expressed as absolute and as % of the grand mean (termed the coefficient of variation) was used in conjunction with the 95% limits of agreement (SD of the difference in scores multiplied by $\pm$ t$_{0.95,\ degrees\ of\ freedom}$) to assess the magnitude by which test 1 and 2 typically differ [15,16]. Finally, Pearson product and intra-class correlation coefficients (test 1 vs. test 2) were determined as a means of assessing how well the rank order of individuals was maintained between trials [16]. The same analyses were used to assess agreement between predicted and actual TTE. Simple linear regression was used to determine the strength of the relationship between MVC and each of fCF$_{impulse}$, fCF$_{peak\ force}$ and W', where all parameters were plotted as the average of the two tests for each subject. Data are expressed as mean $\pm$ standard deviation (SD) unless otherwise indicated. Significance was set at p$\leq$0.05.

Results

Force Profile of fCF Test

All subjects were able to complete the 10 min fCF test. The force decay to a plateau typical of all subjects is represented by the response of a subject in Fig. 1A and B. Within each trial, subjects reached the onset of a plateau somewhere between 420–540 s (Fig. 1C).

Table 2. Forearm critical intensity impulse (fCF$_{impulse}$) and its test-retest repeatability.

Subject	fCF$_{impulse}$ Test 1 (N)	fCF$_{impulse}$ Test 2 (N)	fCF$_{impulse}$ Mean (N)	SD (N)	Difference Score Test 2–Test 1 (N)	CV (%)
1	201.7	223.5	212.6	15.4	21.8	7.2
2	248.6	222.4	235.5	18.5	−26.2	7.9
3	179.3	190.3	184.8	7.8	11.1	4.2
4	123.8	146.8	135.3	16.3	23.0	12.0
5	258.0	287.6	272.8	20.9	29.6	7.7
6	254.6	257.4	256.0	1.9	2.7	0.8
7	229.5	225.3	227.4	2.9	−4.1	1.3
8	225.4	243.5	234.5	12.8	18.1	5.5
9	248.2	222.9	235.5	17.9	−25.3	7.6
10	331.9	303.3	317.6	20.2	−28.6	6.4
Mean	230.1	232.3	231.2	13.5	2.2	6.8
(SD)	(54.9)	(45.0)	(48.9)	(7.0)	(22.2)	–

CV – coefficient of variation. The "mean" CV is the typical error as a % of the grand mean.

Table 3. Individual W′ estimated from maximal effort test, and average contraction impulse above fCF$_{impulse}$ in the constant intensity exercise tests where subjects exercised above fCF$_{impulse}$.

Subject # - Constant Intensity Test	W′ (N+s)	fCF$_{impulse}$ (N+s)	Impulse in Excess of fCF$_{impulse}$ (N+s)	Impulse in Excess of fCF$_{impulse}$ (%)
1 – Above fCF$_{impulse}$	6277	212.9	28.1	13.2
2 – Above fCF$_{impulse}$	10053	236.9	99.0	42.8
3 – Above fCF$_{impulse}$	5477	186.4	28.4	15.2
4 – Above fCF$_{impulse}$	10551	138.6	86.7	62.6
5 – Below fCF$_{impulse}$	6133	276.0	114.9	41.6
5 – Above fCF$_{impulse}$	6133	276.0	57.3	20.8
6 – Above fCF$_{impulse}$	11815	256.6	44.4	17.3
7 – Above fCF$_{impulse}$	6075	231.2	20.7	9.0
Mean	7814	217.8	59.9	27.7
(SD)	(2536)	(46.2)	(36.0)	(18.8)

Above and Below fCF$_{impulse}$ – data from constant load test where target force was 10% above or 10% below the highest fCF$_{peak\ force}$ of the two maximal effort tests. Subject 5 exercised above his fCF$_{impulse}$ during the constant intensity 10% below test and therefore these data have been included.

Repeatability of the fCF Estimate

fCF$_{peak\ force}$ and fCF$_{impulse}$ repeatability is shown in Table 1 and 2 respectively. There was no systematic effect of trial on fCF$_{peak\ force}$ ($p = 0.11$) or fCF$_{impulse}$ ($p = 0.76$). The typical error expressed as absolute and % was small for fCF$_{peak\ force}$ (15.3 N, 5.5%) and fCF$_{impulse}$ (15.7 N·s, 6.8%). 95% limits of agreement were ±43.2 N with a bias of $+12.3$ for fCF$_{peak\ force}$, and ±44.5 N·s with bias of $+2.2$ for fCF$_{impulse}$ (Fig. 4B and 5B). Test-retest correlations using Pearson and intra-class correlations revealed strong positive relationships for both fCF$_{peak\ force}$ ($r = 0.91$, ICC = 0.94, $p<0.01$) and fCF$_{impulse}$, ($r = 0.92$, ICC = 0.95, $p< 0.01$) (Fig. 4A and 5A).

Constant Intensity Tests

For the constant intensity test 6 of 7 subjects were able to complete 20 min of rhythmic forearm exercise when the target force was 10% below fCF$_{peak\ force}$, whereas only 1 of 7 could complete 20 min exercise when the target force was 10% above fCF$_{peak\ force}$ (TTE 18.0±5.0 min vs. 10.3±5.9, $p<0.01$). Table 3 presents W′ and the contraction impulse data from the constant intensity tests where target force was 10% above fCF$_{peak\ force}$ as well as the data for subject 5 where the target was 10% below fCF$_{peak\ force}$ but his average contraction impulse during this constant intensity test actually exceeded the fCF$_{impulse}$, and therefore resulted in TTE well below 20 min. The actual constant exercise intensity contraction impulses performed for tests used in obtaining predicted TTE exceeded fCF$_{impulse}$ by 59.9±36.0 N·s (27.7±18.8%).

Time to Exhaustion (TTE): Predicted vs. Actual

Agreement between predicted TTE calculated as per equation [3], and actual TTE during constant intensity exercise is shown in Table 4 and Figure 6. Subject 5 exercised above his fCF$_{impulse}$ during the 10% below fCF$_{peak\ force}$ target constant intensity test and therefore their TTE data from this test is included. Subject 7 reached the 20 minute end test point during their 10% above fCF$_{peak\ force}$ target constant intensity test at which point they were stopped. They are therefore not included in the analysis of predicted vs actual TTE agreement. There was no difference at the group level between predicted and actual TTE ($p = 0.25$). The

typical error was 0.98 min (12%) and the limits of agreement were; bias 1.38±1.87 min. Pearson and intra-class correlations were strong ($r = 0.97$, ICC = 0.97, $P<0.01$). For the regression fit, the slope was 0.99 and the y-intercept was not significantly different from 0 (1.12 min, $p = 0.31$).

Relationship of MVC to fCF, W′ and Incremental Exercise Peak Intensity

There was no statistically significant relationship between MVC and fCF$_{impulse}$ ($r^2 = 0.06$, $p = 0.490$), fCF$_{peak\ force}$ ($r^2 = 0.10$, $P = 0.37$) or W′ ($r^2 = 0.37$, $p = 0.15$) (see Fig. 7). Five subjects in this study also performed incremental ramp test to failure as part of another study, and again MVC was not related to their incremental ramp test peak exercise intensity ($r^2 = 0.006$, $p = 0.9$).

Discussion

The novel findings of this study were: 1) forearm maximal effort exercise resulted in the same type of force decay to a stable plateau as previously demonstrated for single-leg all out exercise [13], 2) the stable force plateau had good repeatability both as fCF$_{peak\ force}$ and fCF$_{impulse}$, 3) predicted TTE for the constant supra-fCF$_{impulse}$ intensity exercise test based on the fCF test W′ showed good agreement with actual TTE, 4) MVC showed no association with fCF. Taken together, these findings support the reliability and validity of the single bout maximal effort handgrip test in identifying fCF as well as W′ and argue for its use instead of MVC for identification of exercise intensity when considerations of aerobic metabolism are important in studies using the forearm exercise model.

Characteristics of fCF Test Force

The force decay profile for the single bout maximal effort handgrip exercise test was consistent with previous maximal effort tests used to estimate critical torque or CP [11,13]. The longer time to plateau in our study is expected, since duty cycle was less than in cycling or single knee extension [11,13] and less frequent contractions would result in more time required to deplete W′.

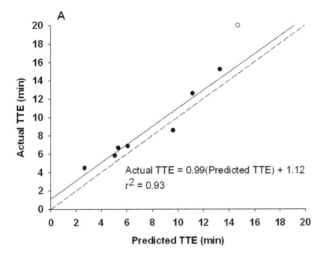

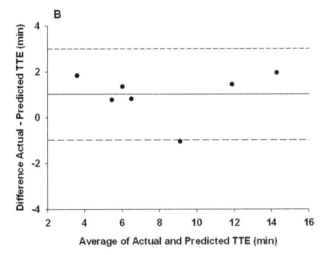

Figure 6. Predicted vs. actual time to exhaustion (TTE) in constant supra-fCF$_{impulse}$ intensity exercise tests. Panel A: Regression of predicted vs. actual TTE (closed circles), excluding data for subject 7 whose actual TTE was constrained by the 20 min limit of test duration (open circle). **Panel B:** Bland-Altman plot of TTE. Mean difference between predicted and actual TTE (solid line). ±1.97 min 95% limits of agreement (dashed lines).

Repeatability of Single Bout fCF Test

Our repeatability analysis demonstrated small within-subject test-retest variation, small change in the test-retest group mean, and a high test-retest correlation, all indicators of good repeatability [17,18]. To allow direct comparison between our study and others that used different parameters and demonstrating widely varying magnitude of response [17] we expressed our indices of repeatability in percent. Our findings were similar to previous findings during maximal effort cycling (CV 3%, ICC 0.99) and a meta-analysis of CP (maximum aerobic power, running or cycling exercise) estimates derived from time-to-exhaustion tests (CV, −0.5–7.6%, Δ mean, −2.2–5.8%) [17,19]. However, CP estimates from traditional multiple bout time-to-exhaustion tests have not always been found to be reliable [20]. Large CV's (>15%) for time-to-exhaustion tests at a given exercise intensity have been previously reported [21,22]. If each data point of a multiple time-to-exhaustion test has considerable variability, then a curve fit

based on those points would be susceptible to increased variability. The single bout maximal effort test eliminates this problem.

Validity of the Single Bout fCF Test

Traditionally, curve fitting of data from three to five fixed power output time-to-exhaustion tests in order to identify the asymptote of the power-duration relationship has been used to identify CP. Therefore, the approach to validating single maximal effort test identification of CP has been to compare results between the two tests in the same individuals [11,13].

As identified by Barker et al. [23], CP is a metabolic rate. Furthermore, it is a metabolic rate that can be sustained because of stabilization of PCr, $\dot{V}O_2$, and pH as identified by Jones et al. [8]. As cleverly proposed by Burnley et al. [19], the basis for a single maximal effort test to result in power output plateauing at CP is the relationship between W′, power output of the task, and CP:

$$P = (W'/t) + CP \qquad (4)$$

such that during continued maximal effort exercise, W′ would "reduce to zero, at which point the highest possible power output would be equal to CP" [19]. Consistent with this, work from this group went on to confirm that a single "all-out" exercise test in both knee extension [13] and cycle ergometer [11] exercise modalities yielded CP estimations that were in excellent agreement with those identified from the traditional multiple fixed power output time-to-exhaustion trial approach. As summarized by Jones et al. [24], the amount of work that can be performed above CP is "not dependent on the chosen work rate above CP". This means that whether W′ is depleted over the course of an all-out exercise bout, or a constant intensity exercise bout above CP, it will be quantitatively the same. This is the basis for being able to utilize W′ to predict time to failure during exercise at a constant intensity above CP.

Based on this we reasoned that, if the contraction impulse plateau in our single bout maximal effort forearm exercise test was a valid estimate of fCF$_{impulse}$, then an estimation of W′ from that test would necessarily allow prediction of time-to-exhaustion (TTE) during exercise at a constant intensity above the impulse plateau. It is necessary to use the contraction impulse rather than contraction peak force, as exercise intensity has both a force and a time domain. Therefore, to assess validity, we calculated a predicted TTE for the constant intensity test that was based on a W′ calculated from the excess force impulse during the maximal effort fCF testing and compared it with actual TTE in the constant intensity test.

For this TTE analysis we included all constant intensity exercise tests where exhaustion occurred before 20 minutes. This was the case for subject 5′s constant intensity test where the target contraction force was 10% below fCF$_{peak\ force}$. The subject actually performed exercise at an intensity that was above his fCF$_{impulse}$. This resulted in task failure before 20 minutes as a consequence of W′ depletion. Likewise, we excluded data from subject 7′s constant intensity exercise test where the target contraction force was 10% above fCF$_{peak\ force}$, because they reached the 20 minute mark where exercise was stopped for all subjects (see Fig. 6) and therefore their data point does not represent the actual TTE during their test. This was considerably greater than his predicted time to exhaustion of 14.7 minutes. It is not clear why in this one instance there was such disagreement between predicted and actual TTE, since the average recorded contraction force impulse during this test was greater (see Table 3 Subject 7) than the fCF$_{impulse}$ determined from the maximal effort

Table 4. Predicted and actual time to exhaustion (TTE) for constant intensity exercise tests where subjects ended up exercising above fCF$_{impulse}$.

Subject # - Constant Intensity Test	TTE$_{predicted}$ (min)	TTE$_{actual}$ (min)	Mean of TTE$_{predicted \text{ and } actual}$	SD (min)	Difference Score TTE$_{actual}$ - TTE$_{predicted}$	CV (%)
1 – Above fCF$_{impulse}$	11.2	12.6	11.9	1.0	1.4	8.3
2 – Above fCF$_{impulse}$	5.1	5.9	5.5	0.5	0.8	10.0
3 – Above fCF$_{impulse}$	9.6	8.6	9.1	0.7	−1.0	8.1
4 – Above fCF$_{impulse}$	6.1	6.9	6.5	0.6	0.8	8.7
5 – Above fCF$_{impulse}$	4.5	2.7	3.6	1.3	−1.8	35.4
5 – Below fCF$_{impulse}$	5.4	6.7	6.0	1.0	1.4	15.8
6 – Above fCF$_{impulse}$	13.3	15.3	14.3	1.4	2.0	9.7
7 – Above fCF$_{impulse}$	14.7	20+	17.4	3.7+	5.3+	21.6+
Mean	7.9	8.4	8.1	0.9	0.5	12.1
(SD)	(3.5)	(4.3)	(3.8)	(0.3)	(1.4)	–

CV – coefficient of variation. The "mean" CV is the typical error as a % of the grand mean. Constant Intensity Test – Above is the test where the target contraction force was 10% >fCF$_{peak force}$. Constant Intensity Test – Below is the test where the target contraction force was 10% <fCF$_{peak force}$. Subject 5 exercised above fCF$_{impulse}$ during the constant intensity test where the target was below fCF$_{peak force}$. Subject 7 data in italics is not included in the Mean±SD.

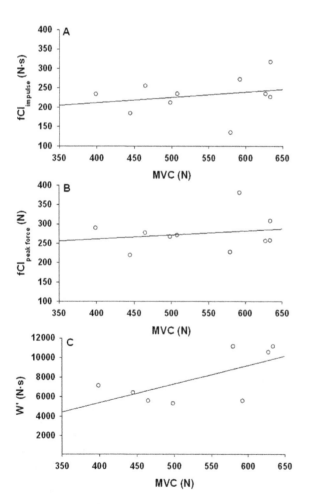

Figure 7. Relationship between Maximum Voluntary Contraction (MVC) and Panel A: fCF$_{impulse}$. $r^2 = 0.06$, p = 0.490, **Panel B:** fCF$_{peak force}$ $r^2 = 0.10$, P = 0.37 and **Panel C:** W' $r^2 = 0.37$, p = 0.15.

test. There are (at least) three potential interpretations of the TTE data. First, for one subject out of 8, the single bout maximal effort forearm exercise test we developed is unable to provide an estimate of W', and therefore the fCF$_{impulse}$, despite excellent repeatability (CV 1.3%; see Table 1 Subject 7), is not valid. Second, the test we developed does not provide valid estimation of fCF$_{impulse}$ and by chance we had 7 tests out of 8 where agreement between actual and predicted TTE was good. Third, it is possible that the position of the handgripper in the subject's hands was different in the constant supra-fCF$_{impulse}$ test vs. the two single bout maximal effort tests from which fCF$_{impulse}$ was determined. A difference in position of the handgripper can alter the mechanical advantage such that the actual muscle contraction force to achieve a given handgrip force can be different. In the case of subject 7, if mechanical advantage was improved during the constant supra-fCF$_{impulse}$ exercise test, the actual muscle contraction force was less than that quantified from the recorded force tracing. Given that the recorded force tracing indicated this subject was exercising only 9% above fCF$_{impulse}$ it would not require much of a reduction in actual vs. recorded force for the subject to be at or below their fCF$_{impulse}$ during this test. Given that in all other cases the predicted vs. actual TTE was close to the line of identity, this third possibility would seem to be the most likely explanation.

Our predicted vs actual TTE findings are in good agreement with those of Jones et al. [8] who used the traditional multiple bout time to exhaustion protocol for identifying the critical power and quantifying the W' (curvature constant of the hyperbolic relationship between fixed power output vs. time using 3 or 4 TTE tests for each subject). Subjects then performed constant intensity exercise tests on separate days at 10% above and 10% below the critical power estimate. All subjects reached 20 min of exercise at 10% below critical power at which time they were stopped. For the 10% above critical power tests the TTE ranged from 6.9–23.8 min such that predicted TTE was similar to actual TTE (mean of 15.1±3.3 min vs. 14±7.1 min; $r^2 = 0.76$).

We also observed no difference between actual TTE 8.4+/−4.3 vs. predicted TTE 7.9+/−3.5 min, with a strong correlation between predicted and actual TTE of $r^2 = 0.93$. The fact that our single bout maximal effort forearm critical intensity test provided estimates of W' and fCF$_{impulse}$ that allowed as good a prediction of

TTE as the traditional multiple bout TTE derived critical power and W′ estimation further supports the validity of this test.

% MVC vs. fCF as a Measure of Relative Aerobic Metabolic Exercise Intensity

We observed a poor relationship between MVC and fCF. This is consistent with MVC force being a function of the cross-sectional area of muscle fibres involved, the percentage of fast-twitch muscle fibres involved, and the number of motor units recruited/activated, not metabolic demand or oxygen delivery [25–27]. By extension, a given %MVC would not represent exercise intensity relative to aerobic metabolic capacity and therefore could not provide a valid identification of aerobic metabolic exercise intensity domains.

This has been previously confirmed by the work of Saugen et al. [5] and Kent-Braun et al. [6]. Their findings reinforce that myocellular environments and aerobic metabolism can be drastically different between individuals during exercise at the same % MVC. Therefore, selection of exercise intensities relative to an individual's MVC could lead to subjects exercising in different aerobic metabolic exercise intensity domains, confounding interpretation of results. In contrast, CP (in the current study $fCF_{impulse}$) represents an exercise intensity that reflects functional aerobic metabolic capacity and delineates steady state from non-steady state exercise [24,28]. Our findings argue for the abandonment of MVC for establishing exercise intensities in the forearm exercise model, and its replacement by the newly developed fCF test.

Potential Limitations

This study utilized a 1 s contraction: 2 s relaxation rhythmic isometric contraction exercise protocol. That the repeatability we found would also occur if exercise was performed with other duty cycles (eg. 1:1, 2:1 etc...) or with other contraction durations without a change in duty cycle (eg. 2:4, 3:6) cannot be claimed with certainty. However, given that critical intensity of a single all-out test shows excellent agreement with multiple bout time to exhaustion tests in isokinetic knee extension exercise with a 3:2 duty cycle [13], and in cycle ergometer exercise [11], and that critical intensity is a metabolic rate that is consistent between cycle cadences with differing $_1\dot{V}O_2$ cost of power output [23], it would not be expected that contraction protocol would affect repeatability. Likewise for other duty cycles, or contraction durations without change in duty cycle, to result in a single bout maximal effort that does not provide a valid estimate of fCF would require that the nature of the contraction protocol disrupts the physiological underpinning of W′, $fCF_{impulse}$, and of their relationship.

Another important consideration is that of the effect of isometric contraction duration on the $_1\dot{V}O_2$ cost under the same tension-time integral (TTI; representing impulse per unit time). It has been well established in animal models that $_1\dot{V}O_2$ is higher during shorter vs. longer duration rhythmic isometric contractions [29,30] under the same TTI. This is believed to be a function of the increased ATP cost of ion transport with more frequent muscle activation and relaxation events [29]. It has also been shown in a cycle ergometer exercise model using different cycle cadences, where faster cadence results in an increased $_1\dot{V}O_2$ cost at a given external power output, that power output but not $_1\dot{V}O_2$ at CP differs [23,31]. Taken together, these findings raise the possibility that comparison of $fCF_{impulse}$ between contraction protocols that differ in contraction duration may be problematic.

In contrast, if one were to compare $fCF_{impulse}$ between tests where duty cycles differ but contraction duration is the same, then differences in $_1\dot{V}O_2$ cost of a given $fCF_{impulse}$ would not be expected to differ and comparison may be possible. One would simply expect that, when relaxation duration is increased for the same contraction duration, the peak force of the contraction at $fCF_{impulse}$ would be increased.

Finally, it is important to realize that when conducting voluntary isometric handgrip exercise tests that the ability of a subject to perfectly execute a 1 second contraction as a square wave of force production to target force is not possible. Thus, there is the potential for variability between subjects in the actual contraction force amplitude and duration such that the peak force and force impulse varies from the target. Unfortunately, this cannot be determined until offline analysis of the contraction force impulse after completion of the exercise test. The exercise task performance of subject 5 in the 10% above $fCF_{impulse}$ is an example of when this variability can have implications for data interpretation. Familiarization of the subject with the exercise task and ongoing monitoring and correction during the actual exercise can reduce this issue to some degree. Nevertheless, quantification of the peak and impulse performed in an exercise test is essential to account for this potential confound when interpreting findings.

Conclusions

In conclusion, we have established that a single bout 10 min maximal effort handgrip exercise test demonstrates good repeatability of $fCF_{peak\ force}$ and $fCF_{impulse}$ estimated from the last 30 s (or 10 contractions) of the test. The good agreement of predicted and actual TTE supports the validity of the $fCF_{impulse}$ estimate and its usefulness in quantifying W′. The poor relationship of MVC with fCF is consistent with MVC being a poor means for identifying relative aerobic metabolic exercise intensity between subjects. Therefore, the fCF rather than MVC should be utilized in the human forearm exercise model to identify exercise intensity domains, and characterize aerobic metabolic demand when aerobic metabolic considerations are important.

Acknowledgments

We would like to acknowledge the subjects for their time and effort. We would also like to acknowledge Robert Bentley and Daniel Moylan for their technical assistance in data collection.

Author Contributions

Conceived and designed the experiments: JMK MET. Performed the experiments: JMK. Analyzed the data: JMK MET. Contributed reagents/materials/analysis tools: MET. Wrote the paper: JMK MET.

References

1. Casey DP, Curry TB, Wilkins BW, Joyner MJ (2011) Nitric oxide-mediated vasodilation becomes independent of beta-adrenergic receptor activation with increased intensity of hypoxic exercise. J Appl Physiol 110: 687–694.
2. Crecelius AR, Kirby BS, Voyles WF, Dinenno FA (2011) Augmented skeletal muscle hyperaemia during hypoxic exercise in humans is blunted by combined inhibition of nitric oxide and vasodilating prostaglandins. J Physiol 589: 3871–3683.
3. Faisal A, Dyson KS, Hughson RL (2010) Prolonged ischaemia impairs muscle blood flow and oxygen uptake dynamics during subsequent heavy exercise. J Physiol 588: 3785–3797.
4. Casey DP, Joyner MJ (2009) Skeletal muscle blood flow responses to hypoperfusion at rest and during rhythmic exercise in humans. J Appl Physiol 107: 429–437.

5. Saugen E, Vollestad NK, Gibson H, Martin PA, Edwards RH (1997) Dissociation between metabolic and contractile responses during intermittent isometric exercise in man. Exp Physiol 82: 213–226.

6. Kent-Braun JA, Miller RG, Weiner MW (1993) Phases of metabolism during progressive exercise to fatigue in human skeletal muscle. J Appl Physiol 75: 573–580.

7. Dimenna FJ, Jones AM (2009) "LINEAR" Versus "NONLINEAR"; $\dot{V}O_2$ Responses To Exercise: Reshaping Traditional Beliefs. J Exerc Sci Fit 7: 67–84. Review.

8. Jones AM, Wilkerson DP, DiMenna F, Fulford J, Poole DC (2008) Muscle metabolic responses to exercise above and below the "critical power" assessed using P-31-MRS. Am J Physiol (Reg Int Comp Physiol) 294: R585–R593.

9. Poole DC, Ward SA, Gardner GW, Whipp BJ (1988) Metabolic and Respiratory Profile of the Upper Limit for Prolonged Exercise in Man. Ergonomics 31: 1265–1279.

10. Dekerle J, Mucci P, Carter H (2012) Influence of moderate hypoxia on tolerance to high-intensity exercise. Eur J Appl Physiol 112: 327–335.

11. Vanhatalo A, Doust JH, Burnley M (2007) Determination of critical power using a 3-min all-out cycling test. Med Sci Sports Exerc 39: 548–555.

12. Vanhatalo A, Fulford J, Dimenna FJ, Jones AM (2010) Influence of hyperoxia on muscle metabolic responses and the power-duration relationship during severe-intensity exercise in humans: a 31P magnetic resonance spectroscopy study. Exp Physiol 95: 528–540.

13. Burnley M (2009) Estimation of critical torque using intermittent isometric maximal voluntary contractions of the quadriceps in humans. J Appl Physiol 106: 975–983.

14. Saunders NR, Tschakovsky ME (2004) Evidence for a rapid vasodilatory contribution to immediate hyperemia in rest-to-mild and mild-to-moderate forearm exercise transitions in humans. J Appl Physiol 97: 1143–1151.

15. Bland JM, Altman DG (2010) Statistical methods for assessing agreement between two methods of clinical measurement. Int J Nurs Stud 47: 931–936.

16. Hopkins WG (2000) Measures of reliability in sports medicine and science. Sports Med 30: 1–15. Comparative Study.

17. Hopkins W, Schabort E, Hawley J (2001) Reliability of power in physical performance tests. Sports Med 31: 211–234. Review.

18. Schabort EJ, Hawley JA, Hopkins WG, Blum H (1999) High reliability of performance of well-trained rowers on a rowing ergometer. J Sports Sci 17: 627–632.

19. Burnley M, Doust JH, Vanhatalo A (2006) A 3-min all-out test to determine peak oxygen uptake and the maximal steady state. Med Sci Sports Exerc 38: 1995–2003.

20. Taylor SA, Batterham AM (2002) The reproducibility of estimates of critical power and anaerobic work capacity in upper-body exercise. Eur J Appl Physiol 87: 43–49.

21. Jeukendrup A, Saris WHM, Brouns F, Kester ADM (1996) A new validated endurance performance test. Med Sci Sports Exerc 28: 266–270.

22. McLellan TM, Cheung SS, Jacobs I (1995) Variability of Time to Exhaustion During Submaximal Exercise. Can J Appl Physiol 20: 35–51.

23. Barker T, Poole DC, Noble ML, Barstow TJ (2006) Human critical power-oxygen uptake relationship at different pedalling frequencies. Exp Physiol 91: 621–632. expphysiol.2005.032789 [pii];10.1113/expphysiol.2005.032789 [doi].

24. Jones AM, Vanhatalo A, Burnley M, Morton RH, Poole DC (2010) Critical power: implications for determination of $\dot{V}O_2$ max and exercise tolerance. Med Sci Sports Exerc 42: 1876–1890. Review.

25. Herbert RD, Gandevia SC (1996) Muscle activation in unilateral and bilateral efforts assessed by motor nerve and cortical stimulation. J Appl Physiol 80: 1351–1356.

26. Todd G, Taylor JL, Gandevia SC (2003) Measurement of voluntary activation of fresh and fatigued human muscles using transcranial magnetic stimulation. J Physiol 551: 661–671. Clinical Trial.

27. Wilson GJ, Murphy AJ (1996) The use of isometric tests of muscular function in athletic assessment. Sports Med 22: 19–37. Review.

28. Vanhatalo A, Jones AM, Burnley M (2011) Application of critical power in sport. Int J Sports Physiol Perf 6: 128–136. Review.

29. Hogan MC, Ingham E, Kurdak SS (1998) Contraction duration affects metabolic energy cost and fatigue in skeletal muscle. Am J Physiol 274: E397–E402.

30. Hamann JJ, Kluess HA, Buckwalter JB, Clifford PS (2005) Blood flow response to muscle contractions is more closely related to metabolic rate than contractile work. J Appl Physiol 98: 2096–2100. 00400.2004 [pii];10.1152/japplphysiol.00400.2004 [doi].

31. Vanhatalo A, Doust JH, Burnley M (2008) Robustness of a 3 min all-out cycling test to manipulations of power profile and cadence in humans. Exp Physiol 93: 383–390. expphysiol.2007.039883 [pii];10.1113/expphysiol.2007.039883 [doi].

20

Virtual Reconstruction and Prey Size Preference in the Mid Cenozoic Thylacinid, *Nimbacinus dicksoni* (Thylacinidae, Marsupialia)

Marie R. G. Attard[1,2]*, **William C. H. Parr**[1], **Laura A. B. Wilson**[1], **Michael Archer**[3], **Suzanne J. Hand**[3], **Tracey L. Rogers**[1], **Stephen Wroe**[2]

1 Evolution and Ecology Research Centre, School of Biological, Earth and Environmental Sciences, University of New South Wales, Sydney, New South Wales, Australia, **2** Function, Evolution and Anatomy Research laboratory, Zoology, School of Environmental and Rural Sciences, University of New England, New South Wales, Australia, **3** Evolution of Earth and Life Sciences Research Centre, School of Biological, Earth and Environmental Sciences, University of New South Wales, Sydney, New South Wales, Australia

Abstract

Thylacinidae is an extinct family of Australian and New Guinean marsupial carnivores, comprizing 12 known species, the oldest of which are late Oligocene (~24 Ma) in age. Except for the recently extinct thylacine (*Thylacinus cynocephalus*), most are known from fragmentary craniodental material only, limiting the scope of biomechanical and ecological studies. However, a particularly well-preserved skull of the fossil species *Nimbacinus dicksoni*, has been recovered from middle Miocene (~16-11.6 Ma) deposits in the Riversleigh World Heritage Area, northwestern Queensland. Here, we ask whether *N. dicksoni* was more similar to its recently extinct relative or to several large living marsupials in a key aspect of feeding ecology, i.e., was *N. dicksoni* a relatively small or large prey specialist. To address this question we have digitally reconstructed its skull and applied three-dimensional Finite Element Analysis to compare its mechanical performance with that of three extant marsupial carnivores and *T. cynocephalus*. Under loadings adjusted for differences in size that simulated forces generated by both jaw closing musculature and struggling prey, we found that stress distributions and magnitudes in the skull of *N. dicksoni* were more similar to those of the living spotted-tailed quoll (*Dasyurus maculatus*) than to its recently extinct relative. Considering the Finite Element Analysis results and dental morphology, we predict that *N. dicksoni* likely occupied a broadly similar ecological niche to that of *D. maculatus*, and was likely capable of hunting vertebrate prey that may have exceeded its own body mass.

Editor: Kornelius Kupczik, Friedrich-Schiller-University Jena, Germany

Funding: This research was funded by Australian Research Council grants to S. Wroe (DP0666374 and DP0987985), and to M. Archer, and S. J. Hand (LP100200486 and DP1094569). M. Attard is supported by the Postgraduate Writing and Skills Transfer Award sponsored by the Evolution and Ecology Research Centre, University of New South Wales. L. Wilson is supported by the Swiss National Science Foundation (PBZHP3_141470). The funders had no role in study design, data collection and analysis, decision to publish, or preparation of the manuscript.

Competing Interests: The authors have declared that no competing interests exist.

* E-mail: marie.attard@une.edu.au

Introduction

Thylacinids first appear in the Australian fossil record during the late Oligocene (~24 Ma) and include the largest representatives of the Dasyuromorphia, i.e., families Thylacinidae, Dasyuridae and Myrmecobiidae [1–8]. A wide range of feeding ecologies are known within the order. They include omnivores, insectivores, small prey specialists, hypercarnivores and osteophageous species [9]. Variation in the dentition, skull shape and body size (~1–60 kg) of thylacinids suggests considerable trophic diversity within the family [10,11]. In addition to the recently extinct thylacine or Tasmanian 'tiger' (*Thylacinus cynocephalus*), eleven extinct species of thylacinid have been described [4,12–18]. Up to five species may have co-existed in the Riversleigh World Heritage Area, north-western Queensland between the late Oligocene (~24 Ma) to middle Miocene (16-11.6 Ma) [12,16]. See Table S1 for the temporal and geographic distribution of all thylacinid species.

The Riversleigh thylacinids inhabited forests [19,20]. These regions were also occupied by an assortment of other carnivorous/omnivorous taxa, including 'giant' carnivorous rat-kangaroos (*Ekaltadeta* spp.), crocodiles (Mekosuchinae, e.g. *Baru darrowi* and *Trilophosuchus rackhami*), flightless dromornithid birds, marsupial lions (Thylacoleonidae), bandicoots (Peramelemorphia), dasyurids (Dasyuridae), pythons (Pythonidae), madtsoiid snakes and the world's oldest known venomous snakes [21–23]. Subsequent drying of the Australian continent from the late Miocene (11.6–5.3 Ma) led to the gradual replacement of forest environments with open woodlands, shrublands and grasslands [19–21]. These changes appear to broadly correlate with declining thylacinid diversity [24].

To date, interpretations of the ecology and feeding behavior of fossil thylacinids have been largely qualitative. This is, at least in part, because most extinct species are known only from jaw fragments and teeth. The near-complete skull of *Nimbacinus dicksoni* [4,14,18], a medium-sized thylacinid, provides an opportunity to more fully investigate feeding ecology in an extinct thylacinid.

Nimbacinus dicksoni was approximately 5 kg in body mass [10]. Fossils of *N. dicksoni* have been recovered from Oligocene-Miocene

(~24–5.3 Ma) deposits in the Riversleigh World Heritage Area, northwestern Queensland and Bullock Creek, Northern Territory [12,14,16,18]. Its dentition is less specialized than that of the species of *Thylacinus*, but broadly similar to that of the living dasyurid, the spotted-tailed quoll (*Dasyurus maculatus*) in the arrangement and geometry of molar shearing crests typically associated with carnivory [18,25].

To date conflicting evidence has been presented regarding the body size of prey *N. dicksoni* may have hunted. Predictions of bite force adjusted for body mass, based on application of 2D beam theory, have suggested that *N. dicksoni* may have taken relatively large prey, as does the slightly smaller *D. maculatus* [26]. However, shape analysis of the cranium has suggested that the species may have been restricted to smaller prey and/or included a higher proportion of invertebrate food in its diet [11].

The loads imposed on an animal during prey acquisition and feeding play an important role in the evolution of its skull morphology [27]. Testing hypotheses regarding the relationship between the form and function of skulls from extinct species requires an understanding of this relationship in living animals [28]. A comparative biomechanics approach involving living analogues has increasingly been applied to predict the feeding ecology and predatory behavior of extinct species [29–34]. To gain further insight in the feeding ecology of *N. dicksoni*, here we perform a biomechanical analysis of the skull of *N. dicksoni* to predict its mechanical behavior in response to loads simulating the capture and processing of prey.

Finite Element Analysis (FEA) is a computer modeling approach now commonly used by biologists and paleontologists to examine and compare mechanical performance in biological structures in comparative contexts [35–41]. In FEA, continuous structures, such as the skull, are divided into discrete, finite numbers of elements, allowing the prediction of mechanical behavior for complex geometric shapes. The structure is analyzed in the form of a matrix algebra problem that is solved with the aid of a computer [42].

Studies of feeding ecology for thylacinids have primarily focused on the most recently extinct member of the family, *T. cynocephalus*, which survived in Tasmania until 1936 [43]. Our understanding of the ecology of *T. cynocephalus* is chiefly based on morphological comparisons and 2D beam theory [11,26,44,45], as well as anecdotal accounts of their behavior in the wild [46,47]. Elbow joint morphology of *T. cynocephalus* evidently most closely resembles that of extant ambush predators, a compromise between efficient distance locomotion and the ability to manipulate and grapple with prey [48]. Three-dimensional biomechanical modeling of the skull of *T. cynocephalus*, extant dasyurids and an introduced Australian predator (*Canis lupus dingo*) have suggested potential limitations in prey body size [32,35].

Morphological and biomechanical comparisons including sympatric native predators in Tasmania indicate that the diet of *T. cynocephalus* may have overlapped considerably with the two largest extant marsupial carnivores, the Tasmanian devil (*Sarcophilus harrisii*) and spotted-tailed quoll (*D. maculatus*) [35,44,49]. These species represented the three largest marsupial carnivores in Tasmania at the time of European settlement.

Sarcophilus harrisii is the largest living marsupial carnivore (mean adult male weight 8.7 kg, female 6.1 kg) [50]. They are the only specialized scavengers among living marsupials, filling a broadly similar ecological niche to that of osteophagous hyenas [44]. They are also opportunistic hunters and are known to prey on mammals that may exceed their body mass [51,52]. Relative to its body size, its predicted bite force is greater than that of any other extant mammal studied to date [26].

Quolls are represented by four extant species in Australia and two in New Guinea [53]. The largest quoll, *Dasyurus maculatus* (maximum weight 7 kg) has a broad diet mainly consisting of mammals and insects, but will occasionally feed on birds and reptiles [54,55]. Larger prey species constitute a higher proportion of the diet of adult male *D. maculatus*, while females and immature *D. maculatus* more frequently feed on smaller bodied mammals and invertebrates [56,57]. The northern quoll (*Dasyurus hallucatus*) is the smallest and most arboreal of the four Australian quolls, weighing up to 1.2 kg [58,59]. Although primarily insectivorous, this active hunter can feed on a variety of foods: fruits, small mammals, birds, reptiles, frogs and carrion [60–62].

In this study we aim to determine whether *N. dicksoni* was capable of killing large prey relative to their body size, or was restricted to catching relatively small bodied species. By digital reconstruction of its skull and applied 3D FEA, we compare its mechanical performance with that of three extant marsupial carnivores; *S. harrisii*, *D. maculatus* and *D. hallucatus*. We use previously applied scaling procedures [31] to account for differences in body mass, allowing for comparison of results between species. We predict that *N. dicksoni* will show similar distributions and magnitudes of craniomandibular stress to that of *D. maculatus* due to similarities in their dental morphology and size [18]. We also include *T. cynocephalus* to establish whether the biomechanical performance of *N. dicksoni* more closely resembles that of this larger, more derived thylacinid than dasyurids. A general assessment of the phylogenetic relationships of dasyuromophians, including taxa examined in this study is shown in Figure S1. We test if the biomechanical patterns and the inferred feeding aspects in *T. cynocephalus* in a recent study [35] are derived. We hypothesize that the relatively long rostrum of *T. cynocephalus* will result in higher stresses in the skull during biting and prey procurement than *N. dicksoni* and other dasyuromorphians.

Materials and Methods

Specimens

The skull of *Nimbacinus dicksoni* (QMF36357) was recovered from AL90 Site on the Gag Plateau of the Riversleigh World Heritage area in northwestern Queensland. Precise locality details can be provided on application to the Queensland Museum. This specimen was collected under permits issued by Queensland Department of Environment and Heritage and Environment Australia, and registered in the paleontological collections of the Queensland Museum, Brisbane, Australia. All necessary permits were obtained for the described study, which complied with all relevant regulations.

The biomechanical performance of the *Nimbacinus dicksoni* skull was compared with that of four dasyuromorphian species covering a range of craniodental morphologies and feeding ecologies. These comprized three extant dasyurids [*Dasyurus hallucatus* TMM M-6921; *D. maculatus* UNSW Z20; *Sarcophilus harrisii* AM10756] and one thylacinid (*Thylacinus cynocephalus* AM1821). Institutional abbreviations are QMF (Queensland Museum Fossil, Queensland), TMM (Texas Memorial Museum, Austin), UNSW (University of New South Wales, Sydney) and AM (Australian Museum, Sydney).

We generated 3D finite element models (FEMs) of each skull on the basis of computed tomography X-ray (CT) scan data. Digimorph (University of Texas; http://www.digimorph.org) was the source of CT data of a *D. hallucatus* skull (0.0784 mm slice thickness, 0.0784 mm inter-slice distance). Permission to use Digimorph derived CT scan data was granted by Dr. Timothy Rowe, Project Director of Digimorph. Other skulls were scanned in a Toshiba Aquillon 16 scanner (ToshibaMedical Systems Corporation, Otawara, Tachigi, Japan) at the Mater Hospital, Newcastle, NSW (1 mm slice thickness, 0.8 mm inter-slice distance, 240 mm field of view). The Australian Museum, Queensland Museum and University of New South Wales granted the loan of specimens to obtain CT data for this study.

We used the same specimen CT scans of *T. cynocephalus*, *D. maculatus* and *S. harrisii* as examined by Attard et al. [35], but constructed the FEMs again using a higher resolution mesh than that used by Attard et al. [35]. More specifically, the 3D surface meshes which formed the bases of the FEMs were computed using the High Quality as opposed to Medium Quality option in Mimics (ver. 13.2). The generated surface meshes were then converted to FEMs in STRAND7 (ver. 2.4) following previously established protocols [31,35,63]. Additionally, 3D objects of *T. cynocephalus* and all dasyurid skulls were exported as separate stl files for the creation of interactive 3D pdf documents that can be viewed using Adobe Reader (Figure S2, S3, S4, S5).

Digital Reconstruction of *Nimbacinus dicksoni*

For detailed descriptions of *N. dicksoni* see Muirhead and Archer [14] and Wroe and Musser [18]. Previous analysis has suggested that, within the family, the dentition of *N. dicksoni* is less derived than the recent *Thylacinus cynocephalus* for at least 12 features, but that relatively few cranial specializations in *T. cynocephalus* distinguish the two species. These two taxa share at least three cranial features not present in the most generalized thylacinid known from significant cranial material, the late Oligocene *Badjcinus turnbulli* [14,18].

The skull of *N. dicksoni* is well preserved, although some regions are absent or damaged. Specifically, some damage/deformation is present at the postorbital processes, frontal, maxillary and nasal bones, which are compressed dorsoventrally (Figure 1). These damaged regions were reconstructed according to the morphology of surrounding bone regions once the damaged areas had been isolated and deleted [64]. Regions of bone that showed only minor damage were smoothed to create a coherent surface mesh for later solid meshing.

The right and left dentaries were largely intact but missing the superior regions of the coronoid processes, the temporomandibular joints (TMJ), condyles and angular processes (Figure 1). The anterior of the mandible is broken, separating both dentaries. We used the right dentary as a basis for reconstruction because its dentition was more complete, with only the incisors missing (Figure 1). We used a surface mesh of the right dentary of *D. maculatus* to reconstruct posterior regions of the right dentary of *N. dicksoni*. *Dasyurus maculatus* was chosen as its mandible was most similar in shape to that of *N. dicksoni* [11], thereby minimizing the extent of warping needed (and see below).

Reconstruction involved scaling the dentary of *D. maculatus* to the same size as that of *N. dicksoni* on the basis of skull length (condylo-basal). The missing posterior region of the *N. dicksoni* specimen was then isolated on the *D. maculatus* specimen and the mesh fitted to the existing structure in the mesh of *N. dicksoni* using Iterative Closest Point (ICP) registration. ICP is an algorithm that revises the transformation needed to minimize the distance between the points of two partially overlapping meshes. This process re-oriented the *D. maculatus* dentary in accordance with the morphology of the *N. dicksoni* dentary [65]. The anterior region of the *D. maculatus* dentary was deleted and the posterior region 'warped' so that overlapping regions of the coronoid process and angular process from the *D. maculatus* mesh matched the existing morphology of *N. dicksoni*. The manual warping method was used as much of the target (fossil) morphology was missing, making it

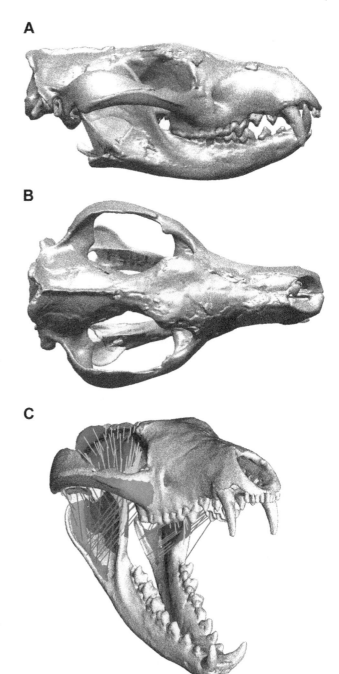

Figure 1. Digital reconstruction of *Nimbacinus dicksoni*. Original (grey) and reconstructed 3D (yellow) in (A) lateral view and (B) dorsal view. (C) Pre-processed Finite Element model of *N. dicksoni*, showing jaw musculature represented by trusses.

impossible to apply homologous landmarks on both complete (*D. maculatus*) and incomplete fossil (*N. dicksoni*) specimens. Procedures to warp overlapping skull regions followed established protocols used by Oldfield et al. and Parr et al. [38,66]. Manual warping works by establishing a grid of control points around the complete model (note that at this stage the incomplete fossil model has been ICP registered with the scaled complete model by matching the orientations of the regions of the jaw that are present in both models). These control points are then manipulated so that the surface morphology of the complete model matches that of the

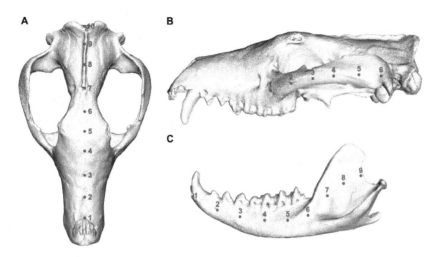

Figure 2. Position of nodes selected on each model to measure von Mises stress. Nodes were selected at equidistant points along the (A) mid-sagittal plane, (B) zygomatic arch and (C) mandible to measure the distribution of von Mises stress for each loading case.

target (fossil). This is another variation of Template Mesh Deformation [66], but with the template points being the grid control points around the complete model rather than homologous anatomical points on both models.

Similarly, the TMJ of the complete (*D. maculatus*) model was warped so that the condyle articulated with and fitted the *N. dicksoni* cotyle of the cranium, again by using the manual template mesh deformation warping method. The left dentary was created by mirroring the reconstructed right dentary. These were positioned so that the condyles articulated with the cranium, the outer surfaces of the lower molars made contact with the inner surface of the upper molars, and the tips of the lower canines aligned with their 'sockets' in the cranium (see Figure 1).

It is important to note that the shape of the warp was determined by the existing regions of the *N. dicksoni* dentary; the need for the condyle to articulate with the cotyle to form the TMJ and for the coronoid process to fit between the cranium and the zygomatic arch. These requirements act as restraints on the warp such that the shape of the starting mesh (*D. maculatus* in this case) is not important in the sense that the warping process would always end with a similarly shaped posterior region of the mandible regardless of which taxon was used. We reiterate that *D. maculatus* was used because it was the most similar in shape [11] and therefore required less 'warping'.

The *N. dicksoni* cranium was missing the following teeth: left I1-4, right I1, 3-4, both right and left C1 and right LDP2. The existing I2 and LDP2 on *N. dicksoni* were mirrored. All incisors were missing from the mandible. Incisors from *D. maculatus* were isolated, scaled and fitted into the empty tooth sockets on *N. dicksoni*. Figure 1 displays the completed reconstruction of *N. dicksoni*.

Finite Element Models

The assembly of FEMs largely follows previously published procedures [30,31,35]. As the skull of *N. dicksoni* was not fully preserved, we were unable to assign multiple material properties to the digital reconstruction without introducing additional assumptions. Consequently, as in most FEA incorporating fossil material [30,39,67], all FEMs were homogeneous and assigned a single material property for cortical bone ($E = 13.7$ GPa, $v = 0.3$, where E is Young's modulus of elasticity and v is Poisson's ratio) [68] to enable direct comparisons between species. Poisson's ratio and

Young's modulus are fundamental metrics in the comparison of stress or deformation for any material when strained elastically, including homogeneous materials [69]. Young's modulus is a measure of stiffness in the material, whereas Poisson's ratio is the negative ratio between transverse strain and longitudinal strain in an elastic material subjected to uniaxial stress [70].

Each homogeneous model was comprized of four-noded tetrahedral elements or 'bricks' (tet4). FEMs for QMF36357, AM1821, AM10756, UNSW Z20 and TMM M-6921 were comprized of 1564048, 1429714, 1799292, 1402103 and 1956942 bricks respectively. Tet4 models are theoretically less accurate than models comprized of tet10 elements. However, the models used in this study are large and any difference in accuracy between results from tet4 versus tet10 models will diminish as the number of elements is increased. Comparable analyses comparing tet4 and tet10 based models much smaller than those used here (<252000 elements) found differences of <10% [27].

Modeling Masticatory Muscle Forces

Jaw elevators were modeled as seven muscle subdivisions: *temporalis superficialis*, *temporalis profundus*, *masseter superficialis*, *masseter profundus*, *zygomatico mandibularis*, *pterygoideus internus* and *pterygoideus externus* [32]. Proportions used for each jaw muscle division were based on muscle mass proportions from a dissected Virginia opossum (*Didelphis virginiana*) [71]. Muscle forces were predicted on the basis of maximum cross-sectional areas (CSA) using the 'dry skull' method [72]. To improve the accuracy of our CSA measurements, we used our FEMs to record the co-ordinates of ~100 nodes at the perimeter of each muscle cross sectional area [73]. The FEM was moved to the correct orientation described by Thomason [70] to select nodes outlining the CSA. The node co-ordinates were then plotted in plane geometry software, GEUP 5 (version 5.0.3) and connected to form a multi-sided polygon. The area of the polygon was measured to estimate the CSA of each major jaw closing muscle. To minimize the incidence of artefacts at bite points and muscle origin and insertion areas, surface regions at these sites were tessellated using a network of stiff beam elements [74].

Restraints, Loading Conditions and Scaling

Dasyurids frequently use a penetrating canine bite to kill prey [44,75–78] which involves the application of a bending load [79].

Table 1. Predicted body mass and masticatory muscle forces for modeled dasyuromorphians.

Species	Predicted body mass (kg)	Temporalis muscle force (N)	Masseteric muscle force (N)	Total muscle force (N)
Dasyurus hallucatus	0.78	67.60	55.89	123.49
Dasyurus maculatus	2.88	211.01	178.67	389.67
Nimbacinus dicksoni	5.25	282.38	368.33	650.71
Sarcophilus harrisii	14.20	300.46	384.73	685.19
Thylacinus cynocephalus	32.49	706.64	843.21	1,549.85

Predicted body mass (kg) calculated using the regression equation for dasyuromorphians provided by Myers [76] based on lower molar row length. Temporalis and masseteric muscle forces (N) were calculated based on cross-sectional area [67].

We simulated bilateral canine biting (intrinsic load) and four extrinsic loads to simulate loads generated by struggling prey (axial twist, lateral shake, pullback and dorsoventral) for all models using protocols described by Attard et al. [35] and following McHenry et al. [31]. Extrinsic loads were modeled without applying bite forces so as to clearly reveal the different influences of each separate loading [31]. A gape angle of 35° was applied in all linear static load cases.

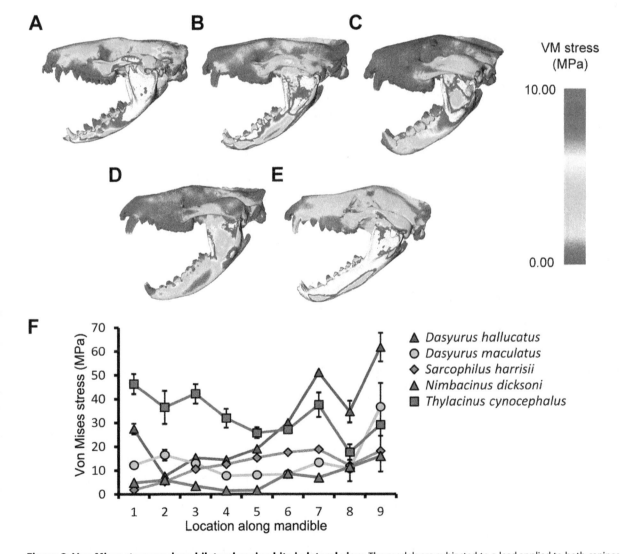

Figure 3. Von Mises stress under a bilateral canine bite in lateral view. The models are subjected to a load applied to both canines, with bite force scaled based on theoretical body mass. Species modeled were (A) *Dasyurus hallucatus*, (B) *Dasyurus maculatus*, (C) *Sarcophilus harrisii*, (D) *Nimbacinus dicksoni* and (E) *Thylacinus cynocephalus*. White colored regions of the skull represent VM stress above 10 MPa. (F) Distribution of von Mises stress was measured from anterior to posterior along the mandible.

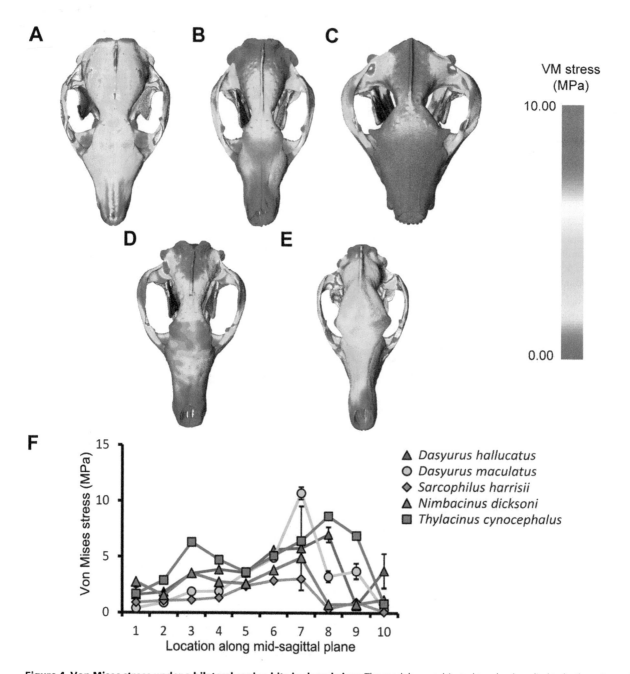

Figure 4. Von Mises stress under a bilateral canine bite in dorsal view. The models are subjected to a load applied to both canines, with bite force scaled based on theoretical body mass. Species modeled were (A) *Dasyurus hallucatus*, (B) *Dasyurus maculatus*, (C) *Sarcophilus harrisii*, (D) *Nimbacinus dicksoni* and (E) *Thylacinus cynocephalus*. White colored regions of the skull represent VM stress above 10 MPa. (F) Distribution of von Mises stress was measured from anterior to posterior along the mid-sagittal plane.

A considerable size range exists between specimens considered in the present study. The relationship between bite force and body mass is negatively allometric [26,80]. To account for differences in body mass, a second series of load cases were solved following the scaling procedures of McHenry et al. [31]. Here, for each model, an estimate of bite force was made based on regression of body mass to predicted bite force for dasyuromorphians [$z = 0.6998$ (log y)+1.8735, where and y = mass (g) and z = bite force at canines (N)] [26], with body mass for each specimen predicted using the equation based on lower molar row length [log $y = -1.075+3.209$(log x), where x = lower molar length (mm), and y = mass (g)] as presented by Myers [81]. Muscle forces were then scaled for

each specimen to achieve bite forces predicted on the basis of body mass. FEMs were solved using these scaled muscle forces. Prediction of bite force based on body mass using the regression equation provided in Wroe et al. [26] is close to that which would be expected following a 2/3 power relationship, whereby muscle force is proportional to area while body mass is proportional to volume [82]. The maximum bite force measured in Newtons (N) was also estimated for intrinsic loads (Table S2) using FEMs with un-scaled, specimen-specific estimated muscle forces (Table S3). Three dimensional approaches are likely to be more accurate than 2D based approaches [83].

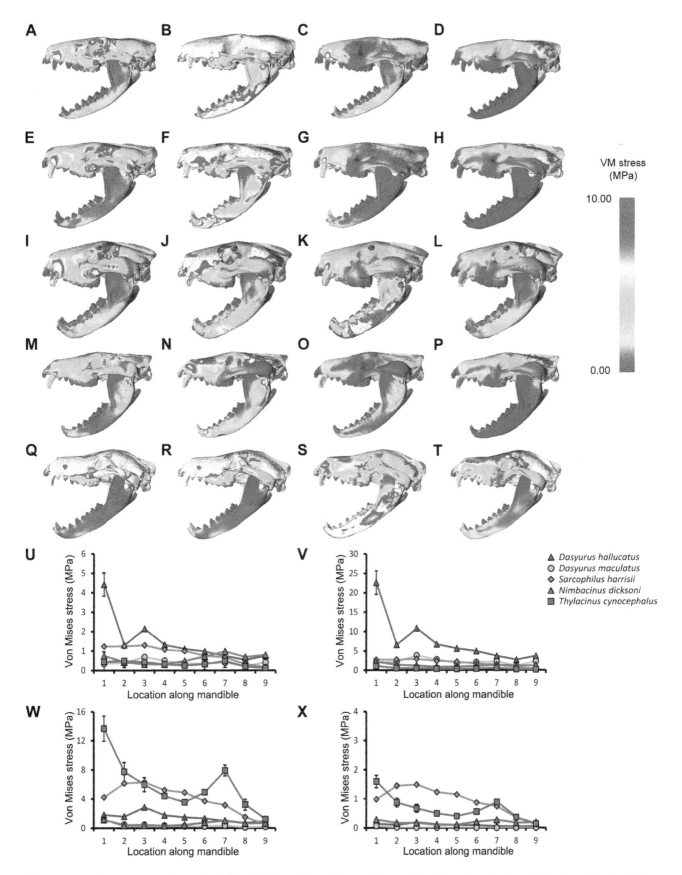

Figure 5. Von Mises stress under extrinsic loads in lateral view. The models are subjected to various loads applied to the canines, including a (A, E, I, M, Q) lateral shake, (B, F, J, N, R) axial twist, (C, G, K, O, S) pullback and (D, H, L, P, T) dorsoventral. The force applied was equivalent to 100 times the animal's estimated body mass for an axial twist, and 10 times the animal's estimated body mass for a lateral shake, pullback and dorsoventral

shake. Species compared were (A–D) *Dasyurus hallucatus*, (E–H) *Dasyurus maculatus*, (I–L) *Sarcophilus harrisii*, (M–P) *Nimbacinus dicksoni* and (Q–T) *Thylacinus cynocephalus*. White colored regions of the skull represent VM stress above 10 MPa. Distribution of von Mises (VM) stress was measured from anterior to posterior along the mandible for a (U) lateral shake, (V) axial twist, (W) pullback and (X) dorsoventral.

A H-frame connecting the canines of the upper and lower jaws was used to apply extrinsic forces, with forces applied at the center of the frame [32,35]. The force (N) applied to extrinsic loads was an arbitrary figure, applied for strictly comparative purposes, equivalent to 100 times the animal's estimated body mass for an axial twist, and 10 times the animal's estimated body mass for a lateral shake, pullback and dorsoventral shake [81]. Each simulation in which forces are applied with the anterior teeth (canines) restrained is a test for the hypothesis that stress will be highest for species with the longest rostrum.

Von Mises (VM) stress is a good predictor of failure in ductile materials such as bone [84,85] and VM stress is used here as a metric for comparison between models following Attard et al. [35]. Nodes were selected at equidistant points along the mid-sagittal plane, zygomatic arch and mandible (Figure 2) following Attard et al. [35] and at each node values were calculated by averaging VM stress recorded in the surrounding elements to assess changes in stress magnitudes and distributions under different loadings.

Principal component analysis (PCA) was used to visualize differences between species in average VM stress values for equidistant nodes along the mid-sagittal plane (N = 10). PCA is an ordination technique that summarizes the maximum variation among a set of variables on few, uncorrelated axes (principal components) [86]. PCA was performed separately on VM stress values for each extrinsic load (axial twist, lateral shake, pullback and dorsoventral) and for a bilateral canine bite. All VM stress values were log transformed prior to PCA.

Differences in VM stress values between species were compared using a Kruskal-Wallis test, which is regarded as a multiple-group extension of the Man-Whitney test [87]. Significance values were corrected for multiple comparisons using Bonferroni corrections, as a conservative approach.

Results

The predicted body mass (kg) of each species was generally within the expected range for each of the extant species (Table 1). Body mass estimates ranged from 0.78 kg for *D. hallucatus*, up to 32.49 kg for *T. cynocephalus*. However, the body mass estimated for *S. harrisii* of 14.20 kg was slightly above the upper limit observed for males (13 kg) [88], possibly because the teeth and skull are relatively large in this species. The robust craniodental morphology and relatively large teeth in *S. harrisii* are probably related to its habitual osteophagy, as has been observed in bone-cracking carnivorans [89]. To obtain body mass estimates for these taxa using simple or multiple regressions adjusted from cranidental variables may lead to overestimates of body mass. Predicted maximum muscle forces for *N. dicksoni* (651 N) were relatively high, approaching those of the larger *S. harrisii* (685 N) (Table 1).

Thylacinus cynocephalus displayed comparatively high levels of VM stress in the cranium and mandible for most simulations (Figure 3– 6, S3). This is consistent with results of Attard et.al. [35]. *Dasyurus hallucatus* showed relatively high levels of stress in the posterior of the mandible for a canine bite (Figure 3A), and along the ventral surface of the ramus for most extrinsic loads (Figure 5A–C).

The regions of highest stress along the dentary of *N. dicksoni* were located at the coronoid fossa and condylar process (Figure 3D). These regions of peak stress may be in part artifacts of reconstruction. Otherwise the dentary of *N. dicksoni* revealed

similar stress patterns for a bilateral bite to *D. maculatus* (Figure 3). The distribution of stress for *N. dicksoni* in the cranium in response to a bilateral bite was intermediate between *S. harrisii* and *D. maculatus* (Figure 4). The magnitudes of stress along the mid-sagittal plane of *N. dicksoni* were slightly higher than for *S. harrisii* and lower than for *D. maculatus* (Figure 4F).

The highest stress in the cranium occurred at the zygomatic arch for all species in response to a bilateral canine bite (Figure 4). Von Mises stress along the zygomatic arch during a bilateral canine bite gradually increased posteriorly in *S. harrisii*, while stress peaked at node 3 in *T. cynocephalus* followed by a gradual decrease posteriorly (Figure S6A). The three other species displayed two peaks in stress along the zygomatic arch during a bilateral canine bite; one at the middle and the other at the posterior region of the zygomatic arch. *Thylacinus cynocephalus* was the only species to show two distinct peaks in stress for a bilateral bite along the mid-sagittal crest (Figure 4F). These stress points occurred at the temporal ridge and at the most narrowed region of the nasal (Figure 4E). Von Mises stress measured along the mid-sagittal crest for a bilateral bite revealed one point of peak stress halfway along the frontal of *D. maculatus*, *S. harrisii* and *N. dicksoni* and at the temporal ridge for *D. hallucatus* (Figure 4).

Stress was quite evenly distributed along the dentaries for all species in response to lateral shaking and axial twisting, with the exception of *D. hallucatus*, wherein stresses peaked anteriorly (Figure 5U–V) resulting in significantly higher VM stress values for that species compared to all others ($\chi^2 = 32.87$, $P<0.0001$). An axial twist resulted in much higher levels of stress along the mid-sagittal crest for *D. hallucatus* compared to all other species, and peaked at the anterior of the nasal and at the frontal (Figure 6B). *Sarcophilus harrisii* and *T. cynocephalus* showed higher levels of stress along the mandible for a pullback and dorsoventral shake than other species included in this study (Figure 5W–X). Comparisons of mandible VM stress values revealed significant differences between species after Bonferroni correction for both pullback ($\chi^2 = 33.28$, $P<0.001$) and dorsoventral shake ($\chi^2 = 35.61$, $P< 0.0001$), with the exception of *T. cynocephalus* and *S. harrisii*. Two points of peak stress were apparent along the dentary for *T. cynocephalus* in these two simulations; one at the most anterior point, and the second at the coronoid fossa. Stress distribution along the dentary of *S. harrisii* followed a similar trend for a pullback and dorsoventral shake; peaking at the ramus inferior to M1 then gradually decreasing posteriorly.

PCA results for mid-sagittal node VM stress values (Figure 7) showed that a high proportion of variance could be explained in all cases by two Principal Component (PC) axes (>85%). These plots provide an appreciation of interspecific differences across all 10 mid-sagittal nodes and bite simulations. PCA results indicate that the main axes of interspecific variance for all bites were explained by either nodes 1 and/or 7–10. *Thylacinus cynocephalus* and *S. harrisii* differed significantly for VM stress values under a bilateral bite at the canines ($\chi^2 = 12.95$, $P= 0.04$) and PCA results indicated separation of those two species along PC1 (60.6%), which largely explained variance in node 8 and node 10 (Figure 7A). PC1 for a bilateral canine bite revealed close similarities between *N. dicksoni* and *D. maculatus*, whereas PC2 (28.9%) clearly separated *N. dicksoni* from *D. maculatus* and reflected differences in node 7 (as seen in Figure 4).

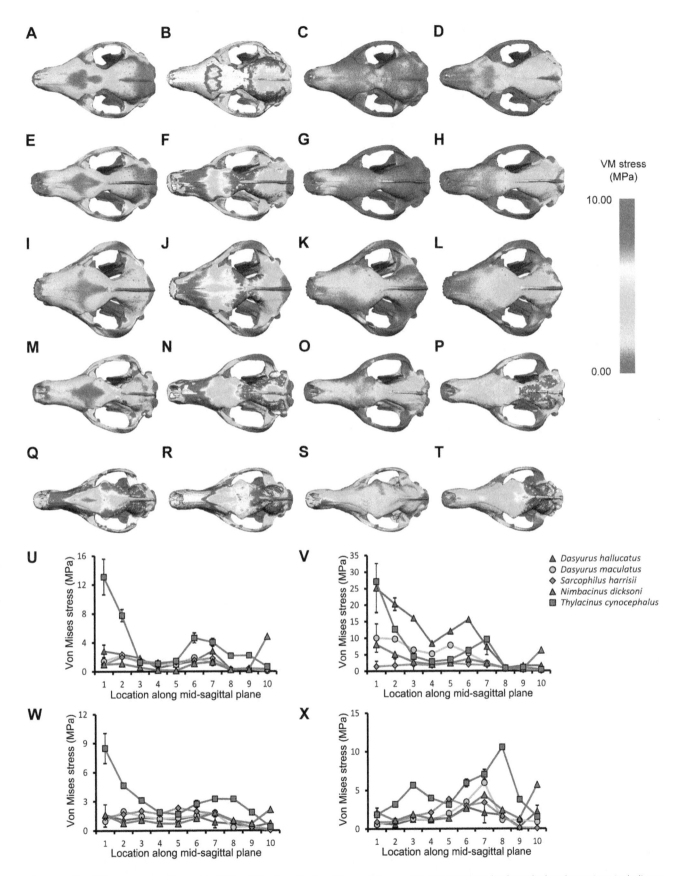

Figure 6. Von Mises stress under extrinsic loads in dorsal view. The models are subjected to various loads applied to the canines, including a (A, E, I, M, Q) lateral shake, (B, F, J, N, R) axial twist, (C, G, K, O, S) pullback and (D, H, L, P, T) dorsoventral. The force applied was equivalent to 100 times the animal's estimated body mass for an axial twist, and 10 times the animal's estimated body mass for a lateral shake, pullback and dorsoventral

shake. Species compared were (A–D) *Dasyurus hallucatus*, (E–H) *Dasyurus maculatus*, (I–L) *Sarcophilus harrisii*, (M–P) *Nimbacinus dicksoni* and (Q–T) *Thylacinus cynocephalus*. White colored regions of the skull represent VM stress above 10 MPa. Distribution of von Mises (VM) stress was measured from anterior to posterior along the mid-sagittal plane for a (U) lateral shake, (V) axial twist, (W) pullback and (X) dorsoventral.

For a lateral shake, PC1 (51.0%) explained change at nodes 1 and 10 and separated *T. cynocephalus* from *N. dicksoni* (Figure 7B), as also seen in Figure 6U. PC2 (42.0%) for a lateral shake revealed differences among all species for nodes 7 and 10, with *T. cynocephalus* closely resembling *N. dicksoni* compared to other species (Figure 7B). Interspecific differences were not significant for a lateral shake after Bonferroni correction, and before correction those distinguished *T. cynocephalus* from *N. dicksoni*, *D. maculatus* and *S. harrisii* ($\chi^2 = 9.27$, $P = 0.01$–0.03). PCA for an axial twist

(Figure 7C) showed that the extremes of PC1 (66.1%) were delimited by *S. harrisii* and *D. hallucatus*, and the remaining taxa were located in between those two species. PC1 mainly accounted for differences among species for node 1 values (as seen also in Figure 6V), which were high for *D. hallucatus* and low for *S. harrisii*, whereas PC2 (26.1%) largely summarized node 10 values. Pairwise comparisons of VM stress values were not significant for an axial twist, however before Bonferroni correction, differences between *S. harrisii* and *D. hallucatus* ($\chi^2 = 10.73$, $P = 0.03$), *N. dicksoni*

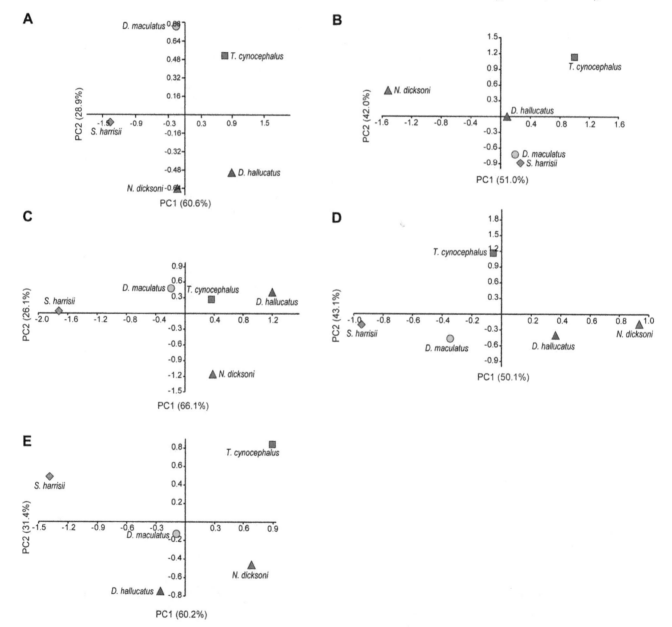

Figure 7. Principal components one and two of von Mises stress along mid-sagittal plane. Results of principal components analysis to compare stress among species along mid-sagittal nodes for each loading case, including (A) bilateral canine bite, (B) lateral shake, (C) axial twist, (D) pullback and (E) dorsoventral. Key to symbols: (pink square) *Thylacinus cynocephalus*; (red triangle) *Nimbicinus dicksoni*; (orange diamond) *Sarcophilus harrisii*; (green circle) *Dasyurus maculatus*; (purple triangle) *Dasyurus hallucatus*.

$(\chi^2 = 10.73, \ P = 0.01)$ and $T. \ cynocephalus$ $(\chi^2 = 10.73, \ P = 0.04)$ could be distinguished from one another. For a pullback bite, PC1 (50.1%) mainly explained interspecific differences for node 10, and PC2 (43.1%) explained change at nodes 1 and 8 (Figure 7D). VM stress values for $T. \ cynocephalus$ were different from those for $D. \ hallucatus$ $(\chi^2 = 14.37, \ P = 0.02)$ and $D. \ maculatus$ $(\chi^2 = 14.37, \ P = 0.04)$ for a pullback bite. For the dorsoventral shake, PC1 explained 60.2% of variance and reflected differences between $T. \ cynocephalus$ and $S. \ harrisii$, whereas values across nodes were more similar among the remaining three species, located toward the middle of PC1 (Figure 7E). PC2 (31.4%) separated $D. \ hallucatus$ from $T. \ cynocephalus$, and pairwise comparisons revealed node values to be different between those two species $(\chi^2 = 14.78, \ P = 0.01)$.

Discussion

Differences in biomechanical performance between the three extant dasyurids included in this study appear consistent with their respective known feeding behaviors. *Dasyurus hallucatus* showed comparatively higher levels of stress in most simulations than *S. harrisii* and *D. maculatus*. *Dasyurus hallucatus* eats invertebrates and other relatively small prey [60–62], which may not require adaptation to sustain the full range of extrinsic loads simulated here. This species shows particularly high VM stress in axial twisting, especially in contrast to *S. harrisii* However, it performs relatively well under pull-back loading, which may be linked to a capacity for pulling invertebrates from the ground. Observational studies on wild *D. hallucatus* will be required to confirm the functional role of their skull in prey acquisition. Future work on the comparative musculoskeletal anatomy and collection of in vivo or ex vivo biomechanical data of the extant species would likely improve the predictive power of current bite force and muscle force estimations. Overall consistencies found between known prey size and biomechanical performance for extant dasyuromorphians underscore the potential value of projections based on comparative FEA for extinct/fossil taxa.

Our comparative biomechanical modeling of dasyuromorphian skulls suggests considerable differences in predatory behaviors between the two thylacinids considered here. Our 3D based results indicate that the Oligocene to Miocene *N. dicksoni* had a high bite force for its size, comparable to that of extant dasyurids known to take relatively large prey, *D. maculatus* and *S. harrisii* [48,60]. In light of similar levels of 'carnassialization' (development of relatively long, high amplitude vertical shearing crests) in the cheektooth dentition with *D. maculatus*, and a lack of obvious dental specialization consistent with regular bone-cracking, our results suggest a predominantly carnivorous diet for *N. dicksoni* that may have included relatively large prey. *Dasyurus maculatus* are opportunistic hunters, varying their diet in response to environmental disturbances and short-term fluctuations in prey abundance [54,56]. They will prey on vertebrate species up to and sometimes exceeding their own body mass. Prey includes bandicoots, smaller dasyurids, possums, smaller macropodoids, snakes, lizards, birds and frogs, as well as invertebrates. Potential prey for a fox-sized thylacinid living in the closed forest communities of Riversleigh likely included many small to medium-size birds, frogs, lizards and snakes, as well as a wide range of marsupials, including bandicoots (peramelemorphians), dasyurids (dasyuromorphians), kangaroos (macropodoids), thingodontans (yalkiparidontians), marsupial moles (notoryctemorphians) and wombats (vombatoids) [12].

Although our FEA results for *N. dicksoni* suggest a capacity to kill prey approaching or exceeding its own body mass, its prey range may have been limited by competition with sympatric carnivores. The extent of niche overlap and competition within this ancient, medium-large sized carnivore community may have been partially alleviated by occupying different habitats and specializing in different hunting strategies. The recovery of a near complete skeleton of *N. dicksoni* [14] will provide further information on the locomotion and predatory behavior based on postcranial material; for example, was *N. dicksoni* as arboreal as the extant *D. maculatus*?

Differences in mechanical performance suggest that *T. cynocephalus* is unusual relative to other dasyuromorphians, including, *N. dicksoni*, as indicated by distinctly higher VM stresses than all other species in response to each loading case. *Thylacinus cynocephalus*, in contrast to *N. dicksoni*, has completely lost the metaconid on the lower molars and has a proportionately much larger postmetacrista on the upper molars. On the basis of traditional beam theory we predicted that taxa with longer rostra would exhibit higher stress [90], as evident in the long-snouted *T. cynocephalus* relative to shorter-snouted dasyuromorphians. Differences between *T. cynocephalus* and other species were also significant for three out of five simulations examined after conservative Bonferroni correction for multiple testing. These results further support the contention by Attard et al. [35] that niche breadth in *T. cynocephalus* may have been more limited and that it likely preyed on relatively small to medium-sized vertebrates such as wallabies, possums and bandicoots.

Although measures of skull performance in response to forces imposed by struggling prey revealed closer similarity between the fossil thylacinid *N. dicksoni* and large extant carnivorous dasyurids, than with *T. cynocephalus*, there were differences. Our reconstruction suggests that the TMJ was more elevated in *N. dicksoni* than in *D. maculatus*, and higher relative to the height of the cheektooth row. The TMJ is a complex joint and is important for occlusion and mastication [91,92]. The position of the TMJ can influence bite strength and muscle activation [93]. The position of the TMJ along the anterior-posterior axis tends to lie closer to the plane of the tooth row in carnivorous taxa [11]. Conclusive determination of the precise position and morphology of the TMJ in *N. dicksoni* must await the discovery of more complete cranial material.

Morphological evidence from past studies further demonstrates diversity within this family. The smallest thylacinid, *Muribacinus gadiyuli*, is believed to have fed on relatively small vertebrates and invertebrates because it lacks a number of dental features present in large prey specialists (e.g., robust protoconids and brachycephalization) such as similarly sized *D. maculatus* [17]. The variety of feeding behaviors among thylacinids may have helped facilitate their co-existence within different ecological niches that were later filled by diversifying carnivorous dasyurids.

Supporting Information

Figure S1 Phylogenetic tree of dasyuromophians investigated in this study. One of several recent assessments of the phylogenetic relationships of dasyuromorphians, including taxa that have been examined in this study (Wroe & Musser 2001).

Figure S2 Interactive 3D pdf showing the digitally segmented cranium and mandible of *Thylacinus cynocephalus*.

Figure S3 Interactive 3D pdf showing the digitally segmented cranium and mandible of *Sarcophilus harrisii*.

Figure S4   Interactive 3D pdf showing the digitally segmented cranium and mandible of *Dasyurus maculatus*.

Figure S5   Interactive 3D pdf showing the digitally segmented cranium and mandible of *Dasyurus hallucatus*.

Figure S6   Von Mises stress along zygomatic arch for all loading cases. Distribution of von Mises (VM) stress was measured from anterior to posterior along the zygomatic arch for a (A) bilateral canine bite, (B) lateral shake, (C) axial twist, (D) pullback and (E) dorsoventral.

Table S1   Temporal and geographic distribution of thylacinid species. Abbreviations: Aust, Australian mainland; E., Early; L., Late; M., Middle; Mio, Miocene; NG, New Guinea; NT, Northern Territory; Oligo, Oligocene; Plio, Pliocene; Qld, Queensland; Tas, Tasmania.

Table S2   Maximum bite forces (N) for un-scaled homogeneous models for a bilateral canine bite.

Table S3   Muscle forces used for each jaw muscle division in un-scaled intrinsic models. Species studied were *Dasyurus hallucatus*, *Dasyurus maculatus*, *Sarcophilus harrisii*, *Nimbacinus dicksoni* and *Thylacinus cynocephalus*. These were calculated using muscle mass proportions from dissected *Didelphis virginiana* (Turnbull 1970). Muscle forces were scaled for a bilateral canine bite by multiplying the muscle force by the ratio between bite force estimated using body mass regressions and maximum bite force estimated from the un-scaled model.

Acknowledgments

We thank Sandy Ingleby from the Australian museum for providing several comparative specimens and the makers of Digimorph for access to CT scan data.

Author Contributions

Conceived and designed the experiments: MRGA SW. Performed the experiments: MRGA WCHP. Analyzed the data: MRGA LABW WCHP. Contributed reagents/materials/analysis tools: SW. Wrote the paper: MRGA WCHP LABW MA SJH TLR SW.

References

1. Krajewski C, Buckley L, Westerman M (1997) DNA phylogeny of the marsupial wolf resolved. Proc R Soc Lond, Ser B: Biol Sci 264: 911–917.

2. Krajewski C, Driskell AC, Baverstock PR, Braun MJ (1992) Phylogenetic relationships of the thylacine (Mammalia: Thylacinidae) among dasyuroid marsupials: evidence from cytochrome b DNA sequences. Proc R Soc Lond, Ser B: Biol Sci 250: 19–27.

3. Lowenstein JM, Sarich VM, Richardson BJ (1981) Albumin systematics of the extinct mammoth and Tasmanian wolf. Nature 291: 409–411.

4. Muirhead J, Wroe S (1998) A new genus and species, *Badjcinus turnbulli* (Thylacinidae: Marsupialia), from the late Oligocene of Riversleigh, northern Australia, and an investigation of thylacinid phylogeny. J Vert Paleontol 18: 612–626.

5. Sarich V, Lowenstein JM, Richardson BJ (1982) Phylogenetic relationships of the thylacine (*Thylacinus cynocephalus*, Marsupialia) as reflected in comparative serology. In: Archer M, editor. Carnivorous Marsupials. Sydney: Royal Zoological Society of New South Wales. pp. 445–476.

6. Szalay FS (1982) A new appraisal of marsupial phylogeny and classification. In: Archer M, editor. Carnivorous Marsupials. Sydney: Royal Zoological Society of New South Wales. pp. 621–640.

7. Thomas RH, Schaffner W, Wilson AC, Paabo S (1989) DNA phylogeny of the extinct marsupial wolf. Nature 340: 465–467.

8. Wroe S, Archer M (2006) Origins and early radiations of marsupials. In: Merrick JR, Archer M, Hickey GM, Lee MSY, editors. Evolution and Biogeography of Australasian Vertebrates. Sydney: Australian Scientific Publishing. pp. 517–540.

9. Goswami A, Milne N, Wroe S (2011) Biting through constraints: cranial morphology, disparity and convergence across living and fossil carnivorous mammals. Proceedings of the Royal Society B: Biological Sciences 278: 1831–1839.

10. Wroe S (2001) *Maximucinus muirheadae*, gen. et sp. nov. (Thylacinidae: Marsupialia), from the Miocene of Riversleigh, north-western Queensland, with estimates of body weights for fossil thylacinids. Aust J Zool 49: 603–614.

11. Wroe S, Milne N (2007) Convergence and remarkably consistent constraint in the evolution of mammalian carnivore skull shape. Evolution 61: 1251–1260.

12. Archer M, Arena DA, Bassarova M, Beck RMD, Black K, et al. (2006) Current status of species-level representation in faunas from selected fossil localities in the Riversleigh World Heritage Area, northwestern Queensland. Alcheringa 30: 1–17.

13. Muirhead J (1997) Two new thylacines (Marsupialia: Thylacinidae) from early Miocene sediments of Riversleigh, northwestern Queensland and a revision of the family Thylacinidae. Mem Queensl Mus 41: 367–377.

14. Muirhead J, Archer M (1990) *Nimbacinus dicksoni*, a plesiomorphic thylacine (Marsupialia: Thylacinidae) from Tertiary deposits of Queensland and the Northern Territory. Mem Queensl Mus 28: 203–221.

15. Murray PF (1997) *Thylacinus megiriani*, a new species of thylacine (Marsupialia: Thylacinidae) from the Ongeva local fauna of central Australia. Rec S Aust Mus 30: 43–61.

16. Murray PF, Megirian D (2000) Two new genera and three new species of Thylacinidae (Marsupialia) from the Miocene of the Northern Territory,
Australia. The Beagle, Records of the Museums and Art Galleries of the Northern Territory 16: 145–162.

17. Wroe S (1996) *Muribacinus gadiyuli*, (Thylacinidae: Marsupialia), a very plesiomorphic thylacinid from the Miocene of Riversleigh, northwestern Queensland, and the problem of paraphyly for the Dasyuridae. J Paleontol 70: 1032–1044.

18. Wroe S, Musser A (2001) The skull of *Nimbacinus dicksoni* (Thylacinidae: Marsupialia). Aust J Zool 49: 487–514.

19. Archer M, Hand S, Godthelp H (1991) Riversleigh: The Story of Animals in Ancient Rainforests of Inland Australia. Sydney: Reed Books. 264 p.

20. Travouillon KJ, Legendre S, Archer M, Hand SJ (2009) Palaeoecological analyses of Riversleigh's Oligo-Miocene sites: implications for Oligo-Miocene climate change in Australia. Palaeogeogr, Palaeoclimatol, Palaeoecol 276: 24–37.

21. Archer M, Brammal J, Field J, Hand SJ, Hook C (2002) The Evolution of Australia: 110 million years of change. Sydney: Australian Museum. 91 p.

22. Wroe S (2002) A review of terrestrial mammalian and reptilian carnivore ecology in Australian fossil faunas and factors influencing their diversity: The myth of reptilian domination and its broader ramifications. Aust J Zool 49: 603–614.

23. Wroe S, Myers TJ, Wells RT, Gillespie A (1999) Estimating the weight of the Pleistocene marsupial lion, *Thylacoleo carnifex* (Thylacoleonidae: Marsupialia): implications for the ecomorphology of a marsupial super-predator and hypotheses of impoverishment of Australian marsupial carnivore faunas. Aust J Zool 47: 489–498.

24. Wroe S (2003) Australian marsupial carnivores: an overview of recent advances in palaeontology. In: Jones M, Dickman C, Archer M, editors. Predators with Pouches: The Biology of Carnivorous Marsupials. Collingwood: CSIRO Publishing. pp. 102–123.

25. Wroe S, Brammall J, Cooke BN (1998) The skull of *Ekaltadeta ima* (Marsupialia, Hypsiprymnodontidae?): an analysis of some marsupial cranial features and a re-investigation of propleopine phylogeny, with notes on the inference of carnivory in mammals. J Paleontol 72: 738–751.

26. Wroe S, McHenry C, Thomason J (2005) Bite club: comparative bite force in big biting mammals and the prediction of predatory behaviour in fossil taxa. Proc R Soc Lond, Ser B: Biol Sci 272: 619–625.

27. Dumont ER, Piccirillo J, Grosse IR (2005) Finite element analysis of biting behavior and bone stress in the facial skeletons of bats. Anat Rec 283: 319–330.

28. Ross CF (2005) Finite element analysis in vertebrate biomechanics. Anat Rec A Discov Mol Cell Evol Biol 283A: 253–258.

29. Tseng ZJ (2009) Cranial function in a late Miocene *Dinocrocuta gigantea* (Mammalia: Carnivora) revealed by comparative finite element analysis. Biol J Linn Soc 96: 51–67.

30. Wroe S, Ferrara TL, McHenry CR, Curnoe D, Chamoli U (2010) The craniomandibular mechanics of being human. Proc R Soc Lond, Ser B: Biol Sci 277: 3579–3586.

31. McHenry CR, Wroe S, Clausen PD, Moreno K, Cunningham E (2007) Supermodeled sabercat, predatory behavior in *Smilodon fatalis* revealed by high-resolution 3D computer simulation. Proc Natl Acad Sci USA 104: 16010–16015.

32. Wroe S, Clausen P, McHenry C, Moreno K, Cunningham E (2007) Computer simulation of feeding behaviour in the thylacine and dingo as a novel test for convergence and niche overlap. Proc R Soc Lond, Ser B: Biol Sci 274: 2819–2828.

33. Young MT, Rayfield EJ, Holliday CM, Witmer LM, Button DJ, et al. (2012) Cranial biomechanics of *Diplodocus* (Dinosauria, Sauropoda): testing hypotheses of feeding behaviour in an extinct megaherbivore. Naturwissenschaften 99: 637–643.

34. Bell PR, Snively E, Shychoski L (2009) A comparison of the jaw mechanics in hadrosaurid and ceratopsid dinosaurs using finite element analysis. Anat Rec (Hoboken) 292: 1338–1351.

35. Attard MRG, Chamoli U, Ferrara TL, Rogers TL, Wroe S (2011) Skull mechanics and implications for feeding behaviour in a large marsupial carnivore guild: the thylacine, Tasmanian devil and spotted-tailed quoll. J Zool 285: 292–300.

36. Chamoli U, Wroe S (2011) Allometry in the distribution of material properties and geometry of the felid skull: Why larger species may need to change and how they may achieve it. J Theor Biol 283: 217–226.

37. Moazen M, Curtis N, Evans SE, O'Higgins P, Fagan MJ (2008) Combined finite element and multibody dynamics analysis of biting in a *Uromastyx hardwickii* lizard skull. J Anat 213: 499–508.

38. Oldfield CC, McHenry CR, Clausen PD, Chamoli U, Parr WCH, et al. (2012) Finite element analysis of ursid cranial mechanics and the prediction of feeding behaviour in the extinct giant *Agriotherium africanum*. J Zool 286: 163–170.

39. Rayfield EJ, Norman DB, Horner CC, Horner JR, Smith PM, et al. (2001) Cranial design and function in a large theropod dinosaur. Nature 409: 1033–1037.

40. Slater GJ, Figueirido B, Louis L, Yang P, Van Valkenburgh B (2010) Biomechanical Consequences of Rapid Evolution in the Polar Bear Lineage. PLoS ONE 5: e13870.

41. Strait DS, Grosse IR, Dechow PC, Smith AL, Wang Q, et al. (2010) The structural rigidity of the cranium of *Australopithecus africanus*: implications for diet, dietary adaptations, and the allometry of feeding biomechanics. Anat Rec (Hoboken) 293: 583–593.

42. Thresher RW, Saito GE (1973) The stress analysis of human teeth. J Biomech 6: 443–449.

43. Paddle R (2000) The Last Tasmanian tiger: the History and Extinction of the Thylacine. Oakleigh, VIC: Cambridge University Press. 273 p.

44. Jones ME, Stoddart DM (1998) Reconstruction of the predatory behaviour of the extinct marsupial thylacine (*Thylacinus cynocephalus*). J Zool 246: 239–246.

45. Jones ME (2003) Convergence in ecomorphology and guild structure among marsupial and placental carnivores. In: Jones ME, Dickman C, Archer M, editors. Predators with Pouches: The Biology of Carnivorous Marsupials. Collingwood: CSIRO Publishing. pp. 285–269.

46. Guiler ER (1985) Thylacine: The tragedy of the Tasmanian tiger. Melbourne: Oxford University Press. 207 p.

47. Bailey C (2003) Tiger Tales: Stories of the Tasmanian Tiger. Sydney: HarperCollins Publishers. 164 p.

48. Figueirido B, Janis CM (2011) The predatory behaviour of the thylacine: Tasmanian tiger or marsupial wolf? Biol Lett 7: 937–940.

49. Jones ME, Barmuta LA (1998) Diet overlap and abundance of sympatric dasyurid carnivores: a hypothesis of competition? J Anim Ecol 67: 410–421.

50. Bradshaw CJA, Brook BW (2005) Disease and the devil: density-dependent epidemiological processes explain historical population fluctuations in the Tasmanian devil. Ecography 28: 181–190.

51. Guiler E (1970) Observations on the Tasmanian devil, *Sarcophilus harrisii* (Marsupialia : Dasyuridae) I. Numbers, home, range, movements and food in two populations. Aust J Zool 18: 49–62.

52. Taylor RJ (1986) Notes on the diet of the carnivorous mammals of the upper Henry River region, Western Tasmania. Pap Proc R Soc Tasman 120: 7–10.

53. Groves CP (2005) Order Dasyuromorphia. In: Wilson DE, Reeder DM, editors. Mammal Species of the World: A Taxonomic and Geographic Reference. 3rd ed. Baltimore: Johns Hopkins University Press. pp. 23–37.

54. Edgar R, Belcher C (1995) Spotted-tailed quoll, *Dasyurus maculatus*. In: Strahan R, editor. The Mammals of Australia. Sydney: Reed. pp. 67–69.

55. Glen AS, Dickman CR (2006) Diet of the spotted-tailed quoll (*Dasyurus maculatus*) in eastern Australia: effects of season, sex and size. J Zool 269: 241–248.

56. Jones ME (1997) Character displacement in Australian dasyurid carnivores: size relationships and prey size patterns. Ecology 78: 2569–2587.

57. Dawson JP, Claridge AW, Triggs B, Paull DJ (2007) Diet of a native carnivore, the spotted-tailed quoll (*Dasyurus maculatus*), before and after an intense wildfire. Wildl Res 34: 342–351.

58. Braithwaite RW, Begg RJ (1995) Northern quoll *Dasyurus hallucatus* Gould, 1842. In: Strahan R, editor. The Mammals of Australia: National Photographic Index of Australian Wildlife. Sydney: Reed Books. pp. 65–66.

59. Strahan R (1995) The Mammals of Australia. Sydney: New Holland Publishing Pty Ltd.

60. Belcher CA (1995) Diet of the Tiger quoll (*Dasyurus maculatus*) in East Gippsland, Victoria. Wildl Res 22: 341–357.

61. Oakwood M (1997) The ecology of the northern quoll, *Dasyurus hallucatus* [PhD thesis]. Canberra: Australian National University. 556 p.

62. Pollock AB (1999) Notes on status, distribution and diet of northern quoll *Dasyurus hallucatus* in the Mackay-Bowen area, mideastern Queensland. Aust Zool 31: 388–395.

63. Wroe S (2008) Cranial mechanics compared in extinct marsupial and extant African lions using a finite-element approach. J Zool 274: 332–339.

64. Benazzi S, Bookstein FL, Strait DS, Weber GW (2011) A new OH5 reconstruction with an assessment of its uncertainty. J Hum Evol 61: 75–88.

65. Besl PJ, McKay ND (1992) A method for registration of 3D shapes. IEEE Transactions on Pattern Analysis and Machine Intelligence. pp. 239–256.

66. Parr WCH, Wroe S, Chamoli U, Richards HS, McCurry MR, et al. (2012) Toward integration of geometric morphometrics and computational biomechanics: New methods for 3D virtual reconstruction and quantitative analysis of Finite Element Models. J Theor Biol 301: 1–14.

67. Rayfield EJ (2007) Finite element analysis and understanding the biomechanics and evolution of living and fossil organisms. Annu Rev Earth Planet Sci 35: 541–576.

68. Cook SD, Weinstein AH, Klawitter JJ (1982) A three-dimensional finite element analysis of a porous rooted Co–Cr–Mo alloy dental implant. J Dent Res 61: 25–29.

69. Dumont ER, Grosse IR, Slater GJ (2009) Requirements for comparing the performance of finite element models of biological structures. J Theor Biol 256: 96–103.

70. Greaves G, Greer A, Lakes R, Rouxel T (2011) Poisson's ratio and modern materials. Nat Mater 10: 823–837.

71. Turnbull WD (1970) Mammalian masticatory apparatus. Fieldiana: Geology 18: 149–356.

72. Thomason JJ (1991) Cranial strength in relation to estimated biting forces in some mammals. Can J Zool 69: 2326–2333.

73. Chamoli U (2011) Biomechanics of the felid skulls: A comparative study using finite element approach [Masters thesis]. Sydney: University of New South Wales. 144 p.

74. Clausen P, Wroe S, McHenry C, Moreno K, Bourke J (2008) The vector of jaw muscle force as determined by computer-generated three dimensional simulation: a test of Greaves' model. J Biomech 41: 3184–3188.

75. Jones ME (1995) Guild structure of the large marsupial carnivores in Tasmania [PhD thesis]. Hobart: University of Tasmania. 176 p.

76. Pellis SM, Nelson A (1984) Some aspects of predatory behaviour of the quoll *Dasyurus viverrinus* (Marsupialia: Dasyuridae). Aust Mammal 7: 5–15.

77. Pellis SM, Officer RCE (1987) An analysis of some predatory behaviour patterns in four species of carnivorous marsupials (Dasyuridae), with comparative notes on the Eutherian cat *Felis catus*. Ethology 75: 177.

78. Fleay D (1932) The rare dasyures (native cats). Vic Nat 49: 63–69.

79. Dumont ER, Herrel A (2003) The effect of gape angle and bite point on bite force in bats. J Exp Biol 206: 2117–2123.

80. Christiansen P, Wroe S (2007) Bite forces and evolutionary adaptations to feeding ecology in carnivores. Ecology 88: 347–358.

81. Myers TJ (2001) Marsupial body mass prediction. Aust J Zool 49: 99–118.

82. Wroe S, Chamoli U, Parr WCH, Clausen P, Ridgely R, et al. (2013) Comparative biomechanical Modeling of Metatherian and Placental Saber-Tooths: A Different Kind of Bite for an Extreme Pouched Predator. PLoS ONE 8: e66888.

83. Ellis JL, Thomason JJ, Kebreab E, France J (2008) Calibration of estimated biting forces in domestic canids: comparison of post-mortem and in vivo measurements. J Anat 212: 769–780.

84. Nalla RK, Kinney JH, Ritchie RO (2003) Mechanistic fracture criteria for the failure of human cortical bone. Nat Mater 2: 164–168.

85. Tsafnat N, Wroe S (2010) An experimentally validated micromechanical model of a rat vertebra under compressive loading. J Anat 218: 40–46.

86. Mitteroecker P, Gunz P (2009) Advances in geometric morphometrics. Evol Biol 36: 235–247.

87. Zar JH (1996) Multiple regression and correlation. Biostatistical Analysis 3rd ed Upper Saddle River, NJ: Prentice Hall: 353–360.

88. Owen D, Pemberton D (2005) Tasmanian Devil: A Unique and Threatened Animal. Crows Nest, NSW: Allen and Unwin. 225 p.

89. Figueirido B, Tseng ZJ, Martin-Serra A (2013) Skull shape evolution in durophagous carnivorans. Evolution 67: 1975–1993.

90. Walmsley CW, Smits PD, Quayle MR, McCurry MR, Richards HS, et al. (2013) Why the long face? The mechanics of mandibular symphysis proportions in crocodiles. PLoS ONE 8: e53873.

91. Hylander WL (1979) An experimental analysis of temporomandibular joint reaction force in macaques. Am J Phys Anthropol 51: 433–456.

92. Breul R, Mall G, Landgraf J, Scheck R (1999) Biomechanical analysis of stress distribution in the human temporomandibular-joint. Ann Anat 181: 55–60.

93. Hickman DM, Cramer R (1998) The effect of different condylar positions on masticatory muscle electromyographic activity in humans. Oral Surg Oral Med Oral Pathol Oral Radiol Endod 85: 18–23.

Permissions

All chapters in this book were first published in PLOS ONE, by The Public Library of Science; hereby published with permission under the Creative Commons Attribution License or equivalent. Every chapter published in this book has been scrutinized by our experts. Their significance has been extensively debated. The topics covered herein carry significant findings which will fuel the growth of the discipline. They may even be implemented as practical applications or may be referred to as a beginning point for another development.

The contributors of this book come from diverse backgrounds, making this book a truly international effort. This book will bring forth new frontiers with its revolutionizing research information and detailed analysis of the nascent developments around the world.

We would like to thank all the contributing authors for lending their expertise to make the book truly unique. They have played a crucial role in the development of this book. Without their invaluable contributions this book wouldn't have been possible. They have made vital efforts to compile up to date information on the varied aspects of this subject to make this book a valuable addition to the collection of many professionals and students.

This book was conceptualized with the vision of imparting up-to-date information and advanced data in this field. To ensure the same, a matchless editorial board was set up. Every individual on the board went through rigorous rounds of assessment to prove their worth. After which they invested a large part of their time researching and compiling the most relevant data for our readers.

The editorial board has been involved in producing this book since its inception. They have spent rigorous hours researching and exploring the diverse topics which have resulted in the successful publishing of this book. They have passed on their knowledge of decades through this book. To expedite this challenging task, the publisher supported the team at every step. A small team of assistant editors was also appointed to further simplify the editing procedure and attain best results for the readers.

Apart from the editorial board, the designing team has also invested a significant amount of their time in understanding the subject and creating the most relevant covers. They scrutinized every image to scout for the most suitable representation of the subject and create an appropriate cover for the book.

The publishing team has been an ardent support to the editorial, designing and production team. Their endless efforts to recruit the best for this project, has resulted in the accomplishment of this book. They are a veteran in the field of academics and their pool of knowledge is as vast as their experience in printing. Their expertise and guidance has proved useful at every step. Their uncompromising quality standards have made this book an exceptional effort. Their encouragement from time to time has been an inspiration for everyone.

The publisher and the editorial board hope that this book will prove to be a valuable piece of knowledge for researchers, students, practitioners and scholars across the globe.

List of Contributors

Haruo Sugi
Department of Physiology, School of Medicine, Teikyo University, Tokyo, Japan

Shigeru Chaen
Department of Integrated Sciences in Physics and Biology, College of Humanities and Sciences, Nihon University, Tokyo, Japan

Takakazu Kobayashi, Takahiro Abe and Kazushige Kimura
Department of Electronic Engineering, Shibaura Institute of Technology, Tokyo, Japan

Yasutake Saeki and Yoshiki Ohnuki
Department of Physiology, School of Dentistry, Tsurumi University, Yokohama, Japan

Takuya Miyakawa and Masaru Tanokura
Department of Applied Biochemistry, Graduate School of Agriculture and Life Sciences, University of Tokyo, Tokyo, Japan

Seiryo Sugiura
Graduate School of Frontier Sciences, University of Tokyo, Tokyo, Japan

Stewart I. Head, Bronwen Greenaway and Stephen Chan
School of Medical Sciences, University of New South Wales, Sydney, New South Wales, Australia

Neil Curtis, Michael J. Fagan and Junfen Shi
Medical and Biological Engineering Research Group, Department of Engineering, University of Hull, Hull, United Kingdom

Marc E. H. Jones and Susan E. Evans
Research Department of Cell and Developmental Biology, University College London, London, United Kingdom

Paul O'Higgins
Hull-York Medical School, University of York, York, United Kingdom

Patricia Ann Kramer
Departments of Anthropology and Orthopaedics and Sports Medicine, University of Washington, Seattle, Washington, United States of America

Adam D. Sylvester
Max Planck Institute for Evolutionary Anthropology, Leipzig, Germany

Lilian Lacourpaille, Franc͟ois Hug and Antoine Nordez
University of Nantes, Laboratory "Motricité, Interactions, Performance" (EA 4334), Nantes, France

Geoffrey A. Power
Canadian Centre for Activity and Aging, School of Kinesiology, Faculty of Health Sciences, The University of Western Ontario, London, Ontario, Canada

Charles L. Rice
Canadian Centre for Activity and Aging, School of Kinesiology, Faculty of Health Sciences, The University of Western Ontario, London, Ontario, Canada
Department of Anatomy and Cell Biology, The University of Western Ontario, London, Ontario, Canada

Anthony A. Vandervoort
Canadian Centre for Activity and Aging, School of Kinesiology, Faculty of Health Sciences, The University of Western Ontario, London, Ontario, Canada
School of Physical Therapy, Faculty of Health Sciences, The University of Western Ontario, London, Ontario, Canada

Hsiao T. Yang and Ronald L. Terjung
Department of Biomedical Sciences, College of Veterinary Medicine, The University of Missouri, Columbia, Missouri, United States of America

Jin-Hong Shin, Chady H. Hakim, Xiufang Pan and Dongsheng Duan
Department of Molecular Microbiology and Immunology, School of Medicine, The University of Missouri, Columbia, Missouri, United States of America

Pauline Gerus
Centre for Musculoskeletal Research, Griffith Health Institute, Griffith University, Gold Coast, Australia

Guillaume Rao and Eric Berton
Institute of Movement Sciences E-J Marey, Aix-Marseille Université , Marseille, France

Arpana Sali, Gina M. Many, Heather Gordish-Dressman, Jack H. van der Meulen, Aditi Phadke, Avital Cnaan, Eric P. Hoffman and Kanneboyina Nagaraju
Center for Genetic Medicine Research, Children's National Medical Center, Department of Integrative Systems Biology, George Washington University School of Medicineand Health Sciences, Washington, DC, United States of America

Christopher F. Spurney
Center for Genetic Medicine Research, Children's National Medical Center, Department of Integrative Systems Biology, George Washington University School of Medicine and Health Sciences, Washington, DC, United States of America
Division of Cardiology, Children's National Medical Center, Washington, DC, United States of America

Graham M. Donovan and James Sneyd
Department of Mathematics, University of Auckland, Auckland, New Zealand

Merryn H. Tawhai
Auckland Bioengineering Institute, University of Auckland, Auckland, New Zealand

Killian Bouillard, Antoine Nordez and Franc‚ois Hug
University of Nantes, Laboratory «Motricité, Interactions, Performance» (EA 4334), Nantes, France

Barbara H. Janssen, Christine I. Nabuurs, Jacky W. J. de Rooy and Arend Heerschap
Department of Radiology, Radboud University Medical Center, Nijmegen, The Netherlands

Nicoline B. M. Voet and Alexander C. Geurts
Department of Rehabilitation, Radboud University Medical Center, Nijmegen, The Netherlands

Hermien E. Kan
Department of Radiology, Radboud University Medical Center, Nijmegen, The Netherlands
Department of Radiology, Leiden University Medical Centre, Leiden, The Netherlands

George W. Padberg and Baziel G. M. van Engelen
Department of Neurology, Radboud University Medical Center, Nijmegen, The Netherlands

Jeffrey B. Thuma, Kevin H. Hobbs, Helaine J. Burstein, Natasha S. Seiter and Scott L. Hooper
Department of Biological Sciences, Ohio University, Athens, Ohio, United States of America

Philip Clausen
School of Biological, Earth and Environmental Sciences, University of New South Wales, Sydney, NSW, Australia

William C. H. Parr
School of Engineering, University of Newcastle, Callaghan, NSW, Australia

Stephen Wroe
School of Biological, Earth and Environmental Sciences, University of New South Wales, Sydney, NSW, Australia
School of Engineering, University of Newcastle, Callaghan, NSW, Australia

Uphar Chamoli
School of Engineering, University of Newcastle, Callaghan, NSW, Australia
St. George Clinical School, University of New South Wales, Sydney, NSW, Australia

Ryan Ridgely and Lawrence Witmer
Department of Biomedical Sciences, Heritage College of Osteopathic Medicine, Ohio University, Athens, Ohio, United States of America

Kiril L. Hristov, Serge A. Y. Afeli, Shankar P. Parajuli, Qiuping Cheng
Department of Drug Discovery and Biomedical Sciences, South Carolina College of Pharmacy, University of South Carolina, Columbia, South Carolina, United States of America

Eric S. Rovner
Medical University of South Carolina, Charleston, South Carolina, United States of America

Georgi V. Petkov
Department of Drug Discovery and Biomedical Sciences, South Carolina College of Pharmacy, University of South Carolina, Columbia, South Carolina, United States of America
Medical University of South Carolina, Charleston, South Carolina, United States of America

Alain Varray
Movement To Health Laboratory, Euromov, University of Montpellier1, Montpellier, France

Nelly Heraud and Nicolas Oliver
Clinique du Souffle La Vallonie, Fontalvie, Lodéve, France

Francois Alexandre
Movement To Health Laboratory, Euromov, University of Montpellier 1, Montpellier, France
Clinique du Souffle La Vallonie, Fontalvie, Lodève, France

David A. Milder, Emily J. Sutherland, Simon C. Gandevia and Penelope A. McNulty
Neuroscience Research Australia, Sydney and University of New South Wales, Sydney, Australia

Yen-Ting Lin
Physical Education Office, Asia University, Taichung, Taiwan
Department of Sports Sciences, University of Taipei, Taipei, Taiwan

Chia-Hua Kuo
Department of Sports Sciences, University of Taipei, Taipei, Taiwan

Ing-Shiou Hwang
Department of Physical Therapy, College of Medicine, National Cheng Kung University, Tainan, Taiwan
Institute of Allied Health Sciences, National Cheng Kung University, Tainan, Taiwan

J. Mikhail Kellawan and Michael E. Tschakovsky
School of Kinesiology and Health Studies, Queen's University, Kingston, Ontario, Canada

William C. H. Parr, Laura A. B. Wilson and Tracey L. Rogers
Evolution and Ecology Research Centre, School of Biological, Earth and Environmental Sciences, University of New South Wales, Sydney, New South Wales, Australia

Stephen Wroe and Marie R. G. Attard
Evolution and Ecology Research Centre, School of Biological, Earth and Environmental Sciences, University of New South Wales, Sydney, New South Wales, Australia
Function, Evolution and Anatomy Research laboratory, Zoology, School of Environmental and Rural Sciences, University of New England, New South Wales, Australia

Michael Archer and Suzanne J. Hand
Evolution of Earth and Life Sciences Research Centre, School of Biological, Earth and Environmental Sciences, University of New South Wales, Sydney, New South Wales, Australia

Index

CPSIA information can be obtained
at www.ICGtesting.com
Printed in the USA
BVHW02*0448020218
506942BV00003B/27/P

9 781632 414519